the mother of all baby books

PRAISE FOR
ANN DOUGLAS AND HER PREVIOUS BOOKS

About *The Mother of All Pregnancy Books*

"[I]f you're looking for the perfect book to address all of your pregnancy concerns, check out Ann Douglas's new book, *The Mother of All Pregnancy Books*."

—Todaysparent.com

"Comprehensive, informative, up-to-date, and brazenly neutral. . . . A must-have primer."

—*Toronto Star*

"Not preachy and bossy . . . it's upfront and fun."

—*Toronto Sun*

About *The Unofficial Guide to Having a Baby*

"Probably the best reference book on the market, giving non-judgemental and fairly exhaustive information on [a variety of] hot-button topics . . . . The book lays out as much information as possible and leaves the decision-making to the parents—a surprisingly rare gambit in the bossy world of pregnancy books."

—Amazon.com Parenting Editor

"Whether you are looking for the latest information on high-tech resources or down-to-earth everyday suggestions, this book has it all. There are money-saving tips and charts and checklists to help you through the pregnancy months and get you ready for the delivery; the comments are honest and often touching, as moms talk about disappointments and highs that were part of their experience. A great resource to have on hand."

—*Valleykids Parent News*

"Anyone who wants to become a parent may very well be overwhelmed by all the decisions to be made. Fortunately, *The Unofficial Guide* does a good job of explaining it all. When there is conflicting data (will it be breast or bottle?), the authors present both sides of the argument. There's even a frank discussion about the pros and cons of having a baby, including the truth about the mommy track."

—Lisa N. Burby, *Newsday*

"There may be better books on individual pregnancy topics, but few can touch the excellent overview of nearly every pregnancy-related issue this book offers. It should answer all the panicky, late-night questions of most expectant couples."

—Wendy Haaf, *Great Expectations*

About *The Unofficial Guide to Childcare*
"The childcare bible."

—*Chicago Tribune*

"A lot of practical information. . . . This clearly written tome discusses working-parent stress, evaluating out-of-home and in-home childcare options, finding care for a special-needs child, breastfeeding, and part-time care."

—*LA Parent*

"*The Unofficial Guide to Childcare* explains how to do a foolproof appraisal of childcare professionals, with plenty of insider secrets and time-saving tips."

—*Newsday*

About *Baby Science*
"With candid photos and a warm, conversational text, *Baby Science* describes the first extraordinary year of life."

—*Children's Book of the Month Club*

"A clearly written, factual book aimed at young children. Peppered with interesting little facts and simple explanations about a baby's first year, it addresses many of the questions kids have about babies."

—*Peterborough Examiner*

"Engagingly educational in focus, *Baby Science* . . . explains how to guess what babies are trying to say, why their bodies look the way they do, how to hold them, and how much they eat and sleep."

—*Publishers Weekly*

About *Trying Again: A Guide to Pregnancy after Miscarriage, Stillbirth, and Infant Loss*
"The authors cover every topic (from how to cope when there's no known medical reason for a baby's death to how to prepare physically and emotionally for a complicated pregnancy) with expertise, candor, and compassion."

—*Publishers Weekly*

"With grace, warmth, and a touch of humour, Ann Douglas and Dr. John Sussman tackle the myths and truths about miscarriage, stillbirth, and infant death. Presented in a style that feels more like a chat across the kitchen table than an analytical medical discussion, their book offers practical advice balanced with accounts of loss and success of more than one hundred parents."

—Preconception.com

"*Trying Again* extends a helping hand to couples [who are] coping with their loss and at the same time contemplating future pregnancies."

—*Genesee Valley Parent*

ANN DOUGLAS

the mother of all *baby* books

An All-Canadian Guide to Your Baby's First Year

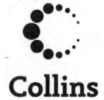
Collins

Mother of All Baby Books
Copyright © 2012 by Ann Douglas

THE MOTHER OF ALL and THE MOTHER OF ALL SOLUTIONS are trademarks owned by Page One Productions Inc. and used under license.

Published by Collins, an imprint of HarperCollins Publishers Ltd.

Originally published by John Wiley & Sons Canada, Ltd., in both print and EPUB editions: 2012

First published by Collins in an EPUB edition and in this trade paperback edition: 2013

Care has been taken to trace ownership of copyright material contained in this book. The publisher will gladly receive any information that will enable them to rectify any reference or credit line in subsequent editions.

This publication contains the opinions and ideas of its author(s) and is designed to provide useful advice in regard to the subject matter covered. The author(s) and publisher are not engaged in rendering medical, therapeutic, or other services in this publication. This publication is not intended to provide a basis for action in particular circumstances without consideration by a competent professional. The author(s) and publisher expressly disclaim any responsibility for any liability, loss, or risk, personal or otherwise, which is incurred as a consequence, directly or indirectly, of the use and application of any of the contents of this book. Please also see Medical Disclaimer on following page.

No part of this book may be used or reproduced in any manner whatsoever without the prior written permission of the publisher, except in the case of brief quotations embodied in reviews.

HarperCollins books may be purchased for educational, business, or sales promotional use through our Special Markets Department.

HarperCollins Publishers Ltd
2 Bloor Street East, 20th Floor
Toronto, Ontario, Canada
M4W 1A8

www.harpercollins.ca

Library and Archives Canada Cataloguing in Publication Data

Douglas, Ann, 1963–
The mother of all baby books : an all-Canadian guide to your baby's first year / Ann Douglas. — 2nd ed.

Includes bibliographical references and index.

Issued also in electronic formats.

ISBN 978-1-44342-794-4

1. Pregnancy—Popular works. 2. Childbirth—Popular works. I. Title.

RG525.D68 2011   618.2   C2011-900857-2

Cover and interior text design: Sun Ngo

Printed in Canada
DWF 9 8 7 6 5 4 3 2 1

MEDICAL DISCLAIMER

Please note: This book is designed to provide you with general information about pregnancy so that you can be a better-informed health consumer. It does not contain medical advice. This book is not intended to provide a complete or exhaustive treatment of this subject; nor is it a substitute for advice from your physician or midwife, who know you best. Seek medical attention promptly for any specific medical condition or problem that you may be experiencing. Do not take any medication without obtaining medical advice. All efforts were made to ensure the accuracy of the information contained in this publication as of the date of writing. The author and the publisher expressly disclaim any responsibility for any adverse effects arising from the use or application of the information contained herein. While the parties believe that the contents of this publication are accurate, a licensed medical practitioner should be consulted in the event that medical advice is desired. The information contained in this book does not constitute a recommendation or endorsement with respect to any company or product.

To Neil, Julie, Scott, Erik, and Ian—the mother of all families

CONTENTS

ACKNOWLEDGEMENTS • xvii

INTRODUCTION • 1

CHAPTER 1: A STAR IS BORN • 5
  Meeting Your Baby • 6
  Getting to know your baby • 7
  What Newborns Really Look Like • 13
  Size • 13; Head • 13; Muscle weakness • 14; Face • 14; Eyes • 15;
  Ears • 16; Skin • 16; Umbilical cord stump • 19; Hands and feet • 20;
  Legs and arms • 20; Genitalia • 20
  What to Expect if Your Baby Is Premature • 22
  Newborn Reflexes • 24
  Rooting reflex • 24; Sucking reflex • 25; Extrusion reflex • 25;
  Grasping reflex • 25; Moro reflex (startle reflex) • 25;
  Stepping reflex • 25; Tonic neck reflex (fencer's reflex) • 26;
  Placing reflex • 26; Crawling reflex • 26; Doll's eye reflex • 26
  The Apgar Test • 27
  The Newborn Exam • 28
  Other tests • 32; Jaundice • 36

CHAPTER 2: YOUR BODY AFTER THE BIRTH • 41
  Your Postpartum Body: The Official Tour • 41
  Heavy vaginal bleeding • 41; Perineal pain • 46; Changes to
  the tone and feel of your vagina • 48; Difficulty urinating • 49;
  Incontinence • 50; Difficulty having a bowel movement • 51;
  Afterpains • 52; A flabby belly • 53; A separation of the
  abdominal muscles • 53; Stretch marks • 54; Breast changes • 54;

Headaches • 57; Fatigue • 57; Faintness • 58; Shivers and shakes • 58; Sweating • 59; Hair loss • 59; Other postpartum body changes • 59
Caesarean Recovery • 60
Weight Loss • 62
Nutrition after Baby • 64
Getting Back into Shape • 66
Sex after Baby? • 70

CHAPTER 3: THE POSTPARTUM SURVIVAL GUIDE • 77
    Life after Baby • 77
    On your mind after baby • 83
    Coming through Postpartum Depression • 89
    What has helped other moms • 91

CHAPTER 4: CARING FOR YOUR NEWBORN • 97
    Breastfeeding: What Every New Mom Needs to Know • 97
    Getting started • 98
    Coping with Sleep Deprivation • 111
    Comforting Your Crying Baby • 114

CHAPTER 5: BECOMING PARENTS • 123
    Why the Early Weeks of Parenthood Can Be Such a Challenge • 124
    First Comes Love • 144
    Intuitive Parenting: Reading Your Baby's Cues • 145

CHAPTER 6: BOSOM BUDDIES • 149
    The Science of Breastfeeding • 151
    Prolactin, not Prozac • 153
    The Art of the Latch • 155
    What Breastfeeding Feels Like • 157
    Your Top Breastfeeding Questions Answered • 158
    Breastfeeding and Working • 191
    Finding a breastfeeding-friendly caregiver • 191; Choosing a breast pump • 193; Pumping 101 • 193
    Troubleshooting Common Problems • 196
    Breast engorgement • 196; Sore nipples • 199; Flat or inverted nipples • 200; Leaking • 201; Plugged ducts • 202; Mastitis (breast infection) • 203; Thrush (oral candidiasis) • 204

    Breastfeeding under Special Circumstances • 206
    Breastfeeding a premature baby • 206; Breastfeeding a baby with a congenital problem • 208; Breastfeeding after adoption • 209; Breastfeeding after breast enhancement or reduction surgery • 209; Breastfeeding multiples • 210

CHAPTER 7: THE OWNER'S MANUAL: NEW BABY CARE • 213
    The Care and Handling of Babies • 214
    The Dirt on Diapers • 215
    Rash decisions • 219; Elimination communication (diaper-free) • 222
    Caring for a Circumcised Baby • 222
    Umbilical Cord Care • 223
    A Baby for All Seasons • 224
    Nail Care • 227
    Dental Care • 227
    Before your baby's teeth come in • 228; Once your baby's teeth come in • 230
    Dressing the Part • 230
    Bath Time Basics • 235
    How to sponge-bathe a baby • 235; Your baby's first real bath • 237; Moving up to the "big tub" • 239
    Infant Massage • 240

CHAPTER 8: THE HEALTH AND SAFETY DEPARTMENT • 243
    How Often Should Your Baby See the Doctor? • 244
    What happens at a well-baby checkup • 244
    The Facts on Immunizations • 245
    How immunizations work • 246
    How Will I Know if My Child Is Sick? • 253
    Respiratory symptoms • 254; Gastrointestinal symptoms • 255; Skin changes • 256; Other symptoms • 256
    More about Fever • 257
    Fever is not the bad guy: The illness is • 257; This does not compute • 258; What type of thermometer to use • 259; What you need to know about febrile convulsions • 260; When to call the doctor • 261; Treating a fever • 263

Coping with Common Childhood Illnesses and Infections • 266
Respiratory and related conditions • 267; Skin and scalp conditions • 277; Gastrointestinal conditions • 285; Other conditions • 295

Babyproofing 101 • 298
Every room • 298; Halls and stairways • 301; Nursery • 301; Bedroom • 303; Bathroom • 303; Kitchen • 304; Family room • 306; Living room • 307; Laundry room • 308; Basement • 308; Garage • 308; Backyard • 308; Miscellaneous • 310

Safety on the Road • 310
Rear-facing infant car seats • 310; Front-facing car seats • 311; Other car safety tips • 312

Be Prepared • 314

Welcoming a Premature Baby or a Baby with Health Problems • 319

Reducing the Risk of SIDS • 324
Coping with SIDS-related fears • 328

Every Parent's Worst Nightmare • 328
Surviving the unthinkable • 329

CHAPTER 9: EATING AND SLEEPING REVISITED • 337

Introducing Solid Food • 337
Baby, give me a sign • 340; Baby's first feeding • 341; And after that first feeding... • 344; Added tastes and textures • 345

Making Your Own Baby Food • 346

Sippy Cup Skills • 352

Food Allergies and Food Intolerances • 354

Sleeping through the Night • 356
The facts about older babies and sleep • 358; Sleep training versus sleep learning • 360

Common Sleep Concerns about Older Babies • 364
Nightwaking • 364; Difficulty settling down at bedtime • 365; Early rising • 365

CHAPTER 10: THE INCREDIBLE GROWING BABY • 367

Baby Geniuses • 367

Baby Love • 388
The power of play • 389; Reading to your baby • 392; Pink versus blue • 400

The Childcare Crunch • 401
Returning to work: The first week survival guide • 402; The Great Canadian Maternity-Leave Cash Crunch • 404
The Secrets of Less-Stressed-Out Parents • 405
Growing with Your Baby • 407

APPENDIX A: GLOSSARY • 409
APPENDIX B: ONLINE RESOURCES • 419

INDEX • 427

ACKNOWLEDGEMENTS

While my name may be the one that's splashed on the front cover of this book, *The Mother of All Baby Books* was anything but a solo effort. Writing a book of this size and scope requires assistance from a huge number of people—people I'd like to take a moment to thank right now.

First of all, I'd like to thank the parents who agreed to be interviewed for this book: Molly Acton, Lenore Allen, Stephanie Anderson, Rita Arsenault, Claudia E. Astorquiza, Sadia Baig, Aubyn Baker, Christina Barnes, Kristi-Anna Beaudry, Althea Blackburn-Evans, Janet Bolton, Carolin Botterill, Vicky Boudreau, Lanny Boutin, Jennifer Brasch, Elisa Brook, Cheryl Carew, Robyn Chalmer, Karen Chamberlain, Michele Claeson, Brandi Conlin, Jennifer J. Conquergood, Stacey Couturier, Carole Anne Crump, Marguerite Daubney, Michelle Davidson, Brenda Davie, Chonee Dennis, Julie Dufresne, Jane Fletcher, Jennifer Fong, Cyndie Forget, Angela Francoeur, Anne Gallant, Leslie Garrett, Danielle Gebeyehu, Monique Gibbons, Jo-Anne Goertzen, Douglas Granter, Melodie Granter, Joyce Gravelle, Sandra Grocock, Sue Guebert, Brande Guisbert, Line Hamelin, M.T. Hare, Terri Harten, Lorna Harvey, Claudia Hawkins, Karen Hayward, Maureen Hill, Mary Ann Hodgson, Anne Hoover, Andrea Illman, Karen Jacksteit, Debbie Jeffery, Sandra Jenkins, Mindy Johnson, Kevin Kee, Dan Kelly, Shauna Kennedy, Trish Kennedy, Jennifer Kilburn, Karen Kozma, Christine Lawson, Mary E. Leblanc, Cindy Legare, Carola Lind, Karen Loutan, Angela MacDonald, Jennifer MacDonald, Stephanie MacDonald, Lara MacGregor, Kathryn MacLean, Jackie Madigan, Heather Martin, Jill Martin, Theresa Maurice, Kelly McClatchey, Debbie McCoy, Dawn

McCoy-Ullrich, Allison McDonald, Kimberly McIntyre-de-Montbrun, Melanie McLeod, Dana Merrett, Colleen Mielen, Alyson Miller, Beth Mindes, Diana Monteith, Kimlee Wong Morrisseau, Samantha Murray, Beverley North, Dee O'Connor, Lusanna O'Shea, Tammy Oakley, Lana Parsons, Diane Pepin, Tina Phelps, Maria Phillips, Tina Pilon, Gwyn Pinto-D'Mello, Catharine Piuze, Heather Polan, Rose Ann Punnett, Julie Pyke, Angelina Quinlan, Kerri Quirt, Christopher Reid, Jennifer Reid, Elli Richardson, Myrna MacDonald Ridley, Lisa Roberts, Lisa Rouleau, Cynthia Sargeant, Krista Schnittker, Kim Selin, Kimberlee Smit, Holly Smith, Janice Smith, Janie Smith, Jennifer Smith, Jeannine St. Amand, Jenna Stedman, Helena Steinmetz, Kelly Steiss, Bevin Stephenson, Nancy Swart, Karen Taillon, Lynda Timms, Melinda Tuck, Lori Voth, Jane Walden, Darci Walker, Lianne Werner, Judith White, Lynn Woodford, Laura E. Young, Susan Yusishen, and Jacqueline Zender.

I'd also like to thank the book's two technical reviewers, Richard Whatley, M.D. (undoubtedly Canada's best-loved family physician) and Laura Devine, R.N. (mother of four and parenting expert extraordinaire), who read all 170,000 words of the manuscript and lived to tell! Thanks for your tremendously insightful comments on the book and for being such a pleasure to work with.

I am grateful to Fiona Chapman of the Canadian Foundation for the Study of Infant Deaths, lactation consultant Flo Levia, and early childhood educator Lorrie Baird for their helpful comments on the manuscript; adoption expert Christine Adamec and grief expert Deborah Davis, for allowing me to quote them extensively in the book; and Tracy Keleher of Canadian Parents Online and Jan Pearce of Perinatal Bereavement Services Ontario, who helped me find large numbers of parents to interview for the book.

I am forever indebted to my husband, Neil, for the countless hours he spent holding down the fort and entertaining a tribe of wild children so that I could (almost) meet my book deadline. And I owe a huge thank you to my friend and mentor Barbara Florio Graham for all the insights she has given me into the always-weird-and-mostly-wonderful world of book publishing.

Finally, I'd like to thank all the people who played an important role behind the scenes while I was researching and writing this book: my research assistants, Janice Kent and Christi Soltermann; the numerous unsung heroes on the editorial, production, and marketing teams at CDG Books; and—last but not least—two very special people who are responsible not just for this book but for my entire career as an author: Robert Harris, who gave me the opportunity to write my very first book and who's still one of my greatest supporters, even as I put book number 17 to bed; and Joan Whitman, who has championed the Mother of All series right from day one and cut me more slack in terms of book deadlines than any editor has the right to do. (Don't worry, Joan. It's our little secret.)

And to anyone else I might have forgotten to thank as a result of deadline-induced dementia, a million thank yous. Writing this book has been one of the highlights of my publishing career. My heartfelt thanks to everyone who made that possible.

• • •

ACKNOWLEDGEMENTS FOR THE SECOND EDITION:

As I put this second edition to bed, my children are a decade older, I'm a decade wiser (or at least I hope I am!), and I am astounded by how much the world of mothers and babies has changed in such a relatively short period of time. The last time I worked on the pages of this book, only techies knew what blogging was, Facebook hadn't even been imagined, and phones weren't smart; people were! Now moms are connected to other moms—and to health and parenting resources—in ways we weren't even thinking about 10 years ago. It makes you wonder what the world of moms and babes will be like by the time I sit down to work on the third edition. (Wait. I'm not ready to think about that quite yet.)

I've got some thank yous to say before I officially slip into post-book relaxation mode (a rather glorious place to be). I need to thank the five technical reviewers who provided me with invaluable feedback as they reviewed the manuscript for the second edition of this book: Virginia Collins, a childbirth educator and doula who specializes in high-risk pregnancy support; Michael Dickinson, head of pediatrics and chief of staff at the Miramichi Regional Hospital in New Brunswick, pediatric faculty member at Dalhousie University in Halifax and Memorial University in St. John's, and an advocate for children's health through his involvement with the Canadian Paediatric Society; Cathy Kerr, a mother of two with an MA in psychology who works with parents and teachers of children with special needs; Teresa Pitman, a La Leche League Leader for more than 30 years and the co-author of three books on breastfeeding as well as nine other books on parenting topics; and Wendy Cohen Reingold, a private practice dietician in Thornhill. Thanks also to everyone at Wiley Canada and to my amazing literary agent Hilary McMahon of Westwood Creative Artists, The Mother of All Agents.

I also need to thank every reader who took the time to write to me to pass along a parenting experience (your stories were all so great to read) or to let me know that something I wrote helped you through a difficult time.

I hope you'll enjoy the revised second edition of *The Mother of All Baby Books*. But, much more than that, I hope you and your baby will have an amazing first year together—that the first chapter in the story of your life as a family will be sweet and tender and filled with love.

INTRODUCTION

"Motherhood is like Albania—you can't trust the descriptions in the books, you have to go there."
—MARNI JACKSON, *THE MOTHER ZONE*

Becoming a parent is like taking a trip to a foreign country: you have no way of knowing beforehand what you'll encounter once you get there. If you're lucky, the maps and guidebooks that you turn to for information will be packed with nitty-gritty insider advice from others who've already walked the same path—fellow travellers who can tell you about both the attractions and the roadblocks you can expect to encounter along the way.

The Mother of All Baby Books is the parenting world's equivalent to just such a guidebook: a book that will help you to find your way as you make the once-in-a-lifetime journey to parenthood. Like all good guidebooks, it is packed with real-world advice from fellow travellers—other moms and dads who've been through the late-night crying marathons and 3 a.m. feedings and somehow lived to tell.

The one thing the book can't tell you, of course, is the very thing you'd most like to know: exactly what the first year of parenthood is going to be like for you and your baby. That's because there's no such thing as a one-size-fits-all parenting experience or a typical baby. Still, even if I can't produce a detailed itinerary and map out your route for you, I can certainly draw your attention to some of the key attractions. And what a lot of attractions there are to take in during Baby's awesome and inspiring first year.

MADE IN CANADA

Guidebook comparison aside, there's something else that sets this book apart from the literally hundreds of other baby books that you'll find on the bookstore shelves. Unlike most parenting books, this book is 100 per cent Canadian made.

While some might argue that there's no need for a Canadian baby book, I happen to disagree on this important point. Allow me to explain why. If you flip through the pages of a typical American baby book, you'll find pages and pages of material that simply doesn't apply to Canadian parents: chapters on coping with health insurance nightmares (a U.S. phenomenon, thank heavens) or your rights under the Family and Medical Leave Act (the American government's watered-down version of our more generous maternity and parental leave legislation). Even the chapters that are relevant to Canadian parents suffer from a major shortcoming: the expert sources cited time and time again are almost exclusively American.

What Canadian parents want and need is a book that reflects what it's like to raise a baby in Canada—a book that addresses the unique challenges that Canadian parents face (the doctor shortage that plagues many communities across the country, for example) and that contains up-to-the-minute advice from such respected Canadian health authorities as the Canadian Paediatric Society and Health Canada. (Believe it or not, health authorities on opposite sides of the border don't always see eye to eye on key pediatric health issues.)

Of course, it wouldn't be possible—or even advisable—to write a baby book that completely ignores what's happening south of the border. After all, some of the most significant breakthroughs in pediatric health research in recent years have occurred in research laboratories in the United States. What Canadian parents need, however, is a baby book that looks at that information through Canadian eyes and interprets it for a Canadian audience.

A ONE-OF-A-KIND BABY BOOK

As you've no doubt noticed by now, books on Baby's first year tend to fall into one of two distinct categories: those that focus so much on the experience of becoming a mother that they almost forget there's a baby involved, and those that focus so much on the ins and outs of feeding and caring for a baby that they neglect to talk about how becoming a parent changes your life. And, boy, does it change things . . .

The Mother of All Baby Books avoids falling into either of those all-too-common traps. Because the book focuses only on the first year of life (rather than attempting to cover a three- to five-year time span, as many other parenting books are inclined to do), it is able to double as both a parenting book and a pediatric health resource. That's why we chose to call it *The Mother of All Baby Books*: this is one comprehensive book, after all.

If you take a quick flip through the book, you'll find a lot of valuable information packed between its covers, including

- mom-proven strategies for caring for yourself while you're caring for your baby;
- advice on what you can do to make the transition to parenthood as smooth as possible for yourself and your partner;
- need-to-know information about the physical and emotional highs and lows of the postpartum period, including how to spot the warning signs of a perinatal mood disorder such as postpartum depression;
- practical tips on getting breastfeeding off to the best possible start for yourself and your baby;
- reassuring answers to your most pressing baby-care questions, with a special emphasis on helping your baby to sleep and soothing your baby;
- a no-worry guide to starting your baby on solid foods, featuring recipes for some of the most popular and easy-to-make baby food purées;
- sensible guidelines on coping with fevers and other infant health concerns that can have you hitting the panic button at 3 a.m.;
- the lowdown on infant development and baby milestones;
- up-to-date information on the issues that parents are talking about at playgroup and online: forming healthy attachments, emotional self-regulation, learning through play, and more;
- advice on choosing age-appropriate books and toys, and tips on games and activities babies of various ages love;
- a detailed glossary of baby-care terms; and
- a directory of online resources of interest to Canadian parents.

What makes this book really special, however, is the fact that it was based on interviews with more than 150 Canadian parents. These parents passed on their best tips on weathering the sometimes tumultuous first year of parenthood—everything from practical tips on getting the baby food into the baby (rather than just in the general vicinity) to creative strategies for finding stolen moments to nurture your relationship with your partner (arguably the Mother of All Challenges).

You'll also find a few other bells and whistles as you make your way through the book.

mom's the word: insights and advice from new parents.

mother wisdom: little-known facts about babies and parenthood—including some fun pop culture tidbits.

baby talk: research updates and other important baby-related information.

the baby department: leads on resources that will be of interest to parents with babies.

As you've no doubt gathered by now, *The Mother of All Baby Books* is unlike any other "baby's first year" book you've ever encountered. It's comprehensive, it's fun to read, and—best of all—it's made in Canada.

Enjoy!

ANN DOUGLAS

P.S. If you have any comments to pass along about this book, please contact me via my website: www.having-a-baby.com.

chapter 1
A STAR IS BORN

"I remember falling in love with my firstborn three days after he was born. I was just looking into his face and feeling so awful because I was just numb after the birth and didn't feel that gushing Mama-love that I thought I was supposed to be feeling. Then he opened his tiny eyes and I realized they looked just like mine. I looked at his ears and they were mine, too. I realized that this was the first person in my life I had looked like. I had been adopted and had longed for those 'you have your mother's eyes' comments my whole life. I realized that for the first time ever I would get to have that. He started to root around to nurse and the tears just started to flow. I was just filled with wonder knowing that he was mine. Those feelings came rushing in all at once and I felt so intensely in love with him."

—KIMBERLY, 28, MOTHER OF THREE

The dress rehearsal for parenting is finally behind you. It's opening night and the curtain is going up. You can practically hear the announcer's voice in your head as your baby makes her grand entrance into the world: "Ladies and gentlemen, a star is born!"

As wonderful as it is to finally have the chance to meet your baby, you may find that you are hit with a bad case of opening night jitters. After all, you're about to take on an unspeakably important role—that of parent. And unlike most actors who have scripts to rely on when they're playing a new role, you have to improvise.

In this chapter, we're going to talk about the joys and challenges of the first few hours of parenthood—how you may feel about that new little person who's just entered your life. We'll also talk about what newborn babies really look like and what you can expect to see the first time you catch a sideways glance at your postpartum body in a mirror.

MEETING YOUR BABY

There are few moments in life that are more memorable than when you have the chance to meet your newborn baby for the first time. Even decades after the fact, you'll find yourself able to recall minute details about these early moments: what time of day it was, what the sky looked like outside, and how the entire world seemed to grind to a halt as you and your baby made eye contact for the very first time.

Don't be surprised, however, if you don't end up feeling sideswiped by maternal love right away. You may be exhausted from the birth and more interested in sleeping and recovering than in spending a lot of time bonding with the new arrival. A lot of women find that it takes a while for their maternal feelings to kick in—something that may be more than a little disconcerting.

"I felt surprised and upset and perhaps even a bit guilty that I did not fall in love with my son the moment I first saw him," confesses Helena, a 31-year-old mother of one. "I was exhausted from the labour and delivery and did not feel up to holding him right away. I think that Cupid's arrow finally struck when all the visitors had left and we fell asleep together. My mother took a picture of the two of us and we used it for our birth announcement. Everyone commented on how much they liked the picture and how peaceful the two of us looked together."

Kimberly, a 28-year-old mother of three, also found that it took time for her to start feeling connected to each of her newborn babies, even though she had started bonding with each of them many months before they were born. "I always fell in love with my babies while I was still pregnant," she explains. "I loved to feel them move. I would grab and stroke the little feet, knees, and elbows that poked out the sides of my belly. After they were born, it took me a little while longer to feel this same flood of emotions. They seemed like different babies altogether."

Like these other mothers, Jane, 31, found that it took time for her maternal feelings to kick in. She clearly remembers the first time she experienced powerful feelings of love for her new son. The mother of two explains: "I didn't get to be alone with my son until the day after he was born. When I finally got him to myself in my hospital room, there was an amazing thunderstorm raging outside over the river. I stood holding him so he could 'see' the beauty of it and I just felt the love for my son enter my heart."

Some women find that it takes weeks rather than days to get used to the idea of being someone's parent. Samantha, 34, confesses to still feeling like a bit of an imposter, even though her son is now 8 weeks old: "I still feel like I'm the babysitter—that my baby's real parents are going to come and pick him up soon."

Whether you are flooded with maternal feelings from the very first moment you lock eyes with your baby or during the hours, days, or weeks that follow is unimportant: what matters is that you respect your feelings and allow them to emerge naturally. Just as you can't fake romantic love, you can't force yourself to feel maternal love before you're ready. But rest assured that your concerns about not feeling "motherly" enough will become a non-issue: one day soon, you'll realize to your delight and amazement that you've fallen head over heels in love with your baby.

mom's the word

"I did not bond instantly. There were no tears of joy. To be honest, while I loved her dearly, it took a couple of weeks for me to realize that she belonged to me. I wasn't just babysitting! It was the oddest sensation, really."

—JANE, 30, CURRENTLY PREGNANT WITH HER SECOND CHILD

Getting to know your baby

The earliest moments of your baby's life are a magical time—the climax of nine months' worth of anticipation. Finally, you get to meet your baby and to drink in everything about her.

And just as you're fascinated by your baby, your baby is fascinated by you. A newborn baby experiences a period of tremendous alertness shortly after the birth, most of which is spent quietly studying her mother's face. Your baby already recognizes your voice and the unique scent of your body. Now she's eager to discover everything else about you.

While your baby will likely appear distressed during the first few minutes after the birth—she may have a disgusted-looking facial expression, a wrinkled forehead, puffy eyes, tightly flexed limbs, and clenched fists, and she may be wailing at the top of her lungs—she will settle down almost as soon as her body comes into contact with yours. Studies have shown that infants who are placed in skin-to-skin contact with their mothers seldom cry during their first 90 minutes of life, while infants who are immediately shuttled over to a bassinet tend to cry for 20 to 40 seconds during each five-minute period over the next 90 minutes. Enjoying skin-to-skin contact is the ideal way to welcome your baby to the world: your body helps to keep your baby warm, and your scent, your voice, and your heartbeat are comfortingly familiar to her.

---

mother wisdom

"A baby is a question mark and his mother the answer he seeks. Sensitive to every new encounter, the newborn experiences life through the soft filter of mother's embrace, her milk, her lullabies."

—DEBORAH JACKSON, *WITH CHILD: WISDOM AND TRADITIONS FOR PREGNANCY, BIRTH, AND MOTHERHOOD*

Approximately 30 to 40 minutes after the birth, your baby will start making mouthing movements. She may even smack her lips. Saliva will begin to drip down her chin, signalling in no uncertain terms that she's ready to test-drive her sucking reflex on something other than her own hands (something she was doing before birth). Babies placed on their mothers' abdomens are able to find their way to the breast by using a combination of arm and leg movements. (It doesn't always happen quickly, mind you; sometimes it can take the better part of an hour for the baby to make the trek.) Researchers think the baby is guided to the breast at least partly by her sense of smell. Apparently, the baby uses the taste and smell of amniotic fluid on her hands to make a connection to a breast secretion—something that has led some hospitals to decide to delay washing a newborn baby's hands during this initial period of mother/baby bonding.

Not all babies are enthusiastic breastfeeders right from the very beginning, however, so don't worry if your baby is only interested in licking the nipple tentatively rather than sucking vigorously. While some babies dive into breastfeeding with great enthusiasm, others are too sleepy or preoccupied during the first hour or two after the birth to master the art of breastfeeding. No worries. Keep the baby skin-to-skin against your chest or abdomen for at least the first hour or two in order to give him the opportunity to find the breast and latch on. Even if he doesn't, you'll have plenty of additional opportunities to teach your baby to nurse during the hours ahead.

mother wisdom Breastfeeding soon after the birth isn't just good for your baby; it's also good for you. Breastfeeding helps to induce a surge of oxytocin, the hormone responsible for contracting the uterus, expelling the placenta, and closing off the many blood vessels in the uterus—something that can help to reduce bleeding. It also aids in the production of prolactin, the hormone responsible for stimulating milk production, and is responsible for giving you the so-called breastfeeding high (more on that later). The pressure of your baby on your abdomen also helps to trigger uterine contractions—all the more reason to enjoy skin-to-skin contact with your baby in the first hour or two after the birth.

Regardless of whether breastfeeding occurs right away or not, this early contact between mother and baby is very important—so important, in fact, that Health Canada's *Family-Centred Maternity and Newborn Care: National Guidelines* recommends that a newborn baby be placed in physical contact with the mother as soon as possible after the birth, and that routine hospital procedures be delayed until the baby and his or her new family have had a chance to get to know one another: "The mother and newborn should be viewed as an inseparable unit . . . The initial mother/infant bond marks the beginning of all of the infant's subsequent attachments . . . Keeping babies and mothers together should be of higher priority than institutional convenience or adherence to traditional policies."

baby talk Human babies aren't the only ones who need some time to get to know their mothers after the birth. Mother dolphins and their newborns call and whistle to one another over and over again until they learn one another's signature calls. And mother zebras make a point of keeping their babies away from the rest of the herd until their babies are better able to recognize them. (Otherwise, baby zebras have a bad habit of trying to latch on to any large object that comes within nursing distance.)

mother wisdom — Researchers used to focus exclusively on the almost magnetic bond between mother and baby. Over time, they learned to expand their focus to include fathers' fascination with their new babies (a process they described as engrossment) and to study the emerging bond between father and baby.

It only makes sense to try to take advantage of your baby's period of quiet alertness after the birth. But if you're not able to do so, don't become overly concerned that you've somehow missed out on the opportunity to bond with your baby. Bonding is not a "use it or lose it" proposition. In the meantime, your partner can enjoy some time with the new baby while you focus on recovering from the birth.

a tour of your newborn — If you haven't spent much time around newborns before, you could be in for a bit of a surprise when yours first arrives on the scene. Newborns have a number of distinctive characteristics that make them look very different from older babies. If you know what to expect in advance, you'll be a lot less likely to worry when you notice these characteristics in your newborn.

- √ **Irregular head shape.** Your baby has just made a rather gruelling journey through the birth canal. Along the way, his head may have become a little moulded or cone-like in appearance. Don't worry. These changes are temporary. Your baby's head will assume a more rounded appearance within a week or two of the birth as the plates in his skull shift back into their pre-labour positions.

- √ **Strange swelling or an unusual lump on the scalp.** Labour isn't just physically demanding for you: it's hard work for your baby, too. Some babies are born with a *caput succedaneum* (a swelling of the soft tissues of the skull that can occur during labour as the baby's head pushes against the cervix). Fortunately, this swelling tends to subside on its own shortly after the birth. Other babies are born with a *cephalohematoma*—a raised bump that is caused by the pooling of blood between the skull bone and the tough covering of the skull during the birthing process. At first the bump will be soft, but, after several weeks, it will become hard (the result of calcium building up in the tissues underneath the skin). While cephalohematomas can be alarming to look at, they usually go away on their own within a couple of weeks, although some take several months to disappear.

- ✓ **Extra skin on the back of the head.** Your baby may have extra folds of skin on the back of his head—the result of shifts in your baby's body fluid balance as he adjusts to life outside the womb. Don't worry. It won't be long before your newborn grows into his extra skin.

- ✓ **Unusual-looking eyes.** Your baby may be born with puffy, droopy eyelids and eyes that are tightly squeezed together. It'll only be a matter of time before your baby starts flashing his baby blues (or browns) at you. Your baby's eyes may also ooze sticky secretions. This happens because your baby's eyes are not yet capable of producing tears. It doesn't mean your baby has picked up an eye infection. Some babies are born with a flame-shaped red streak on the white of their eye—the result of pressure during the birthing process. The streak will disappear on its own over time.

- ✓ **Unusual-looking ears.** Your baby's ears may be folded over or otherwise misshapen, common side effects of labour that tend to correct themselves.

- ✓ **Vernix caseosa coating.** Your baby is likely to have traces of vernix caseosa (a greasy white substance that protected your baby's skin while he was floating around in the sea of amniotic fluid inside your uterus) remaining in the folds of his skin. Vernix caseosa is made up of cells and glandular secretions and is responsible for that intoxicating newborn baby smell. Some babies are born with a lot of vernix. They may look like they've been coated in hand lotion. Vernix is very good for Baby's skin, so don't be in a hurry to wash it off.

- ✓ **Lanugo.** Your baby may have fine downy hair on her shoulders, back, forehead, and temples. This hair, which is known as lanugo, usually disappears within the first week of life and is more abundant in slightly premature infants.

- ✓ **Swollen genitals.** Your baby's genitals may seem large and swollen—the result of hormonal changes and fluid retention. These effects are temporary and will reverse themselves in the days following the birth.

- ✓ **Bird-like arms and legs.** Your baby's arms and legs may look short and bird-like in comparison to the rest of his body (just as his head appears to be gigantic). This is normal for a newborn. His body proportions will change as he grows.
- ✓ **Oversized hands and feet.** Your baby's feet may look out of proportion to his body, and his feet may turn out or his toes may overlap—all par for the course for this stage of infant development.
- ✓ **Birthmarks.** Some babies are born with birthmarks. Reddish blotches are most common in Caucasians, whereas bluish-grey pigmentation on the back, buttocks, arms, or thighs is more common in babies of Asian, Southern European, or African American ancestry. (See Table 1.2 for more about birthmarks.)
- ✓ **Red marks on the skin or broken blood vessels in the skin.** Your baby may have broken blood vessels or red marks on his skin caused by pressure during the birth. These marks typically disappear within a matter of days.
- ✓ **Minor bumps and bruises.** Don't panic if your baby's face appears swollen or if there are patches of bluish bruising or flat streaks of broken blood vessels on his face. These changes are all temporary and result from the tight squeeze during birth. If your baby was delivered with the aid of forceps (medical instruments that look like salad tongs), he may arrive with a few minor bumps and bruises. And if he hitched a ride down the birth canal with a vacuum extractor (another type of medical device), he may end up with a temporary suction mark on his head as well. You may also find marks from fetal monitoring, scalp sampling, or amnio-hooks if these obstetrical interventions were ordered during your labour.

Note: Forceps marks typically disappear within a day or two, but if a firm, flat lump develops as a result of damage to the underlying tissue, it could take up to two months for the marks to disappear. Forceps aren't used nearly as often today as they were a decade or two ago. Babies who run into complications that might have resulted in a forceps delivery in days gone by are now more likely to be delivered with a vacuum extractor or via Caesarean section. There are still a few special situations in which a forceps delivery may be required, but these situations tend to be the exception rather than the rule.

WHAT NEWBORNS REALLY LOOK LIKE

After months of waiting, the big moment has finally arrived. You get to meet the tiny little person who's been subletting your uterus! But don't expect your newborn to look like a Gerber Baby right away—most newborn babies are considerably less chubby. In fact, they can look a little scrawny. And that's not all that's different. Let's take a head-to-toe tour of the tiny person who has changed your world overnight.

Size

While babies come in all shapes and sizes from the very small to the almost unimaginably large, the vast majority of newborns—approximately 95 per cent, in fact—weigh in somewhere between 5.5 and 9 pounds (roughly 2.5 to 4 kilograms) and measure between 18 to 22 inches (46 to 55 centimetres) in length. An "average baby" (whoever he or she is!) weighs 7.5 pounds (3.5 kilograms) and is 20 inches (51 centimetres) long.

Newborns are very lean: they have just 16 per cent body fat when they are born. (This is because they have a large surface area as compared to their body weight: three times the ratio found in an adult.) Newborns are born with special stores of brown adipose tissue (BAT)—a type of fat that they can draw upon for heat production. These BAT stores (which are mainly located in the upper body, across the core organs) are gradually depleted during the baby's first year of life.

A number of different factors influence a baby's size: maternal health and lifestyle during pregnancy (especially nutrition), the duration of the pregnancy, and whether or not the baby has any congenital problems. Women who suffer from chronic hypertension (high blood pressure), vascular or renal disease, or pre-eclampsia or who smoke during pregnancy tend to give birth to lighter babies than other women, while women who develop gestational diabetes or who are chronically diabetic tend to give birth to larger babies. Newborn girls generally weigh less than boys, and twins or other multiples typically weigh less than singletons.

Head

Most babies show some signs of the moulding that typically happens during a vaginal delivery. This moulding occurs as the baby's skull bones shift to allow for an easier passage through the birth canal. You may feel slight ridges on your baby's head as a result of the skull bones overlapping during labour—nature's way of helping to ease the baby's head out without the baby's head sustaining any permanent damage. Moulding is more noticeable in births in which labour has been prolonged or in which the baby's head is larger than average, and less noticeable with breech births. It doesn't occur at all during a Caesarean birth unless, of course, the mother went through labour before the decision was made to deliver the baby via Caesarean section. Even if your baby did end up with a lot of moulding, there's no need to worry: he won't always have a slightly pointed head. In fact, your baby's head will assume a more rounded shape within a couple of days.

Your baby's scalp is likely to have an unusual appearance, too. Your baby may appear to have more skin on her scalp than she needs, something that can result in a slightly wrinkled appearance. She may also develop a mild case of cradle cap (seborrheic eczema: peeling skin on the head). Don't be alarmed if you're able to see or feel your baby's pulse beneath the fontanelle (the so-called soft spot that appears in the centre of and toward the back of the baby's head). This is perfectly normal. And if you're worried about accidentally injuring your baby's soft spot, try to take comfort in the fact that her fontanelle is covered by an extremely thick membrane that's designed to protect her from injury. As long as you handle her with care, she'll be fine.

Of course, you're going to have a hard time finding your baby's fontanelle if she's born with a full head of hair, as some babies are. It's always fun to see how much variation there is in the hair department when you get together with other parents from your prenatal classes: some have babies with as much hair as a typical 3-year-old, while others have tots that are almost as bald as a bowling ball. But even if your baby does end up with a headful of hair, there's no guarantee that she'll get to keep it or that her permanent hair will even be the same colour: a newborn's hair tends to fall out and is sometimes replaced with hair of an entirely different colour (a dry run for the teen years when your child's hair colour and/or style can vary from week to week).

Muscle weakness

Some parents are alarmed to discover that their baby seems to lack muscle control on one side of the face or in one shoulder or arm. This is a common type of birth injury and is caused by pressure on the nerves and/or stretching of the nerves during the delivery. These problems typically correct themselves within a few weeks, but they can be quite worrisome in the meantime.

Face

Newborn babies typically have swollen faces, flattened noses, and receding chins. They can also have bluish bruising on their cheeks and faint streaks of broken blood vessels on their faces—evidence of the tight squeeze they experienced during the birthing process. Fortunately, your baby's face will look much less puffy and distorted after the first day of life, when the swelling subsides. (Just think of this magical post-birth transformation as the baby-world equivalent of do-it-yourself plastic surgery.)

Eyes

When your baby is born, she's likely to look as if she's suffering from a massive hangover, complete with puffy, drooping eyelids and eyes that are tightly squinted together. It's no wonder she looks like this: she's trying to protect her sensitive eyes from the bright lights. Fortunately, within a matter of minutes, your baby will open her eyes and start checking out her new world, starting with you.

Once she opens her eyes during that amazing period of wide-eyed alertness after the birth, you'll be able to get a peek at their colour. Just don't make the mistake of assuming that this is going to be her eye colour for life. While most babies are born with dark blue or greyish-brown eyes, a baby's final eye colour can't be reliably determined until she is at least 6 months old. (Of course, at this early stage of the game, you may be more struck by the fact that her eyes are bloodshot—the result of the pressures of labour rather than too many late nights inside the womb.)

Don't be surprised if your baby's eyes have sticky secretions during the first few weeks of life, or if one of her eyes appears to wander. The sticky secretions should disappear once the baby's eyes start producing tears in a couple of weeks' time. However, if the discharge becomes copious or greenish, you'll want to check with your baby's doctor to see if she might have developed an infection. And the wandering-eye problem should take care of itself by the time your baby is 6 months old. If it doesn't, or if your baby has a fixed squint (in other words, her eyes are permanently out of alignment with one another), you'll want to talk to your baby's doctor about your concerns.

If you notice that one of your baby's eyes keeps watering, it could be because the tear duct in that eye is blocked. In most cases, the problem resolves itself. If, however, your baby's tear duct is still blocked by the time his first birthday rolls around, your baby's doctor will likely recommend that he have minor surgery to correct the problem (a tiny instrument would be inserted into your baby's tear duct to open it up.) This type of surgery is usually successful.

Ears

Your baby may be born with an ear that is folded over or otherwise misshapen—another common side effect of labour and one that, in most cases, will correct itself over time.

As a general rule, there shouldn't be any discharge from a newborn baby's ears other than wax, so if you notice any other type of discharge, put a call in to your baby's doctor.

Skin

When your baby is born, she'll be covered in all kinds of goop—amniotic fluid, blood, and traces of vernix caseosa (the white, slippery, cheese-like material that protected your baby's skin in the watery pre-birth environment and acted as a lubricant during the delivery). She's also likely to have traces of fine, downy hair known as lanugo, which typically rubs off during the first or second week of a baby's life.

Here are some other things you need to know about your baby's skin.

- Your baby's skin may look dry and flaky, particularly on her hands and feet, during the first few weeks of life. (If her skin cracks, apply thin layers of a non-perfumed, preservative-free emollient or a cold-pressed oil such as olive oil.)
- Some babies are born with skin that is somewhat translucent, which makes the patches of blood vessels on the bridge of the nose, the eyelids, and the nape of the neck more visible than normal.
- While some babies (mainly full-term babies) are born with smooth, wrinkle-free skin, other babies (typically premature and small babies) have loose, wrinkly skin. Don't worry if your baby falls into the second category: she will grow into her skin over time.
- Your baby's skin may take on a flushed appearance when she cries. This is very common in newborn babies and doesn't indicate any serious health problems.
- Some parents notice that their baby's blood tends to pool in the lower half of the body when the baby is held in an upright position, which makes the baby's body look redder in the lower half than in the upper half. This is due to an immature circulation system and will correct itself over time.
- It's not unusual for your baby's hands and feet to be cool and bluish rather than warm and pink. This is because her circulation system is

TABLE 1.1

Newborn Skin Conditions

Milia are little yellow-white bumps that resemble whiteheads. They appear to be raised, but they are actually flat and smooth to the touch. They are typically found on a baby's nose, forehead, and cheeks. They are caused by a buildup of sebum—a skin lubricant that is secreted by your baby's body. Milia (sometimes referred to as "baby acne") will disappear on their own once your baby's oil glands and pores are a little more mature—something that typically occurs within the first two to three weeks of life. They occur in 40 per cent of infants.

Miliaria is a raised rash that consists of small, fluid-filled blisters. The fluid is made up of normal skin secretions and may be clear or milky white. This rash usually disappears on its own with normal washing. It typically occurs during the first 12 hours of life, and will disappear within a week.

Erythema toxicum are red splotches with yellowish-white bumps in the centres. They generally appear within the first one to three days following the birth and disappear on their own within a week or two, although they may fade in and out during that time. They occur in 30 to 70 per cent of infants.

Pustular melanosis is the name given to small blisters that quickly dry up and peel away, leaving dark, freckle-like spots underneath. (Don't worry: the "freckles" typically disappear within a couple of weeks, too.)

Note: All of these skin conditions clear up on their own over time, so resist the temptation to poke at your baby's pimples or otherwise attempt to treat these skin conditions.

still immature and is not yet operating at full capacity. Once again, this problem will fix itself after the first couple of days.

Here's the scoop on the most common types of newborn skin conditions—conditions that may be causing you some concern.

---

baby talk — Harlequin (meaning "in varied colours") colour change is a temporary colour change that causes a baby to appear pale on one half of the body and redder on the other half, divided at the midline. The phenomenon can last from a few minutes to half an hour when it occurs. It is more common in preterm babies than in full-term babies, and is caused by a temporary imbalance in circulation. Babies outgrow this condition within a few days to a few weeks.

TABLE 1.2

Birth Marks

Stork bites (salmon patch hemangioma) are pinkish, irregularly shaped patches that are typically found at the nape of the neck or on the face, although they can also be found on other parts of the body. They are caused by the dilation of small blood vessels. When pressed on, they will turn pale. Stork bites on the face tend to disappear by age 1; ones on the neck tend to be more permanent. They occur in 70 to 75 per cent of newborns.

Port wine stains are large, flat, irregularly shaped patches on the skin ranging in colour from purple to red to jet black. They are caused by a surplus of blood vessels under the skin. They tend to darken with age and can become raised and vulnerable to injury. They can be associated with certain types of genetic disorders. Port wine stains can be removed by either a plastic surgeon or dermatologist when the child gets older, if they happen to be particularly disfiguring. They won't disappear on their own.

Strawberry hemangiomas (capillary hemangiomas) are raised birthmarks with a soft texture. While strawberry hemangiomas may initially be white or pale-coloured, they turn red over time. They come in all sizes: some are smaller than a pea while others are larger than a softball. Strawberry hemangiomas occur when a certain area of the skin develops an abnormal blood supply, causing the affected tissue to enlarge and become reddish blue. Approximately two out of every hundred babies are either born with a strawberry hemangioma or develop one shortly after birth (typically at 2 to 5 weeks of age). Strawberry hemangiomas tend to increase in size over a period of four to nine months, and then disappear during late childhood (between the ages of 5 and 9), leaving behind a small amount of brownish pigmentation, but they can be treated with medication prior to that if they're close to the eye and threatening the child's vision.

Cavernous hemangiomas are similar to strawberry hemangiomas but involve deeper layers of the skin and may grow in size during the first year of a baby's life. A cavernous hemangioma is reddish or bluish red in colour and has a lumpy texture. Cavernous hemangiomas decrease in size after the first year of life. They are typically half gone by age 5 and fully gone by age 12. Treatment is possible if a cavernous hemangioma is particularly unsightly.

Mongolian spots are temporary accumulations of pigment under the skin. They tend to be about 10 centimetres (4 inches) in size or greater and are grey blue without sharp borders. Most common in babies of African American, Native American, or Mediterranean descent, they tend to be found on the buttocks, lower back, and arms and legs. They gradually disappear during the first few years of life.

Café au lait marks are permanent tan-coloured patches that can appear at birth or at any point during the first two years of life. They can show up anywhere on a baby's body. If your baby is born with or develops six or more café au lait marks, be sure to let your baby's doctor know: there is a link between large numbers of café au lait marks and certain types of neurological disorders.

> **Spider nevi** are thin, dilated blood vessels that are spider-like in shape. They typically fade during the baby's first year of life.
>
> **Congenital pigmented nevi**—better known as the common mole—come in a variety of shades ranging from tan to black. Some have hair growing from them. There is only cause for concern if the mole is very large (in which case there is a risk of it becoming malignant) or if the mole bleeds or changes colour, shape, or size (other possible signs of a malignancy). These types of moles tend to grow with the child.
>
> **Skin tags** are small, soft, flesh-coloured or pigmented growths of skin. They can be removed by your baby's doctor if they are irritating or generally unsightly.

No discussion of the appearance of the newborn would be complete without a discussion of birthmarks. While the majority of birthmarks disappear within the first five years of a baby's life, some are there permanently. Here's what you need to know about the most common types of birthmarks.

Umbilical cord stump

If there's one thing about the new arrival that most parents could live without, it's their newborn baby's umbilical cord stump. Not only is it rather unsightly and (in some cases) even a little stinky, it's also a source of tremendous anxiety to many parents.

A newborn baby's umbilical cord is cut and clamped with a plastic clip shortly after the birth. The plastic clip is usually removed 24 hours later, and the cord—which is initially wet and yellowish—gradually becomes dry and brownish black until it falls off entirely (something that typically happens when the baby is 10 to 14 days old, although some take as long as three weeks). The World Health Organization now recommends dry cord care (letting your baby's cord dry out naturally), and using just soap and water to clean visibly soiled cords. There is no evidence that swabbing a baby's umbilical cord with rubbing alcohol or other substances reduces the risk of infection. All it does is increase the length of time it takes for the cord to fall off.

Most umbilical cord stumps fall off naturally on their own with little cause for concern. Sometimes complications do arise, however. You should call your baby's doctor if you notice any redness in the area, the umbilical cord stump becomes moist and foul smelling, there is a lot of drainage from the navel (mucus, pus, or fluid), or you suspect that your baby may be developing an umbilical hernia (his navel looks like it's pushing outward when he cries).

Hands and feet

One of the first things that new parents like to do is examine their baby's fingers and toes. It's hard to believe that these body parts can be so tiny! You may have to pop on a pair of reading glasses to check out the toenail on your newborn's baby toe—it's that small.

Your baby's hands will likely be bluish and wrinkled, and clenched into fists that are pulled up toward his face. (Even before birth, babies like to keep their hands close to their mouths. In fact, some master the fine art of thumb-sucking long before birth.) Don't be surprised if your baby claws at his face and manages to scratch himself even though his fingernails appear to be soft and paper-thin. Babies tend to do this a lot. The best way to prevent him from scratching his face is to keep his fingernails trimmed. You can pick up a special pair of baby-sized nail clippers and some baby-sized emery boards at the drugstore. Or you can bite your baby's nails off while he's breastfeeding.

Like your baby's hands, your baby's feet will likely be bluish and wrinkled. Don't be surprised if his feet are a bit turned in or if his toes overlap slightly. This is very common in newborns and isn't an indication of permanent foot-related problems.

Legs and arms

Your baby's arms and legs will tend to look short and bird-like in comparison with the rest of her body. Don't be surprised if she holds them in a frog-like position, particularly when you place her on her belly. This is the position she got used to in the womb, so it's still very natural for her.

Genitalia

More than a few parents are downright alarmed when they first see their baby's genitals. The vulva of a female newborn and the scrotal sac and testes of a male newborn may appear large and swollen due to both the rush of hormones just prior to the birth and the extra fluid accumulated during the birth. What's more, these body parts may appear red and inflamed. While swelling of the vulva disappears within the first week of life, extra fluid in the scrotal sac may last for weeks or months, leaving a newborn baby boy with a disproportionately large scrotum during the early months of his life.

Here are some other things you need to know about your baby's genitals.

- If you have a baby girl, she may pass some thin white or blood-tinged mucus (pseudomenses) from the vagina during the first week of life. This discharge is triggered by withdrawal from maternal hormones.

- Approximately 1 per cent of baby boys are born with one or more undescended testicles. (The testicles develop in the abdomen, normally descending into the scrotum just before a full-term birth. But, in some cases, the testicles have not yet descended by the time the baby is born.) Some testes spontaneously descend during the first year of life. If this does not occur, hormonal treatment and/or surgery may be required to preserve your son's future fertility.

- Some boys are born with a condition called phimosis (tight foreskin), in which the penis and the foreskin are fused together. In this situation, circumcision may be required. (You don't have to have your son circumcised right away. In fact, there is good reason to wait. Often this condition resolves itself without treatment by the teen years. If it doesn't, then surgery should be considered.)

- Some boys are born with epispadias or hypospadias—penile abnormalities in which the urethral opening is on the upper surface or underside of the penis, respectively. Although these conditions will not cause fertility or sexual-function problems later in life, they can be corrected with surgery when your son is a bit older. In the meantime, because the foreskin is used in the surgery, he cannot be circumcised.

As you can see, your newborn baby is fascinating from head to toe. He or she is also a unique individual right from day one. While your baby will likely share some traits with any future brothers or sisters, none will be an exact carbon copy. He or she is truly one of a kind.

---

baby talk Who can resist the charms of a baby? Not very many people. This is because babies are born with a series of "attachment-promoting" traits—characteristics such as big soulful eyes, chubby cheeks, soft skin, and, of course, that intoxicating newborn scent. Scientists theorize that babies are programmed to be cute so that they'll quickly win the hearts of all the adults around them, thereby maximizing their odds for long-term survival.

---

baby talk — The World Health Organization classifies babies who are born three weeks or more before their due dates and who weigh less than 5 pounds (about 2.5 kilograms) as preterm. Certain babies face a greater risk of being born prematurely than others: babies with abnormal chromosomes or those who have developed an infection prior to birth; twins and other multiples; babies whose mothers have experienced placental problems, uterine abnormalities, or maternal complications such as congenital heart disease or kidney disease that may trigger preterm labour; and babies whose mothers smoke, drink, or take illicit drugs during pregnancy. Babies who are born prematurely face a greater risk of experiencing learning disabilities, attention deficit hyperactivity disorder, problems with visual-spatial concepts, hearing difficulties, and eye problems.

WHAT TO EXPECT IF YOUR BABY IS PREMATURE

Until now, we've been generally focusing on the physical appearance of a healthy, full-term baby. Now let's talk about what your baby may look like if she decides to make her grand entrance a few weeks early. While she'll still have a lot in common with a full-term infant, there are some rather noteworthy differences that you need to know about.

- **Eyes:** If your baby was born before the 26th week of gestation, her eyes may be sealed shut.

- **Genitals:** Your baby's genitals may be immature. In boys, the testicles may be undescended. In girls, the labia majora (the outer lips of the vulva) may not yet be large enough to cover the labia minora (inner lips) and the clitoris, and there may be a tag of skin protruding from the vagina (don't worry, it will disappear over time).

- **Scrawny appearance:** Your baby may look wrinkled and scrawny because his body is lacking the layers of fat that are normally deposited toward the end of pregnancy (after the 30th to 32nd week). As he begins to gain weight, he'll add this layer of fat and start to look more like a full-term infant.

- **Translucent skin:** Your baby's shortage of body fat also affects the appearance of his skin. Veins and arteries are clearly visible through his skin, and his skin has a reddish-purple tint regardless of his ethnic background. (This is because natural pigmentation does not typically appear until around the eighth month of gestation.)

- **Lack of body hair:** Extremely premature babies may not have any body hair at all. The hair on the head may be nothing more than a fine fuzz. On the other hand, babies who are born closer to term may be covered in lanugo (the fine, downy hair that covers a baby's body before birth). This hair may be particularly abundant on the back, upper arms, and shoulders.

- **No nipples:** Nipples don't typically appear until the 34th week of pregnancy, so your baby may lack nipples if he's born before then. Some babies will, however, have a completely formed areola—the darkish circle of skin that normally surrounds the nipple.

- **Poor muscle tone:** Premature babies have less control over their bodies than full-term infants. When they are placed on their backs, their hands, arms, and legs may either shake and startle frequently or go limp. Younger preemies may not move around much at all. Their movements may be limited to gentle stretches or curling their fingers into a fist. Babies born before 35 weeks' gestation lack the muscle tone required to tuck themselves into the fetal position that is typically assumed by a full-term infant.

- **Underdeveloped lungs:** Premature babies have more breathing problems than full-term babies because their lungs are underdeveloped. Fortunately, it's possible for a baby's lungs to continue to mature outside the womb, so breathing problems lessen as a premature baby matures.

---

baby talk Premature babies tend to cry less than their full-term counterparts because they don't have the energy to engage in a lot of crying. Consequently, many premature infants deal with stress by shutting down and doing nothing.

---

baby talk Sometimes the parents of very premature babies are afraid to look at their babies for the first time for fear that they will be shocked or alarmed by what they see. In most cases, what the parent is imagining is far worse than the reality. While it can be shocking to see an infant small enough to fit into an adult's hand being hooked up to tubes and wires, particularly if you're not quite clear about what all those tubes and wires are for, most parents are surprised to see just how fully formed their babies are, even if their babies arrived months ahead of time. As Dana Wechsler Linden, Emma Trenti Paroli, and Mia Wechsler Doron, MD, note in their book, *Preemies: The Essential Guide for Parents of Premature Babies*, "A preemie's parents soon start to find their baby the most graceful and beautiful in the world, and to view full-term newborns as ungainly giants."

If your baby is born between 24 and 28 weeks' gestation, you should be prepared for the fact that your baby may look more like a fetus than a typical newborn. Your baby's eyes may still be fused shut, his skin may look shiny and translucent and be too delicate to touch, and his ears may be soft and folded in places where the cartilage has yet to thicken. You will probably find that your baby changes dramatically during the weeks ahead as his skin becomes thicker and his eyes open for the first time. Suddenly, he'll start looking more like a full-term newborn. Note: A baby who is born before 24 weeks' gestation faces a very difficult struggle. His odds of survival are significantly less than those of a baby born just a few weeks later.

NEWBORN REFLEXES

You already know that newborns are programmed to be cute. (Remember? We talked about those "attachment-promoting" traits earlier on in this chapter.) Now let's talk about the other amazing things that newborn babies are born knowing how to do. Believe it or not, your baby comes pre-wired with a number of important reflexes, including the following.

Rooting reflex
How it works: If you touch your baby's mouth or stroke her cheek on one side, she'll turn her head in that direction and open her mouth, looking for a nipple to latch onto.

How long it lasts: Until about the fourth month.

Sucking reflex
How it works: If you touch your baby's palate (with a nipple or a finger), she uses a sucking motion made up of rhythmic jaw actions and pressure from the tongue to remove milk from the breast and transport milk to the throat, triggering the swallowing reflex. This reflex doesn't begin to develop until the 32nd week of pregnancy and isn't fully developed until the 36th week of pregnancy, which explains why many premature babies have a weak or immature sucking reflex.

How long it lasts: The sucking reflex is slowly replaced by a baby's ability to make a conscious decision to suck. This transition occurs during the first year of life.

Extrusion reflex
How it works: If your baby detects any solid or semi-sold material in the mouth, it is extruded via cottage-cheese-like spit-ups.

How long it lasts: For four to six months.

Grasping reflex
How it works: If you touch your baby's fingers and palm, he'll grasp your finger tightly. (Most new parents are astounded by the strength of a newborn baby's grip.)

How long it lasts: The grasping reflex is at its strongest during the first two months of life, disappearing entirely by the time the baby is 5 to 6 months old.

Moro reflex (startle reflex)
How it works: Your baby reacts strongly to a loud noise or sudden movement. She arches her back, throws open her arms and legs, and may cry before pulling back her arms again. (The best way to deal with this particular reflex is to avoid sudden movements and noises, and to hold your baby close and soothe her if she becomes startled.)

How long it lasts: For five to six months.

Stepping reflex
How it works: If you hold your baby in a walking position with his feet touching a flat surface, he'll start taking steps. Your baby will

exhibit similar reflexes when placed on his stomach: he'll start trying to "swim" forward. This is the reflex that allows the baby to crawl to the breast after birth and latch on by himself.

How long it lasts: Typically subsides around the second month.

Tonic neck reflex (fencer's reflex)

How it works: If a baby is placed on her back, she will turn her head to one side and extend the arm and leg on that same side in a classic fencing position. She'll then turn her head in the opposite direction and extend her other arm and leg in turn.

How long it lasts: About six months.

Placing reflex

How it works: If a baby is held in an upright position in front of the edge of an object, such as a table, he will lift his foot as if to step up onto that object. His arm will react in a similar fashion: if the back of his arm touches the edge of a table, he will automatically raise his arm.

How long it lasts: Throughout the early weeks of life.

Crawling reflex

How it works: If you place a baby on her stomach, she will automatically assume a crawling position with her knees pulled up under her abdomen. She may kick her legs and be able to propel herself in a crawling-like fashion. (It's not real crawling, of course. You'll have to wait quite a few months longer to see that.) Once the crawling reflex disappears, she'll stretch her legs out behind her when she's placed on her belly.

How long it lasts: Throughout the early weeks of life.

Doll's eye reflex

How it works: If you lift a baby and turn him to the right or the left, his eyes will stay fixed on the same object he was looking at before you moved him.

How long it lasts: About 10 days.

While it's easy to figure out why the rooting reflex is useful to a newborn, it's less obvious why newborns come equipped with some of the other reflexes. Still, even if you don't quite understand why your baby responds the way he does to certain stimuli, it's fun to try to observe some of these reflexes in your newborn.

THE APGAR TEST

Your baby is only a minute old and she's already being subjected to her first test—an Apgar test (see Table 1.3).

TABLE 1.3

The Apgar Scoring System

Sign	0	1	2
Heart Rate	Absent	Below 100 beats/minute	100 beats/minute or higher
Respiratory Effort	No spontaneous respirations	Slow; weak cry	Spontaneous, with a strong, lusty cry
Muscle Tone	Limp	Minimal flexion of extremities; sluggish movement	Active spontaneous motion; flexed body posture
Reflex Irritability	No response to suction or gentle slap on soles of feet	Minimal response (grimace) to stimulation	Prompt response to suction and a gentle slap to sole of foot with a cry or active movement
Colour	Blue or pale	Body pink, extremities blue	Completely pink (light skin) or absence of bluish tinge to extremities (dark skin). Note: With dark-skinned babies, doctors examine the colour of the inside of Baby's mouth or the palms of hands/soles of Baby's feet to see if skin is pinkish or bluish in colour.

An Apgar score of 7 to 10 indicates that the baby is adjusting well to life outside the womb, a score of 4 to 6 means that the baby requires some gentle stimulation (such as rubbing the back), and a score of 3 or lower means that the baby needs active resuscitation.

Note: Just as important as the score itself is the overall trend in the baby's Apgar scores: whether he scores higher or lower on the five minute test than he did on the one minute test. If a baby seems to be experiencing greater difficulties at five minutes of age than he did at one minute of age, there could be a serious problem.

The brainchild of anesthesiologist Virginia Apgar, MD, who invented the test back in 1952, the Apgar test is performed one minute and five minutes after birth. The test measures five different attributes: heart rate, respiration, muscle tone, reflex responsiveness, and the baby's skin colour (whether the baby is "pinking up" or still a bit blue). The test isn't designed to function as any sort of intelligence test or to predict which babies will do better over the long term: its sole purpose is to identify babies who may need a little more care and attention initially.

It's not surprising that some babies need a little help during the first few hours after the birth. What's surprising is the fact that the majority of infants make the transition from life inside the womb to life outside the womb with very little trouble at all. It's pretty amazing when you stop and think about it.

---

baby talk Your baby will be weighed and measured shortly after birth. A light blanket or disposable paper will be placed on the scale so that your naked baby won't have to come into contact with the cold metal surface. Once your baby has been weighed, her length and head and chest circumference will be measured to ensure that her various body parts are all in roughly the right proportion.

THE NEWBORN EXAM

Even if your baby manages to sail through the Apgar test with flying colours, she will be carefully examined by members of the health-care team to ensure that she continues to thrive. While her weight, measurements, and vital signs will be taken immediately, her head-to-toe examination might not take place for at least a few hours, although it will take place at some point during her first day of life.

Here's what the doctor conducting the newborn examination will be looking for as he or she checks over your new baby.

- **Overall health:** Does your baby appear to be in good health? Does he have good muscle tone? Is he active, alert, and pinkish rather than bluish in colour? If your baby appears to be experiencing some difficulty adapting to life outside the womb, some medical interventions may be in order.

- **Heart:** Are there any abnormal sounds or beats that might indicate a structural problem with your baby's heart? Note: A heart rate of 120 to 160 beats per minute is normal for a newborn, although the heart rate will be lower if a baby is sleeping and higher if a baby is crying.

- **Body temperature:** Is your baby maintaining her body temperature properly? It's important to ensure that your baby is warm enough because a low body temperature can quickly lead to hypoglycemia (low blood sugar) as the baby draws upon her glucose reserves to keep herself warm. Hypoglycemia can, in turn, cause a baby's temperature to go down—the start of a vicious cycle. Note: Newborn temperatures used to be taken rectally, but these days auxiliary (under the armpit) temperatures are more commonly used. While tympanic (ear) temperatures are used quite often with older babies, they've been proven to be less accurate in newborns.

- **Breathing:** Is the baby having any difficulty breathing? Is she exhibiting any of the symptoms of respiratory distress, such as a bluish tinge to parts of the body other than the hands and feet, flaring nostrils, grunting respirations, rapid breathing, or other breathing irregularities?

---

baby talk Prior to birth, the mother's body regulates the baby's temperature. After birth, that all-important task is handed over to the baby. Newborns can lose heat quickly after the birth as the amniotic fluid on their skin evaporates from their body. The temperature can drop as much as 1 degree Celsius (1.8 degrees Fahrenheit) per minute and glycogen and brown fat stores may become depleted in a matter of hours. That's why it's so important to keep newborn babies warm.

- **Gestational age evaluation:** Does the baby appear to be of the anticipated gestational age? Is the baby's skin thin and transparent (as you would expect from a preterm baby) or is it peeling (as you would expect from a post-term baby)? Is there vernix covering most of the body (as you would expect if the baby was preterm) or only in the baby's creases (as you would expect if the baby was born at term), or is there no vernix left at all (as you would expect if the baby was post term)?

Is there an abundance of lanugo (an indication that the baby might be preterm) or lanugo in just a few places (an indication that the baby is probably term)? Do the baby's ears spring back slowly after being folded toward the lobe (an indication of possible prematurity)? Is there any breast tissue? (If there isn't much, the baby is likely preterm.) Do the genitals appear to be that of a preterm or term infant? Are there creases on the soles of the feet (something that only happens toward the end of pregnancy and that may therefore serve as confirmation that the baby was born on or around her due date)? Is the skin on the baby's feet peeling (a sign that the baby may be post-term or may have experienced growth-related problems inside the womb)?

- **Birth-related injuries:** Are there any birth-related injuries such as bruises, injured muscles or ligaments, or broken bones?
- **Congenital anomalies:** Does the baby appear to have any congenital anomalies?
- **Head:** Does the baby's head exhibit any abnormalities? Is the fontanelle soft and flat? Is the circumference of the baby's head proportionate to the baby's length and weight? Are the baby's facial features and body proportions normal?
- **Eyes:** Does the baby appear to have any eye problems? Are the eyes a normal size?
- **Ears:** Are the baby's ear canals properly formed? Note: Don't be overly concerned if your baby's ears are pinned against his head, folded over, or otherwise sticking out. These types of problems tend to correct themselves over time and, even if they don't, they can be corrected relatively easily.
- **Nose:** Are the nasal passages wide enough to allow for the flow of air?

---

baby talk — Most respiratory secretions are produced within the first few hours after the birth. Fluid and mucus are wiped from the infant's face, and the mouth and nose are suctioned by the birth attendant as soon as the baby's head is born. If your baby is particularly mucous, you may have to turn your baby on his side and pat his back to help him clear the mucus.

- **Mouth:** Is the front of your baby's tongue attached too tightly to the floor of her mouth, something that could interfere with a good latch during breastfeeding? (The tongue of a newborn baby is attached along a greater proportion of its length than the tongue of an older child. If it turns out that your baby's tongue is attached too tightly, your baby's frenulum—the piece of tissue that joins the bottom of the tongue to the floor of the mouth—may need to be clipped.) Are there any loose teeth or teeth that are growing at an unusual angle? (If such teeth exist, they will be removed so that there's no risk of them falling out and being swallowed by the baby.) Is the roof of the baby's mouth fully formed? (If not, the baby may have a cleft palate, which will require reconstructive surgery.)

- **Neck:** Does your baby's neck have any abnormal bumps? Is there evidence of a broken collarbone (a common birth-related injury)?

baby talk Your baby's umbilical cord is examined after it has been cut in order to determine the number and type of blood vessels. A normal umbilical cord has three vessels: two arteries and one vein. Two-vessel cords can be associated with certain types of anomalies, which is why the cord is checked so carefully after the birth.

- **Arms:** Is there a pulse in each arm (an indication that your baby's circulation is functioning as it should)? Do the arms exhibit signs of normal movement and strength? Your baby's doctor will also check her fingers (to see if there are any anomalies) and the creases of her palms (if your baby has only one crease in her hands, your doctor will want to check for some other related physical abnormalities).

- **Legs:** Are your baby's legs the same length? Do they exhibit signs of normal movement and strength? Are there any abnormalities, such as clubfoot—a condition that occurs when the front half of the foot is curved in excessively? The doctor will also hold your baby's thighs and move them around the hip joints to see if your baby has dislocatable hips—a condition that's much easier to treat in newborns than in older babies or toddlers.

- **Abdomen:** Are your baby's liver, spleen, and kidneys the right size and in the correct position? Are there any abnormal growths in the abdomen? Does the baby have an umbilical hernia (a small swelling close to the belly button that becomes more prominent when a baby is crying)? Note: Umbilical hernias are caused by a weakness in the abdominal muscles. In most cases, they repair themselves within a year. Very few babies with umbilical hernias require surgery.
- **Spinal column:** Is there any evidence of spina bifida (a disorder in which the meninges—the membranes that cover the spinal column and brain—are left exposed)?
- **Genitals:** Is the vaginal opening normal? Is the clitoris a normal size? Are the lips of the labia separate (as they should be) or joined? Have the testicles descended into the scrotum? Are there any intestinal protrusions (hernias) beneath the skin of the groin?
- **Anus:** Is the anus open and located in the appropriate position? (If the anus is not open or is otherwise malformed, surgery will be required.) Has the baby passed any meconium (the blackish-green tar-like substance that fills a baby's intestines before birth)? The doctor will also place a finger in the centre of the baby's groin to check for the femoral pulse. The strength of the pulse helps to indicate whether the baby's circulatory system is functioning properly.

Other tests

In addition to conducting the head-to-toe physical examination on your newborn, your baby's health-care providers will perform the following procedures and tests:

- **Cord blood sample:** A sample of umbilical cord blood will be taken so that the baby's blood type and Rh factor can be determined. It's important to find out early on if there are any blood incompatibility problems because such problems can lead to an increased risk of jaundice and other health problems (such as anemia) in the newborn.
- **Vitamin K:** Your baby will receive a vitamin K injection in his thigh within the first few hours of life. Vitamin K is necessary for blood coagulation, and newborns are born with a temporary vitamin K deficiency. (Vitamin K is manufactured by the bacteria in the intestines, and the intestines remain sterile until normal bacteria are

established.) Having this injection helps to promote blood clotting and lessens the risk of abnormal bleeding into vital tissues such as the brain. Note: If you have a strong objection to your baby receiving a vitamin K injection, talk to your doctor about the advisability of having vitamin K administered orally instead. While most caregivers recommend that you go the injection route because it is more effective, it is possible to give a baby a series of oral doses of vitamin K: during the first feeding, at 2 to 4 weeks of age, and at 6 to 8 weeks of age. If you do decide to opt for oral vitamin K rather than injections, it's critically important that your baby receive the follow-up doses. Note: If you're planning to have your baby circumcised, you should opt for the injection rather than the oral dose of vitamin K because you'll want to ensure that your baby's blood is clotting properly before he has any surgical procedure.

- **Eye ointment:** Newborn babies can contract infections such as gonorrhea and chlamydia from the mother during the birth process. Since these sexually transmitted infections are known to cause blindness in newborns, it's standard hospital procedure to apply erythromycin ointment to the baby's eyes within a couple of hours of the birth. Since this treatment leads to blurred vision for a short time after the ointment has been applied, you will want to ask your baby's caregiver to delay treatment until you've had some time to bond with your baby. (Health Canada states that such treatment can be delayed for up to two hours after the birth.) Note: Erythromycin ointment can cause some mild irritation to your baby's eyes for 24 to 48 hours after treatment.

- **Screening tests:** Heath Canada recommends that all babies be screened for potentially serious health problems that may be present at birth. Newborns in Ontario, for example, are now screened for 27 rare disorders that can cause health problems in babies and children. These disorders include metabolic disorders (which occur when the body lacks the ability to break down certain substances in food, a condition that, if undiagnosed and untreated, can lead to organ damage and other serious health problems), endocrine disorders (which occur if the body isn't producing the right balance of hormones, and which can lead to illness or developmental disabilities), and blood disorders (which can lead to severe anemia and serious infections).

A small sample of blood will be taken by pricking your baby's heel and squeezing out some blood. Hypothyroidism (one of the conditions that is tested for)—occurs in one out of every five thousand infants and is caused by an inadequate thyroid gland. It can lead to cretinism (a form of developmental disability) if left undetected and untreated. The sooner treatment with thyroid hormone is started, the more effective the treatment—which explains why early detection is so critical. Likewise, phenylketonuria (PKU)—which occurs in one out of every 15,000 infants—is an inability to metabolize (break down) the protein phenylalanine. This condition can lead to a buildup of protein in the blood, which can result in brain damage if left untreated. Fortunately, if the condition is detected early on and treated with a special diet, the child is able to develop normally. That heel pinprick may not be fun for your baby (or for you) but it yields a lot of valuable—even potentially life-saving—health information.

---

baby talk   A baby who loses a lot of blood through the umbilical cord or the placenta during the delivery faces an increased risk of becoming anemic (having low iron stores). Babies who are anemic may require iron supplements to help them build up the number of red blood cells in their bodies, since these red blood cells play a vital role in transporting oxygen. Because of the threat to the infant's health, severe cases of anemia are treated with blood transfusions.

Note: Delaying umbilical cord clamping until the cord has stopped pulsing allows more blood to remain in the baby's body, reducing the risk of anemia in the newborn. Anemia can also be caused by Rh incompatibility between mother and baby. If you are Rh-negative, your doctor may want to test a sample of umbilical cord blood to determine whether any Rh antibodies have built up in your baby's blood.

- **Hearing check:** The Canadian Paediatric Society now recommends routine hearing screening of all newborns. Many provinces have already adopted this recommendation. The testing is done with a portable machine that detects hearing ability in the newborn. The test is non-invasive. In fact, it can be done while a baby is sleeping.

Note: Some babies face an increased risk of experiencing hearing loss, which typically occurs at a rate of 1.5 to 6.0 per one thousand live births. The risk factors for hearing loss in newborns include a family history of childhood sensorineural hearing loss, congenital infections such as cytomegalovirus (CMV), rubella, syphilis, herpes, and toxoplasmosis, certain types of facial anomalies, severe jaundice requiring blood transfusions, bacterial meningitis, certain instances of perinatal asphyxia, and a birth weight of less than 5 pounds (1.5 kilograms).

---

baby talk Some babies face a higher-than-average risk of experiencing problems during the newborn phase. This includes

- √ babies who were born before 37 weeks' or after 42 weeks' gestation;
- √ babies who are small or large for their gestational age;
- √ babies who required prolonged resuscitation at birth;
- √ babies whose mothers experienced pregnancy-induced hypertension (high blood pressure);
- √ babies whose blood is incompatible with that of their mother;
- √ babies whose mothers were diagnosed as having an exceptionally large or small amount of amniotic fluid during pregnancy; and
- √ babies born to mothers who smoked, drank, or took illicit drugs during pregnancy, took certain types of medications during the delivery, are diabetic, and/or had poor prenatal care.

- **Other screening tests:** If your baby is either very large or very small at birth, is premature, is a twin or other multiple, or has some specific medical risk factors (for example, he has experienced perinatal asphyxia or is showing signs of encephalopathy, is in cardiorespiratory distress, is developing sepsis, or has blood that is incompatible with yours), and/or if you are diabetic, the hospital staff may wish to monitor your baby's blood pressure, blood glucose, and iron levels carefully.

mom's the word

"Personally, I don't enjoy the hospital stay. I find the nights tiring and stressful. You have just given birth and desperately need sleep, and yet you need to care for a newborn and master breastfeeding. I asked my mom to stay with me in the hospital when my third child was born, and that was so much better."
—KAREN, 34, CURRENTLY EXPECTING HER FOURTH CHILD

Once the initial newborn checkup has been completed, your baby will be monitored carefully during the early days of his life. His heart rate, respiratory rate, heart and breathing sounds, temperature, skin colour, and feeding and elimination patterns will be checked regularly to ensure that he is continuing to do well. If a complication arises, your baby can be treated quickly and with a greater likelihood of success.

mom's the word

"We left the hospital roughly 30 hours after Sarah was born. I was so high on adrenaline that I couldn't wait to leave. That night we attended our last prenatal class with our new daughter in tow."
—JENNIFER, 32, MOTHER OF ONE

Jaundice

Your baby's caregivers will also be on the lookout for signs of jaundice, since most newborns develop some degree of jaundice during their first few days of life. This is because newborns are born with more red blood cells than their bodies need now that they are no longer in the womb, and their bodies have to dispose of these blood cells during the first few days of life. As these excess cells are broken down, one of the things they break down into is a substance called bilirubin. If the baby's liver isn't able to get rid of all the bilirubin quickly enough (either because the liver is immature or there are an excessive number of cells for the baby's body to get rid of), the baby's skin and eyeballs will take on a yellowish hue. Excessively high *mother wisdom* — If you decide to exit stage left as soon as possible after the birth (whether because you miss being at home, your roommate's snoring is driving you crazy, or the hospital food is proving to be less than inspiring), make sure that you find out whether your baby will require any follow-up care during his first week of life. If, for example, your baby leaves the hospital before the screening tests have been completed, you'll have to find out what arrangements need to be made for your baby to have these important tests performed. Your doctor or midwife may also want to check on you and your baby in a couple of days' time.

If you gave birth at home, you can expect to be visited by your midwife during the first 24 hours and then twice more during the first week. These visits will take place in your own home. You'll have follow-up visits back at the midwifery clinic at two, four, and six weeks' postpartum to ensure that both you and your baby are continuing to do well.

---

levels of bilirubin can be dangerous (possibly leading to brain damage) so your baby will be monitored closely to ensure that his bilirubin levels aren't getting too high. Babies who were exposed to Pitocin (synthetic oxytocin) during labour are more prone to develop jaundice, as are babies who are born prematurely, babies who experience a lot of bruising during birth, babies whose blood type is incompatible with their mother's, and babies who are not getting enough milk. Traditionally, bilirubin levels were measured by taking a few drops of blood from a baby's heel, but now there is a less invasive alternative: the flash method. With the flash method, a small flashlight-like device is placed against a baby's skin to provide an estimate of the bilirubin level. It isn't as accurate as the heel poke, but it is good for monitoring trends and it makes for a happier baby.

There are different types of jaundice:

- **physiological jaundice**, which typically occurs three to five days after the birth and disappears as the baby's liver matures; and
- **pathological jaundice**, which is due to an underlying medical condition and often begins within 24 hours of the birth, and which can lead to brain damage, deafness, cerebral palsy, or intellectual disability if untreated.

baby talk Your baby's caregivers will want to know if your baby has passed any meconium (the blackish-green tar-like substance that makes up his first stool). Meconium is high in bilirubin, and a delay in passing meconium can lead to jaundice because the bilirubin in the meconium will be returned to the baby's circulation.

Babies with moderate cases of jaundice may be treated with phototherapy (exposing the baby's skin to a special type of light that helps the baby's body to dissolve the extra pigment in the skin) and extra fluids (to help the baby's body flush out the extra bilirubin through urination). If your baby is treated with phototherapy, his eyes will be protected with eye patches or he will be wrapped in a biliblanket (a fibre-optic blanket). Note: Some babies who undergo phototherapy develop skin rashes or loose bowel movements, so you should be on the lookout for these common side effects.

Babies with jaundice may be sleepy and not nursing well, which is a concern because getting plenty of milk is important in removing the bilirubin. (Water or sugar water won't help, since the bilirubin only leaves the body in bowel movements.) In the vast majority of cases, jaundice is brought under control within a week or two of the birth without any harm to the baby. Jaundice is more of a concern for a sick or premature infant than for a healthy, full-term newborn.

baby talk It doesn't take long for the various government authorities to start creating a paper trail for your baby; within a day or two of her birth, you will have already filled out enough paperwork to keep a small army of bureaucrats busy. Here are some government documents that you're likely to find in that rather daunting package of papers you were handed shortly after your child's birth.

√ **A birth registration form.** One of your first jobs as a new parent is to register your child's birth with the Department of Vital Statistics in your province or territory. If you give birth in a hospital, you will be given a form to fill out shortly after your child is born. If you deliver at home, the attending midwife should provide you with a copy of this form or explain what you need to do to obtain one and register your child' birth. In true Canadian fashion, the policies and procedures involved in registering a birth vary from jurisdiction to jurisdiction (who is responsible for registering the birth, how many days you have to register the birth, what options you have in terms of choosing your baby's last name, and so on). Note: Once your baby's birth has been registered, you may wish to order a copy of his birth certificate. In most cases, you will be required to fill out an application form and pay a nominal fee to obtain this additional—but very useful—document. Consult your provincial or territorial Department of Vital Statistics to learn more about the birth registration process in your part of the country.

- **An application for health insurance coverage.** The policies and procedures may vary by jurisdiction, but regardless of where you live in Canada, you'll either need to apply for a health card for your baby or arrange to have her added to your own existing provincial or territorial health insurance coverage. If you give birth in a hospital, you'll be given the necessary forms to fill out before you head home. (In many parts of the country, you'll be required to leave the completed forms with the hospital staff before you and your baby check out.) If you give birth at home, your midwife will either be able to supply you with the necessary paperwork or tell you what you need to do to apply for health insurance coverage for your new baby.

- **Canada Child Tax Benefit.** The CCTB is a tax-free monthly payment from the federal government that is designed to help eligible families offset some of the costs of raising children under the age of 18.

- **Social Insurance Number.** Something else you might want to take care of sooner rather than later is apply for a Social Insurance Number (SIN) on behalf of your baby. If you're planning to set up a Registered Educational Savings Plan (RESP) for her, you'll want her to have her own Social Insurance Number so that all her income can be taxed in her name, not yours. To apply for a Social Insurance Number for your baby, you will need to fill out a Social Insurance Number application form (readily available through any Human Resources Development Canada (HRDC) office).

Note: If your child has dual citizenship, taking care of the documentation early can save you headaches and paperwork later.

chapter 2

YOUR BODY AFTER THE BIRTH

"I was getting dressed one morning right after my milk had come in and my partner walked into the room. I heard a gasp. He stood staring at my breasts. When I looked in the mirror, I understood his amazement. They were huge! Unfortunately, he quickly learned that they were also extremely sore. I guess you have to take the bad with the good."

—TRACEY, 31, MOTHER OF ONE

It's the stuff of pregnant women's fantasies: you'll give birth to your baby and immediately slip back into your pre-pregnancy jeans—or, better yet, you'll be able to step straight into your bikini. (Hey, why not go for the bikini? After all, you're not going to work stretch marks, a Caesarean scar, a saggy abdomen, and leaky, cantaloupe-sized breasts into your fantasies, are you?) If this is the fantasy that's running through your head as you come into the home stretch of pregnancy, I have some sobering news for you: your body still has a lot of work to do in order to return to anything resembling its pre-pregnancy state.

In this chapter, we'll be talking about your body after the birth—what you can really expect.

YOUR POSTPARTUM BODY: THE OFFICIAL TOUR

Here's what you can expect from your body during the first days and weeks after the birth.

Heavy vaginal bleeding

During the postpartum period, your uterus will begin to shrink down to roughly its pre-pregnancy size (a process that is known as "involution").

While this is happening, you'll shed the lining of your uterus—something that results in the postpartum bleeding known as lochia. You'll experience lochia whether you have a vaginal or Caesarean birth.

You may be surprised by the amount of bleeding and the size of the blood clots you pass. "It was a lot heavier than I thought it would be," recalls Tina, a 32-year-old mother of one. "It was much heavier than even the heaviest menstrual period."

all systems check

During the first moments after the birth, you may feel as if you've been hit by a freight train. Or you may feel so excited and euphoric that you swear you could hop off the birthing bed and go run a marathon.

Regardless of how well you're feeling, you can expect to experience your fair share of poking and prodding during the first day or two postpartum as your health-care practitioner checks you over to make sure that your body is successfully making the shift from a pregnant to a non-pregnant state. He or she will be assessing

- √ your general wellness (your energy level, your responsiveness, whether you're experiencing a lot of pain, and, if so, whether the pain relief measures that you've been receiving are proving to be adequate);
- √ your emotional state (whether you're feeling depressed or weepy, how much family support you have, and how you're relating to your new baby);
- √ your vital signs (your pulse, blood pressure, temperature, and breathing);
- √ whether or not you are becoming dehydrated (a possibility if you endured a lengthy labour or threw up a lot when you were in transition);
- √ the consistency, location, and height of the fundus (the top of the uterus) and whether you are experiencing any tenderness that might indicate that you are developing a postpartum infection (endometritis—a uterine infection—is the most common cause of infection up to six weeks postpartum. It is more likely to occur following a Caesarean than a vaginal delivery. Symptoms include fever, lower abdominal pain, uterine tenderness, and foul-smelling lochia.);
- √ your lochia (the character, colour, and amount of postpartum bleeding, and whether or not any clots and/or unusual odour are present);

- ✓ your perineum (to check for signs of swelling, bruising, or other complications, and if you experienced a perineal tear or required an episiotomy, to see how well the incision or tear site is healing);
- ✓ whether you are having problems with hemorrhoids (how large they are and how much discomfort you are experiencing);
- ✓ whether your bowels are functioning properly (whether you've had a bowel movement since the delivery or, in the case of a Caesarean delivery, whether any bowel sounds can be detected—something that may indicate that your bowels are getting ready to starting functioning again);
- ✓ whether you're urinating regularly (to ensure that your bladder is functioning properly and that you aren't experiencing any delivery-related bladder problems caused by trauma to the area during the delivery, the effects of certain anaesthetics, and so on);
- ✓ your breasts (to look for signs of any potential problems such as flat or inverted nipples, breast engorgement that may interfere with breastfeeding, nipple pain, and so on); and
- ✓ your incision site, if you had a Caesarean (the nurse will want to see that the area is clean and dry and that the staples remain intact until they are removed approximately three days after the delivery).

Depending on your situation, you may need some additional care after the delivery. If, for example, you have Rh-negative blood and you give birth to an Rh-positive baby, you will need to receive a dose of Rh immune globulin (RhoGAM) within 72 hours of the birth to prevent problems in future pregnancies.

Don't immediately assume that you're experiencing a postpartum hemorrhage, however, if you feel a sudden gush of blood or fluid when you stand up (which causes the uterus to empty) or breastfeed your baby (which causes the uterus to contract). This is perfectly normal. There is generally only cause for concern if you are soaking more than one heavy-duty pad over the course of an hour, passing blood clots that are larger than lemons (yes, *lemons!*), or your lochia has developed an extremely unpleasant odour, a possible sign of a postpartum infection.

mother wisdom — It's not surprising that postpartum bleeding (lochia) is heavy and lasts for many weeks. You have a lot of uterine tissue to shed. At the time you gave birth, your uterus weighed between 28 and 42 ounces (800 and 1,200 grams). Before you became pregnant, it weighed 1.8 ounces (50 grams). Your uterus will weigh about 2.1 to 2.5 ounces (60 to 70 grams) by the time it is finished contracting and shedding the lining it built up to nurture your baby during pregnancy.

Most women experience lochia for at least a month after the delivery, and, in some cases, for up to six weeks. Lochia tends to last longer with a first baby and with larger babies, and also following a Caesarean birth. Lochia typically tapers down from a bright red flow to a lighter pinkish discharge around the third to tenth day postpartum, to an almost colourless, odourless discharge sometime after the tenth day postpartum.

If your lochia has tapered off to a colourless or yellowish discharge but then suddenly becomes bright red again, call your doctor or midwife. Chances are you've simply been overdoing things a little—which can cause the amount of postpartum bleeding you experience to increase again—but it's always best to err on the side of caution where your reproductive health is concerned. (See Table 2.1 for some guidelines on other postpartum symptoms that warrant a call to your caregiver.)

mother wisdom — It's important to be alert to the possibility of early postpartum hemorrhage (excessive bleeding that occurs within 24 hours of the delivery—something that happens following 4 per cent of births) and late postpartum hemorrhage (excessive bleeding that occurs at any time after that point, but that typically becomes a problem between seven and fourteen days after the delivery—something that happens following 1 per cent of births). Postpartum hemorrhages can be caused by retained fragments of the placenta or the membranes, an infection of the uterine lining, or the failure of the uterus to contract properly and return to its normal size after the birth.

CHAPTER 2 — YOUR BODY AFTER THE BIRTH

TABLE 2.1

When to Call Your Caregiver

You will need to get in touch with your caregiver immediately if you experience one or more of the following symptoms, which may indicate that you are experiencing a postpartum hemorrhage, a postpartum infection, or other postpartum complications:

- sudden, heavy bleeding;
- a large number of blood clots;
- the return of bright red bleeding once your lochia has begun to subside;
- a foul-smelling vaginal discharge;
- severe pain or redness around, or discharge from, an episiotomy, tear, or Caesarean-section incision;
- a fever over 100°F (37.8°C);
- nausea or vomiting;
- blurred vision or dizziness;
- pain, redness, hot spots, or red streaks on your breasts;
- localized swelling or tenderness in your breasts;
- painful, burning urination or urgency when you urinate;
- painful, swollen, or tender legs;
- persistent perineal pain with increasing tenderness;
- vaginal pain that worsens after, or lasts longer than, a couple of weeks;
- a headache that does not go away;
- sharp pains in your abdomen, breasts, or chest;
- crying spells or mood swings that feel out of control; and
- thoughts of harming yourself or your baby.

---

mother wisdom — Some women develop an infection of the reproductive tract during the first six weeks postpartum. The symptoms include fever, pain, and tenderness in the abdomen; a foul-smelling vaginal discharge; difficulty urinating; and—in more severe cases—chills, a loss of appetite, lethargy, and a rapid pulse. If you are diagnosed with such an infection, your doctor will prescribe antibiotics, oxytocin (to keep the uterus contracted), and pain relief (to help you cope with those uterine contractions). You'll also need to rest and to consume plenty of fluids in order to help your body fight off the infection.

Perineal pain

You can expect your perineum to be sore and tender after a vaginal birth, even if you didn't end up having an episiotomy or a tear that required a lot of stitches. After all, the tissues of your perineum got quite a workout as your baby was being born. Stephanie was shocked by how swollen her perineum looked and felt: "I did not recognize parts of my own anatomy, they were so swollen," the 33-year-old mother of one recalls. "The biggest surprise came one day after I delivered. I was going to the bathroom and when I took the toilet paper to wipe, I was in utter shock at how swollen and odd my vaginal area felt. I immediately got a hand-held mirror so I could take a closer look. Between the swelling and the hemorrhoids, I did not recognize myself." You can minimize your discomfort during the postpartum period by keeping these tips in mind.

- The first day is the worst day when it comes to perineal pain. Your body will amaze you by how quickly it heals. Note: If you required any stitches to repair a perineal tear, your stitches should dissolve within five to seven days.

- Get in the habit of squeezing your buttocks together as you sit down and then relaxing your buttocks after you sit down. This will help to reduce a bit of the wear and tear on your perineum. If you still find that sitting down is pure torture, then you might want to send someone to the closest medical supply store in search of a hemorrhoid cushion. (For best results, only partially inflate the cushion.)

- Experiment to find out whether heat or cold provides you with the greatest relief. If it's heat that does the trick, try soaking your perineum in a warm bath (either a full-sized bathtub or a sitz bath) or carefully applying heat from a blow-dryer to your perineum. (Obviously, you'll want to set your blow-dryer on the lowest possible setting and limit the amount of time you spend blow-drying your perineum in order to prevent burns. The same applies to sitting spread-eagled in front of a sun lamp—something your mother or grandmother is sure to recommend but that generally isn't recommended these days. This tender part of your body burns quickly, and getting a sunburn "down there" will add to your postpartum woes immeasurably.) Note: Don't soak in hot water when you're using your sitz bath if you have stitches. This could cause your stitches to dissolve prematurely.

mom's the word "Soak some sanitary pads in water and freeze them. Wear these for the first little while postpartum. They help to soothe the perineum."
— CARRIE, 34, CURRENTLY PREGNANT WITH HER SECOND CHILD

- If cold brings you the greatest relief, place an ice pack on your perineum, add ice to your sitz bath, or try soaking some sanitary pads in water and freezing them (you'll want to mould them to the approximate shape you need) or filling a washcloth or rubber glove with ice and applying it to your perineum. Some women swear that there's no greater relief to be had than from chilled witch hazel pads (you'll find witch hazel at your local health food store). You just tuck the frozen pads between your perineum and your sanitary pad and—voila—relief is on its way.

mother wisdom You can reduce your chances of developing a perineal infection by changing your sanitary pad at least every couple of hours and by wiping your vulva from front to back each time you use the bathroom. (Initially, you may find that it works best to squirt your perineum with warm water using a squirt bottle, and to then pat the area dry using clean tissue or toilet paper.) The fewer bacteria that are hanging out in the area, the lower your risk of infection. Note: Do not use tampons or douche. You could end up giving yourself a serious postpartum infection.

mother wisdom It may take as long as four to six months for your episiotomy site to heal completely, but you'll notice a significant reduction in pain and tenderness after about two to three weeks.

mother wisdom — Either pick up these items ahead of time or on an as-needed basis after the birth. Your body will thank you for it.

- ✓ *Sanitary napkins:* You'll need at least two large boxes of the most absorbent sanitary napkins you can find—ideally ones designed specifically for postpartum or overnight use. Tampons are taboo during the postpartum period, and they'd be next to useless anyway, so forget about simply relying on any old tampons you might have kicking around in the back of your bathroom vanity.

- ✓ *Premoistened wipes for hemorrhoids:* Bet you've always wondered what those premoistened hemorrhoid wipes were for anyhow. Now's your chance to find out. Just in case you end up being blessed with this delightful by-product of both pregnancy and the pushing stage of labour, stock up on wipes before the delivery. That way, they'll be there if you need them.

- ✓ *A bottle of witch hazel lotion or ointment:* There's no denying it: witch hazel is a hemorrhoid-suffering girl's best friend. Pick up a bottle at your pharmacy or health food store and apply it to your tender parts with a cotton ball. It will help to reduce some of the itching and burning.

- ✓ *A hemorrhoid cushion:* These doughnut-shaped pillows can make sitting a little more comfortable if you're dealing with a tender perineum and/or hemorrhoids. Be sure to have one on hand.

- ✓ *Prenatal vitamins:* It's a good idea to continue taking your prenatal vitamins throughout the postpartum period (and even beyond that if you're nursing or planning to get pregnant again in the very near future).

Changes to the tone and feel of your vagina

If you delivered your baby vaginally, your vagina may feel stretched and tender after the delivery. It takes a few days for elasticity to return to the tissue, which feels quite spongy at first. Kegel exercises (pelvic floor muscle exercises, described later in this chapter) will help your vagina to regain its tone and can also help to ward off incontinence and other gynecological problems. Most women regain normal muscular tone and strength within two months of the birth. If you experienced a prolonged pushing stage, perineal trauma, or an episiotomy, or you gave birth to a very big baby, it may take longer than average for your perineal area to heal or to regain tone and strength, or you may have difficulty with incontinence.

If you are breastfeeding, you may experience vaginal dryness—something that can cause discomfort during intercourse unless you use a water-soluble vaginal lubricant. If your problems are particularly severe, you might want to ask your doctor to prescribe a topical estrogen cream to help with lubrication.

---

mom's the word "One problem I experienced postpartum was extreme vaginal dryness, which made intercourse impossible. I ended up going to a gynecologist and getting a topical estrogen cream, which fixed the problem. None of the books I read mentioned estrogen as a remedy. They simply advised additional lubrication, which, in my case, was not enough."

—JANA, 35, MOTHER OF ONE

Difficulty urinating

It's not at all unusual to experience a decreased urge to urinate after you give birth. This can be the result of a number of different factors, including

- a low fluid intake prior to and during labour;
- an excessive loss of fluids during the delivery (think perspiration, vomiting, and bleeding);
- bruising to the bladder or the urethra during labour;
- the effects of drugs and anaesthesia during the delivery (these types of drugs can temporarily decrease the sensitivity of your bladder or interfere with your ability to tell when you need to urinate);
- perineal pain that can cause reflex spasms in the urethra (the tube that transports urine from the bladder); and
- a fear of urinating on your oh-so-tender perineum.

You can encourage the urine to start flowing again by contracting and releasing your pelvic muscles, upping your intake of fluids, and placing hot or cold packs on your perineum (whichever triggers your urge to urinate).

If it's good old-fashioned fear that's holding you back, you might want to try drinking plenty of liquids to dilute the acidity of your urine, straddling the toilet saddle-style when you urinate, urinating while you pour water across your perineum (you can use either a "peri" bottle or a bowl), or—if you get really desperate—urinating while you're standing in the shower.

Don't worry that you'll be stuck with this problem forever: you'll soon find yourself dashing to the bathroom at regular intervals as your body goes about its postpartum "housekeeping," getting rid of all the extra fluids you accumulated during your pregnancy.

If you experience intense burning after urination or an intense, painful, and unusually frequent urge to urinate, it could be because you've developed a urinary tract infection, in which case you'll want to drink plenty of unsweetened cranberry juice and contact your caregiver to arrange for treatment.

---

mother wisdom It's important that you start urinating again soon after the birth because failing to empty the bladder regularly can contribute to urinary tract infections—the last thing you want to be dealing with at this stage of the game—and can prevent the uterus from contracting properly (which may increase your risk of experiencing a postpartum hemorrhage). Sometimes anaesthetics used during the delivery reduce your urge to urinate, so don't be surprised if your nurse asks you to try to urinate even though you swear you don't need to go. Note: If you had a Caesarean, you can expect your urinary catheter to be removed within 24 hours of the delivery.

Incontinence

Some women have the opposite problem when it comes to urination: incontinence. Incontinence usually improves during the first six weeks after the delivery (particularly if you do your Kegels religiously) but it can be rather disconcerting and inconvenient in the meantime. (Thank goodness you're going to be wearing a pad anyway.)

mother wisdom — A 2002 study published in the *Canadian Medical Association Journal* concluded that anal incontinence (stool leakage) is associated with forceps delivery and anal sphincter laceration. Anal sphincter laceration is most likely to occur during a first vaginal birth, when a median episiotomy is performed, and during a forceps- or vacuum-assisted delivery. Neither the weight of the baby nor the length of the pushing stage increase the risk of an anal sphincter laceration. The researchers involved in this study found that 3.1 per cent of new mothers were experiencing anal incontinence and 25.5 per cent were experiencing involuntary flatulence three months after the births of their babies.

Difficulty having a bowel movement

The lack of food during labour, the temporarily decreased muscle tone in your intestines, and any narcotics you were prescribed during or after the delivery may mean that you don't end up having a bowel movement for a few days after the delivery. And when the urge to have a bowel movement finally hits, you may find it hard to relax and let nature take its course, out of fear of hurting your tender perineum and/or painful hemorrhoids, or of popping the stitches on your episiotomy site (you can scratch this last worry off your list, by the way).

The best way to cope with this problem is to increase your intake of fluids (water, milk, soy beverages, and soups are best) and fibre (prune, pear, or apricot nectar; fresh fruit and vegetables; whole grains; and bran muffins are always good bets), to avoid foods and beverages that contain caffeine (coffee, cola, and chocolate), and to remain as active as possible. These steps will help to keep your stools soft and regular.

mother wisdom — Don't be surprised if you experience some problems with constipation during the first few days after the delivery. It tends to be a problem for a number of reasons: the fact that your abdominal muscles may be stretched—which can make it more difficult to bear down and expel stool—and the fact that there are still some pregnancy-related hormones kicking around in your system. (One of those hormones is progesterone—a perennial offender in the constipation department.) And, of course, if your baby was born via a Caesarean section and/or you experienced a lengthy labour, it's probably been a while since you ate a lot of solid food, which may contribute to your difficulties in having that first post-baby bowel movement. In some situations, the effects of certain types of medications taken during or after the delivery are what's causing you grief. In other cases, all that's holding you back is an understandable reluctance to have a bowel movement when you may be dealing with hemorrhoids the size of golf balls and an oh-so-tender perineum. This explains why so many doctors routinely prescribe stool softeners to new mothers—a little something to help Mother Nature along.

---

mom's the word

"After a few days, I had to have a suppository. I found it embarrassing to ask for and doubly embarrassing to have it put in, but that was my own hang-up. The nurse was very professional and caring and, in the end, the relief was worth the embarrassment."

—JENNIFER, 32, MOTHER OF ONE

Afterpains

You can expect to experience afterpains in the days following the birth. These post-labour uterine contractions can range in intensity from virtually unnoticeable to downright excruciating. (Some moms actually have to resort to their labour breathing to cope with the pain.) Afterpains are most intense when you're nursing because your baby's sucking triggers the release of oxytocin, the hormone that causes the uterus to contract.

While afterpains tend to be relatively mild after the birth of your first baby, they can be extremely painful after your second or subsequent birth. "I was shocked by the strength of the afterpains after my second delivery," Marguerite, 36, recalls. "I had vaguely remembered reading about them, but hadn't noticed anything after the first delivery, so I wasn't particularly worried about them. I found them almost as bad as labour the second time around. I couldn't believe they could be so painful!"

If you're experiencing a lot of discomfort from your afterpains, you might want to ask your caregiver to prescribe a pain medication that's safe to take while you're breastfeeding. A heating pad may also provide comfort. Or you can grin and bear it and wait for the afterpains to disappear on their own. (You'll find that the afterpains decrease in both frequency and intensity within 48 hours of the birth, gradually disappearing altogether during the next few weeks.)

A flabby belly

You may also be surprised by the tone (or rather, lack thereof) of your stomach muscles. "I was completely unprepared for the jelly-belly," recalls Carrie, 34, who is currently pregnant with her second child. "It seemed so flabby and fat." You can expect to look approximately five months' pregnant about a week after the birth—great news, if no longer being nine months' pregnant leaves you feeling wonderfully svelte, but bad news if you were counting on having supermodel-like abs by now. Hey, cut yourself some slack: even the supermodels have pot-bellies at this stage of the game. This is because your uterus is just starting to return to its pre-pregnant size (a process known as involution, whereby the uterine muscles alternately relax and contract). By the time you show up for your six-week checkup, however, your uterus, at least, will be back to its pre-pregnant size.

You can check on the progress of your incredible shrinking uterus if you learn how to find the top of your uterus (the fundus). It should feel firm and round (as opposed to the rest of your belly, which will be quite soft and soggy right now). The top of your uterus is normally just below your belly button on the first day or two after you've given birth. The height of your fundus should decrease by one or two finger widths per day. You won't be able to track its progress after about a week because your uterus will have shrunk enough that your fundus will be below your pubic bone.

A separation of the abdominal muscles

Some women experience *diastasis recti abdominis* (a separation of the longitudinal abdominal muscles that extend from the chest to the symphysis pubis). This muscle separation can be corrected by doing abdominal exercises during the postpartum period. (See the section on postnatal fitness later in this chapter.)

You're also likely to be a bit surprised by the appearance and texture of your belly: think wrinkly skin. You've just done some major shrinking overnight. It's going to take a bit of time for your skin to adjust to the new (relatively) slimmer you.

Stretch marks

They've been there all along, but you might not have been able to see the stretch marks on the underside of your belly or your upper thighs. (After all, there was a baby blocking your view.) It can come as a bit of a shock to see all those red-crayon-like lines. While they won't disappear entirely, they will fade from reddish purple to silver over time. (If they don't fade as much as you'd like, you can talk to a dermatologist about ways of reducing their appearance. Or you can simply choose to look at them in an entirely different way and treat them as pregnancy souvenirs!)

Fortunately, there's better news where the linea nigra (the brown line down your belly) and chloasma, the "mask of pregnancy" (the tan-coloured areas on your face), are concerned: as the pregnancy hormones leave your body, these two side effects of pregnancy will disappear (in the case of linea nigra) or fade (in the case of chloasma) spontaneously.

> *mom's the word*
>
> "During my pregnancy, I felt great and sexy. Then came the postpartum period. My body image sank into the sea."
>
> —MARY, 35, MOTHER OF ONE

> *mother wisdom*
>
> The most common postpartum health issues reported by the 6,000+ new moms who participated in the *Canadian Maternity Experiences Survey* were breast pain (16 per cent); pain or discomfort in either the vaginal region or at the Caesarean incision site (15 per cent); and back pain (12 per cent). At the time of the interview (five to fourteen months postpartum), 75 per cent of moms described their health as either excellent or very good.

Breast changes

You can also expect to notice some dramatic changes to your breasts. While your breasts already contain nutrient- and immunity-rich colostrum when you give birth, within two to three days your actual milk will come in. Your breasts may become flushed, swollen, and engorged during the 24 to 48 hours after that. (You can ease the discomfort of engorgement by expressing small amounts of milk. You don't want to express too much milk or you'll end up stimulating your breasts to produce even more milk—something that will *mom's the word* "I hadn't expected to be in such physical distress myself. That made the early days a lot harder than I had anticipated. I thought I'd be able to rebound quickly after giving birth and get used to this new mother thing. Despite my best efforts to do that, things just didn't work quite right. I was struggling against the tide."

—MARY, 35, MOTHER OF ONE

only add to your engorgement woes. And hand-expressing milk—as opposed to using a breast pump—will be more effective at relieving your engorgement. Using a breast pump can pull more fluid—not milk—into the breast.)

Bevin, a 27-year-old mother of one, remembers being surprised by the sheer size of her post-baby breasts: "We had a couple of Christmas parties to go to about a month after the delivery. I wanted to wear a dress, but everything I tried on looked bizarre. I thought I looked like a drag queen with a petite bottom and a huge chest!"

Don't be surprised, by the way, if you find yourself leaking milk both during and between feedings. You may leak milk from one breast when you're nursing on the other side. (The leaking will tend to taper off after a minute or so but, in the meantime, you'll want to keep some breast pads handy.) You may also find yourself leaking milk whenever you think of your baby or if you go for a particularly long stretch between feedings. "I remember thinking that I didn't need breast pads," confesses Jenny, 31, a first-time mother. "Ha! I was soaked in a matter of seconds while walking up Yonge Street. I hadn't ever believed that the sound of a baby crying or just thinking about your baby could make you leak, but it was true!"

Even if you're doing everything "right," you may find that your nipples feel a bit tender during the first week of breastfeeding. The cause of this initial discomfort is obvious: your nipples aren't accustomed to being in use for hours every day. Given how often and how vigorously babies suck, it's hardly surprising that there can be some initial tenderness. Note: There's a difference between some initial tenderness and out-and-out pain. If you find yourself cringing as you put your baby to the breast (or even at the thought of your baby's next feeding), you're dealing with something more than nipple tenderness. The good news is that most breastfeeding problems can be resolved when mothers receive the necessary support as soon as possible. So reach out for help as soon as you think you might need it. It's better to ask for support that you might not need than to fail to ask for help that you desperately needed after all. When breastfeeding is going well, motherhood is a breeze (well, relatively speaking). When it's not, it can feel like everything is going wrong.

"I had no idea how hard a baby can suck. I swear it felt like she was going to suck my toes out through my nipples!" recalls Bevin. The best way to treat sore nipples is to check your latch with a lactation consultant. In the meantime, you may want to expose your nipples to air and sunlight. (You can settle for a heat lamp if you're not into nude sunbathing, but be very careful not to burn your breasts.) Express a little milk, drip it on your nipples, and allow your nipples to air dry. Breast milk promotes healing and prevents infection. Also, to ensure maximum airflow to your nipples, avoid breast pads with plastic backings and clothing made out of synthetic fibres.

Here are some other breast-care tips:

- If your breasts become so engorged with milk that you're in pain, try lying on your back (to elevate your breasts) and applying ice packs made of crushed ice (bags of frozen vegetables, such as peas or corn, work really well, too). Important: Place a towel or face cloth between your breast and the ice pack to prevent tissue damage, and only apply the ice pack for 10 to 15 minutes at a time. If you don't want to go the ice-pack route, try cold, green cabbage leaves instead. Line your bra with the leaves and replace them when they become warm and wilted. Ahhh, relief . . .

- Treat yourself to some new bras. Your breast size has no doubt changed since you embarked on this adventure called motherhood. Look for nursing bras that are easy to operate with one hand (you'll have a baby in the other) and that provide underwire-free support. (Underwires aren't just uncomfortable when you're breastfeeding: they can lead to breastfeeding complications such as blocked ducts.)

---

mother wisdom Not every piece of advice you receive on dealing with sore nipples is necessarily good advice. Here are some home remedies that you're best not to try.

- √ **Vaseline.** Not only does Vaseline keep air away from your nipples (something that interferes with the healing process), it's also a petroleum-based product that should not be ingested by your baby. And there's an added problem: getting the Vaseline off once you've put it on. That requires washing, which can lead to yet more nipple damage.

- √ **Aloe vera.** Aloe vera may be natural, but it can trigger a nasty allergic reaction in some women. The last thing you want is a rash on your nipples. And, what's more, it can lead to cramping and diarrhea if swallowed by your baby.
- √ **Vitamin E.** Vitamin E capsules generally contain more than the recommended daily allowance of this vitamin for an infant.
- √ **Warm, moist tea bags.** The tea bags might feel soothing, but their astringent qualities could cause your nipples to dry out and crack over time.

Headaches

You may find that you experience headaches during the early days postpartum as your body begins flushing out the extra fluids it accumulated during pregnancy. New mothers are also susceptible to tension headaches. These types of headaches tend to be triggered by hormonal changes, nasal congestion, emotional stress, muscle spasms, dehydration, low blood-sugar levels, and fatigue. To treat, massage your neck and shoulder muscles (better yet, get someone else—such as your partner, or a registered massage therapist if you can manage it!—to massage them), apply heat or ice to your neck (whichever you find most effective), rest, take a warm bath, keep healthy snacks and a water bottle in the diaper bag, and take a pain-relief medication such as acetaminophen or ibuprofen (whichever your caregiver suggests for breastfeeding women). Note: Some new mothers develop migraine headaches for the first time during the first two to three months postpartum.

Fatigue

How big an issue is fatigue for new mothers? Important enough that fatigue topped the list of the top-10 postpartum complaints in a 2006 study conducted at the University of Minnesota and published in the *Annals of Family Medicine*. Nearly 64 per cent of mothers listed fatigue as an issue for them. Here's the full list of complaints: fatigue (63.8 per cent), breast discomfort (60.3 per cent), decreased desire for sex (52.4 per cent), nipple irritation or soreness (50.0 per cent), headaches (49.6 per cent), back or neck pain (43.3 per cent), decreased appetite (31.3 per cent), constipation (27.4 per cent), runny or stuffy nose (26.4 per cent), and hemorrhoids (23.6 per cent).

---

mom's the word "I was exhausted when I returned home from the hospital and totally unprepared for the length of the recovery period I needed. Every inch of my body between my waist and my knees was in pain. It took me about 12 weeks to recover. If it hadn't been for my mother's and my grandmother's help, I don't know what I would have done—and I can't imagine what women with no support go through."

—CHONEE, 35, MOTHER OF TWO WHO WAS PRESCRIBED BEDREST FOR THE LAST FEW MONTHS OF HER PREGNANCY AND WHO ALSO EXPERIENCED A DIFFICULT LABOUR AND DELIVERY

Faintness

Don't be surprised if you find yourself feeling a bit faint during the first few days after the delivery. Body fluid levels shift suddenly when pregnancy ends, and it can take a bit of time for your cardiovascular system to adjust. If the faintness continues for more than a few days, ask your caregiver to test you for anemia (iron deficiency). Believe it or not, even moderate blood loss during birth can result in anemia. Fortunately, most cases can be resolved with liquid doses of iron—which tend to have a less-constipating effect than traditional iron supplements.

Shivers and shakes

It's not at all unusual to experience shivers and shakes right after you've given birth. Researchers believe this occurs because of a resetting of the body's temperature as your pregnancy comes to an end. Usually all it takes to stop the shivering and the shaking is a warm blanket and a little time to snuggle up to your newborn.

Sweating

One of the ways your body gets rid of all the extra fluids accumulated during your pregnancy is by sweating. You can expect to perspire more heavily than usual, especially at night. In fact, you might want to cover your sheet and pillow with a towel to soak up some of the excess perspiration. Researchers believe that the sweating may be caused by the sudden decrease in your estrogen levels—something that can have you experiencing menopause-like hot flashes during the first week or two postpartum.

Hair loss

It's not enough that you have to cope with stretch marks, a flabby belly, and hips that mysteriously expanded during pregnancy: you also have to cope with limp hair! Thanks to a crash in estrogen levels after the birth, your body finally gets around to doing a little housekeeping in the hair department, getting rid of all the extra hair it should have been shedding during pregnancy. (During pregnancy, your body stopped shedding hair at its usual rate of 100 hairs per day, leaving your hair looking every bit as lush as the hair on a model in a shampoo commercial.) Since natural regrowth can't possibly keep up with the rate at which you're shedding hair, your hair seems to go from lush to limp overnight. (Talk about a bad hair day!) Fortunately, the hair nightmare that you're experiencing will be relatively short-lived. While your hair won't look quite as lush as it did during pregnancy, it'll look a heck of a lot better about six months down the road. Until then, ask your hairdresser to suggest a cut that will be flattering and easy to maintain. Remember, your days of spending a half hour each day fiddling with a blow-dryer and a container of styling gel are a thing of the past for now.

---

mom's the word

"I was on an emotional high after the birth—something that allowed me to recover quite quickly."

—DEE, 32, MOTHER OF ONE

Other postpartum body changes

Now that you've given birth to your baby, your body is busy morphing from a pregnant to a non-pregnant state, so you'll notice that many of the symptoms that might have been driving you crazy during your pregnancy have disappeared virtually overnight. Other bits of pregnant-body redesign will take a little longer to undo. Here's the lowdown on the timing of some of those changes, information that's helpful to have as you adjust to life in your new postpartum body.

- **Joint laxity:** The very same hormone (relaxin) that encouraged your pelvis to open up during birth is making you ultra-flexible right now. While it sounds great in theory (it would be handy to be able to do contortions while strapping your baby's car seat into your vehicle, for example), you're extra susceptible to injury, so go easy with the back seat limbo.

- **Eyes:** If fluid changes to your eyes prevented you from wearing your contact lenses for part of your pregnancy, here's some good news: your eyes should be back to normal (or normal for you) within the next two to four months.

- **Nasal changes (pregnancy rhinitis) and effects on ears and voice:** You feel like you've had a cold since early pregnancy. You've had a runny nose, stuffy ears, and a husky voice for months. Good news! Your symptoms should disappear any day now, if they haven't already. (They were caused by sky-high levels of estrogen and progesterone, and those levels drop within 72 hours of delivery.)

As you can see, your body has a lot of work to do to recover from the birth. While you might think that your body will never get back to normal, you'll be surprised to see just how much progress it has made by the time your six-week checkup rolls around. By then, you will be ready to do at least a decent impression of your pre-pregnancy self.

CAESAREAN RECOVERY

If you gave birth via Caesarean section, you can expect to experience a few additional discomforts during the postpartum period: extra fatigue, tenderness around your incision, and gas buildup in your upper chest (which you may feel as pain in your shoulder area). Here are tips on coping with these common post-Caesarean complaints.

- If you need to spend the first day or two after your Caesarean recovering in bed (or you are too weak or nauseated to walk during that time), do some leg exercises to prevent blood clots from forming in your legs. Bend and stretch your knees, or press your knees into the bed and then relax your legs.

mother wisdom   Although your incision will heal within six months of the delivery, don't be surprised if you experience some numbness in the area until the nerves regenerate (something that typically happens about six to nine months after the birth). You should also be prepared for the fact that your scar may continue to be bright red for up to a year. (It will fade in time, but sometimes the fading process takes longer than you'd like.)

- Learn how to minimize pain around your incision site. Hold a pillow against your incision when you cough, sneeze, or laugh in order to provide some gentle support to your midsection. Avoid heavy lifting and limit the number of times you trek up and down the stairs in a day. Keep your incision clean and dry, and expose it to air as often as possible.

- Don't be alarmed if you experience pressure and uncomfortable urination for a week or two afterward as a side effect of your surgery. This problem will disappear as your body heals.

- You will likely have a few problems with gas pains, too. Mother Nature's reaction to abdominal surgery is to call all intestinal activity to a halt. That's why it's normal for women who've been through a Caesarean section to experience uncomfortable gas pains during the first three days (until the intestinal tract starts working again). Try taking short walks, changing your position frequently, and rocking in a chair. These techniques will help to get rid of any trapped gas, thereby relieving the gas pains that are causing you so much grief.

- It will take time for your incision site to heal. During that time, you will want to keep tabs on your incision to make sure it is healing normally. Get in touch with your health-care provider right away if you develop a fever or if the incision becomes red or swollen or oozes pus. The internal stitches that you received will dissolve on their own. External staples, on the other hand, are generally removed after four to six days. In the meantime, it's okay to shower with stitches or clips. (Drip plain or soapy water over the incision and gently pat dry with a clean towel.)

Be prepared to take it easy for a while. You need plenty of rest in order to heal properly, so make caring for your baby and caring for yourself your top priorities for at least the first few weeks. It will likely take you four to six weeks to recover from a Caesarean. Don't expect yourself to bounce back as quickly as other mothers you know who have given birth vaginally.

---

mom's the word "I was shocked by how I looked, and I felt disgusting, to be honest. It was very hard and still is to reconcile the 'new' me with the image I had of myself in my mind. I wasn't prepared for how much pregnancy and birth would alter my body and the number of stretch marks I'd get. I also have a huge Caesarean scar on my stomach that's very hard to get over emotionally."
—JENNIFER, 31, MOTHER OF TWO

WEIGHT LOSS

Everyone knows at least one woman who was able to slip back into her pre-pregnancy jeans before she left the hospital, but women like this are the exception rather than the rule. Most of us find that we are left with at least a few extra pounds after the birth. You can expect to lose 10 to 13 pounds (4.5 to 5.9 kilograms) from the baby, the placenta, and fluid and tissue losses associated with the birth itself, another 5 to 8 pounds (2.3 to 3.6 kilograms) through fluid loss, and another 2 to 3 pounds (0.9 to 1.4 kilograms) through postpartum bleeding and discharge (lochia).

How quickly you lose the rest of your pregnancy weight will depend on such factors as how much you gained during pregnancy, your eating habits, how much you exercise, and your metabolism. Weight loss after pregnancy tends to be greater in younger women, women with fewer children, and women who embarked on pregnancy at a lower pre-pregnancy weight.

While breastfeeding can actually help you to lose weight—you'll burn an extra 500 calories per day while you're nursing—some new moms find that they aren't able to lose the last few pounds they put on during their pregnancy until after they stop breastfeeding. (Just plop one of your breasts on the nearest postal scale and you'll see why: breastfeeding mothers are designed to hold on to an extra 5 to 7 pounds of fat reserves for milk production purposes). Some new moms find that they lose weight at a steady rate while they are breastfeeding. Others find that their weight remains stable. A few find that they actually gain weight because they are quite hungry while they are breastfeeding. Here are some important points to bear in mind if you find yourself obsessing about weight loss while you're breastfeeding:

- A combination of healthy eating, regular exercise, and stress reduction generally works best when it comes to achieving a healthier weight.
- Give your body the food it needs to make breast milk, to care for your new baby, and to help you feel your best. Sure, you want to lose those extra pounds, but there's a right way and a wrong way to do it. Crash dieting can reduce the volume of your milk supply, leading to an unhappy baby and a stressed-out you.
- Ease into a fitness routine that meshes well with your lifestyle as a new mom, and that is something you enjoy doing. Being active should feel like something nurturing you do for your body, not one more dreaded task on your to-do list.
- Keep in mind that whatever you eat or don't eat while breastfeeding is transferred to your baby, so it's important to eat well.

mother wisdom Remind yourself that healthy self-esteem is a key ingredient in nurturing your body and achieving full wellness. Make sure you're treating your body with the kindness and respect that it deserves. (For wonderful, body-affirming messages, visit www.fatnutritionist.com.)

mother wisdom Some new moms find that they gain weight while they're breastfeeding because the extra energy requirements of nursing can trigger an increase in appetite. Being sleep deprived can also cause your appetite to increase (your body figures that if it can't get its energy via sleep, it might as well go for another energy source, like food). You may find you have to make a conscious effort to reach for protein- and fibre-rich foods that will help to curb your appetite as opposed to highly appealing processed foods and snack foods that will only leave you craving more.

mother wisdom Wondering if it's safe to lose weight while you're breastfeeding? According to a study conducted at the University of North Carolina at Greensboro, breastfeeding moms can safely lose up to a pound a week without affecting the quality or quantity of their breast milk. That said, there's no one-size-fits-all rule that applies to all moms and all babies. If you're trying to lose weight, pay attention to your body and your baby and be prepared to adjust your caloric intake if it appears your milk production has dropped off.

mom's the word "Women should be taught that giving birth and becoming a mother are life changes. This heavy pressure to be thin again is some bizarre ritual that negates that fact. By returning to that pre-pregnancy figure, we are encouraged to believe that nothing has changed; we've just added a child to the mix and life goes on as before. But, of course, life does not and should not go on as before. Our body changes are a very primal and accurate reflection of the changes that have occurred in the rest of our life. Welcome them."

—MARY, 35, MOTHER OF ONE

NUTRITION AFTER BABY

Your body requires a steady supply of healthy food in order to do all the important postpartum repair work it needs to do to your body, and to meet the ongoing nutritional needs of your baby. Here are some important points to keep in mind.

- **If you don't give your body enough of the nutrients it needs while you're breastfeeding, you force it to choose between you and your baby.** Your body is programmed to meet your baby's needs first, even if that means depleting your body's nutritional stores. That can affect your health and the health of any babies you conceive in future.
- **Stay on track nutritionally while caring for your baby.** It takes an extra 200 to 500 calories a day to make enough breast milk

to feed your baby, which means most breastfeeding moms need between 2,200 and 2,900 calories per day. You also need plenty of fluids (8 to 15 cups (2 to 3.5 litres) per day) in order to combat constipation, assist with digestion, and help to ensure a plentiful supply of milk.

- **Get the maximum nutritional bang for your caloric buck.** Rather than choosing convenience foods that are likely to be high in sugar, fat, salt, and little more, choose nutrient-rich whole foods. Make a particular effort to work calcium (you need even more calcium now than you did while you were pregnant), vitamin C, iron-rich foods, and plenty of fluids into your diet, and to ensure that you're getting the recommended number of servings from each of the food groups in *Canada's Food Guide*. Note: If you haven't got a copy of *Canada's Food Guide* handy, ask your local health unit to send you a copy, or track down a copy of the guide online at www.myfoodguide.ca. It's the one piece of paper that has earned a place of honour on the refrigerators of the nation.

- **Get plenty of iron-rich foods.** Many new moms are slightly anemic by the time they've had their babies, as a result of the blood loss associated with giving birth and the iron depletion that can occur during pregnancy. Because being low in iron leads to fatigue, and you need plenty of energy as a new mom, it's important to focus on rebuilding your iron stores. Build your meals around iron-rich foods such as meat, tofu, beans, lentils, dried fruit, and fortified cereals. Take an iron supplement for at least three months, or continue to take your prenatal vitamin for as long as you continue to nurse your baby. Team iron-rich foods with foods and beverages that are rich in vitamin C (which aids in iron absorption) and avoid consuming coffee and tea with your meals, since these block iron absorption.

- **Food affects mood.** Up to 80 per cent of new moms experience some degree of postpartum blues. Fifteen per cent experience symptoms of postpartum depression that are severe enough to require

---

mother wisdom

Low in iron? Breastfeed your baby. Missing your period for a prolonged amount of time while you're breastfeeding can help you to build up your iron stores again. (Breastfeeding helps to suppress your period.)

professional help. Here are some ways you can use food to ease your symptoms:

- *Boost your intake of iron-rich foods* (or take an iron supplement). Being low in iron may be a risk factor for depression.

- *Eat more carbohydrates* (in moderation). If your diet is too low in carbohydrates and your blood-insulin level drops too low, you may experience some of the symptoms of postpartum depression. You'll also want to be aware that women experiencing postpartum mood disorders have a tendency to crave carbs because of the mood lift they provide. If you find yourself bingeing on crackers and other carbs in order to boost your mood, you may want to talk to your health-care provider about other ways of warding off the postpartum blues and dealing with the stresses of early motherhood.

- *Up your intake of Omega-3 fatty acids* (flax seeds and flax seed oil, walnuts, canola oil and soy oil, fatty fish such as salmon or trout, and eggs containing Omega-3 fatty acids). These foods may help to prevent and reduce symptoms of postpartum depression.

---

mother wisdom Don't expect to automatically feel like a million bucks once you reach the magic six-week mark. A study of more than 1,300 Australian women found that most were still experiencing a variety of aches and pains eight weeks after their babies' births. The most common complaints included exhaustion and extreme tiredness (60 per cent), backache (53 per cent), bowel problems (37 per cent), hemorrhoids (30 per cent), lack of sleep (30 per cent), perineal soreness (22 per cent), problems with sex (19 per cent), urinary incontinence (19 per cent), and frequent migraines or headaches (19 per cent).

GETTING BACK INTO SHAPE

We'd all like to imagine that we'll be able to slip on our skin-tight yoga pants within days of giving birth. What we sometimes forget, however, is that it takes most of us a lot longer than a couple of weeks to get back into shape after giving birth. That's not to say the situation is all doom and gloom, of course. (If it were, those slim-and-trim moms you see carrying babies would be on the endangered species list!) Here are some tips on designing a postpartum fitness program for yourself that will work during this exciting but busy time in your life.

- **Give your body the credit it deserves.** Rather than beating yourself up for being "out of shape," remind yourself that your body is actually in perfect shape for having just had a baby. There's a reason why your abdominal muscles are flabby and you're carrying around a few extra pounds: you've just sublet your uterus to another human being for the last nine months!

- **Be realistic about what you can expect to accomplish at this stage in your life.** It's better to set a series of small, achievable fitness goals for yourself than to aim so high that you throw in the towel after just a couple of days. Besides, studies have shown that people who aim for moderate rather than high-intensity workouts are only half as likely to abandon their fitness programs.

- **Look for fitness activities you can enjoy with your baby in tow.** Walking is a given: you simply pop the wee one into her stroller or baby carrier and hit the pavement. But so are such activities as dancing (with or without a baby in your arms), jogging (provided you buy a decent-quality jogging stroller), and weightlifting. (There are even postnatal fitness workouts that show you how to use your baby as a free weight!) And there are plenty of postnatal classes you can join: yoga, dance, and stroller fitness class, and even mom-and-baby boot camps—all with the added benefit of allowing you to meet other moms in your community.

- **Choose an activity that's easy to fit into your schedule.** If you're breastfeeding a baby who's colicky in the evenings, it may not make sense to sign up for an after-dinner water fitness class at your local gym. On the other hand, if that's the only time you can squeeze in a workout and it's the one thing that's keeping you sane, then go for it.

- **Wear a sports bra or two nursing bras while you're working out to give your breasts the support they need.** If you're nursing, you'll probably feel more comfortable if you breastfeed your baby right before your workout.

- **If you're having trouble with incontinence**, urinate before you start your workout and then wear a panty liner to guard against leakage. (If you make a point of including Kegel exercises in your workout—those much-lauded exercises that can help to tone your pelvic floor muscles—you'll probably find that your incontinence becomes less of a problem.)

- **Don't overdo it.** Joint laxity (looseness) can be a problem for months after you give birth, something that can easily result in twists, sprains, and other injuries. To minimize the risk of hurting yourself, perform all movements with caution and control when you're exercising, and avoid jumping; rapid changes of direction; jerky, bouncing, or jarring motions; and deep flexion or extension of joints. Skip your workout if you're feeling particularly exhausted. The more tired you are, the more likely you are to injure yourself. Being active is about nurturing yourself, not punishing your body.
- **Drink plenty of liquids before, during, and after your workout.** It's important to keep your body fully hydrated.
- **Stop exercising immediately if you experience pain**, faintness, dizziness, blurred vision, shortness of breath, heart palpitations, back pain, pubic pain, nausea, difficulty walking, or a sudden increase in vaginal bleeding. You should report any of these symptoms to your caregiver.
- **Make sure your workout is suitable for someone who's just had a baby.** Most fitness experts advise that you pass on knee–chest exercises, full sit-ups, and double leg lifts during the postpartum period, and to focus on exercises that are designed to get the abdominal and pelvic floor muscles back into shape. (See Table 2.2.)

TABLE 2.2

Postpartum Exercises

The following exercises can be started as soon as your caregiver gives you the go-ahead to embark on a postpartum exercise regime—typically within a day or two of an uncomplicated vaginal delivery, but if you've experienced a Caesarean delivery or a particularly difficult vaginal delivery, your doctor or midwife will likely want you to wait a little longer than that.

Abdominal Tightening

Position: Standing or lying on your back

What to do: Inhale slowly and exhale slowly while contracting your abdominal muscles to a count of 10. Then relax your muscles. Repeat three times initially, but progress to up to five or ten repetitions as your abdominal muscles become stronger. You should also increase the number of sets of abdominal exercises you do from three sets to five sets to ten sets over time.

Head Lift

Position: Lying on your back with your knees bent

What to do: Inhale. Then, while exhaling, lift your head, chin to chest, and look at your thighs. Hold this position to a count of three and then relax. You should feel this exercise in your abdomen and pelvic floor. Repeat this exercise several times. After a few weeks, you can start lifting your shoulders off the ground, too. You should aim to do five to ten sets of head lifts daily.

Pelvic Tilt

Position: Lying on your back in bed with your knees bent and feet flat

What to do: Inhale and exhale, flattening your lower back into the bed and contracting your abdominal muscles. Hold the contracted muscle position to a count of three and then release. Start with five repetitions and work up to ten repetitions daily.

Kegel Exercises

Position: Sitting or standing

What to do: Tighten the muscles of the perineal area as if you were trying to stop the flow of urine, and then relax those muscles. Inhale, tighten for a count of five, exhale, and relax. Aim to do the exercise five times an hour for the first few days after the delivery, gradually increasing to 10 repetitions of 10 seconds each. Caution: Do not do your Kegels when you're urinating because this will increase your chances of developing a urinary tract infection.

Pull-ins (for diastasis recti)

Position: Lying on your back in bed with your head on a pillow and your knees bent and feet flat

What to do: Place your hands on your stomach on either side of your belly button. Gently pull your belly button toward your spine. Hold this position for 10 seconds and then slowly release. Repeat 10 to 20 times.

Don't allow yourself to get into a fitness rut. It's easy to allow boredom to sabotage your workout program. Either rotate fitness activities on a regular basis or find a workout buddy who can help you stay motivated. Your body will thank you for it!

---

mother wisdom — Tune into your body and treat it kindly. Your body will feel less tired and achy if you stand up straight (rather than slouching), gently contract your stomach muscles as you change positions (you'll give your back muscles a break), and release the tension from your neck and shoulder muscles.

- **Spend your fitness dollars wisely.** Before you fork over a small fortune on a gym membership, be realistic about how often you're actually going to make it there to work out. Unless they offer on-site child care or you can work around your partner's schedule, or you have someone who can come into your home a few times a week so that you can get out, you may find that it's such a hassle to get to the gym and back that you rarely step foot in the place.

- **Don't pooh-pooh the benefits of working out at home.** A Stanford University study revealed that people who exercise in their own homes are more likely to stick with their fitness programs than people who work out elsewhere. What's more, a University of Florida study confirmed what many exercise physiologists have long suspected: people who exercise at home tend to lose more weight over the course of a year than people who exercise in other locations.

- **Treat yourself** to some workout clothes, a new workout video, or a new piece of exercise equipment—anything that will inspire you to build on your fitness success.

- **Stick with it.** Fitness should remain a priority for you long after those extra pregnancy pounds are gone. Not only will it help to ensure that your body is in the best possible physical condition, it will also help you to combat some of the day-to-day stresses that seem to go along with the whole motherhood turf and ensure that you become a role model of active living for your child. (When mom is active, kids are more likely to be active. You have the opportunity to raise your child in a family where taking care of your body is the norm.)

SEX AFTER BABY?

While sex may be the last thing on your mind during the first few hours and days after you have your baby, at some point it's going to show up on your radar screen again. (Or at least that's the theory.) But because you'll be contending with a smorgasbord of physical complaints during the early weeks—everything from a sore perineum to heavy bleeding to sleep deprivation—as well as new emotional challenges—body image concerns, relationship adjustments, worries about waking the baby, fears about sex hurting the first time—you may find your libido running on empty a little longer than you'd initially anticipated. A University of Wisconsin study of 570 new parents found that it takes bottle-feeding parents about seven weeks and breastfeeding parents about eight weeks to start having sexual intercourse again. Only 17 per cent of couples involved in the study reported having sexual intercourse during the month after childbirth. While there's typically some sexual contact during the postpartum period—65 per cent of women in the University of Wisconsin study reported engaging in some form of sexual touching and 34 per cent reported having performed oral sex on their partner during the first few weeks after the birth—many women choose to hold off on having sexual intercourse until after their six-week checkup because of maternal fatigue or postpartum discomfort, or because they're eager to get reassurance from their doctor or midwife that their bodies are healing properly after the delivery.

Some women find that they also need time to psychologically process the events of the birth (something that's most likely to be an issue if the delivery was particularly traumatic) and to come to terms with the multitude of changes that have occurred to their bodies during pregnancy, labour, and birth. While you might worry that your partner may no longer find you as attractive as you once were because you're a few pounds heavier than you were nine months ago, or because there's a Caesarean scar on your belly, that's not usually the case. Consider these words of wisdom from Douglas, a first-time father, who wishes that his wife, Melodie, weren't quite so critical of her postpartum body: "She bears the scars of giving life to my child—something that just makes me love her all the more."

---

mother wisdom Has your desire for sex gone AWOL ever since you had your baby? Hey, it happens. According to the Society of Obstetricians and Gynaecologists of Canada, hormonal changes, sleep deprivation, anemia, depression, and anxiety—all common complaints among new mothers—can take their toll on the libido. And there's no reason to feel guilty about it. Talking to your partner—and your doctor—about what you're feeling (or not feeling) is the first step to getting your sex life back on track. That assumes, of course, that you're eager to jump-start your libido right now. Some new moms aren't in any rush to bring the sexy back. They are feeling swept away by baby bliss, or overwhelmed by the demands of early motherhood, or experiencing a mix of both emotions. If that's how you're feeling, talk things through with your partner and try to find some sexual middle ground until your interest in sex revs up again.

> *mother wisdom* Wondering when to expect your first post-baby period? Unless you have a crystal ball, you're going to have a bit of trouble pinpointing the exact date of its arrival. Breastfeeding mothers can expect to get their periods back at any time between two and eighteen months after the birth. Mothers who don't breastfeed menstruate on average 55 to 65 days after giving birth. Even more importantly, they ovulate 40 to 55 days after delivery. There have been cases of women conceiving within two weeks of giving birth. Ovulation precedes menstruation. Make that your mantra.

Some partners find that there is a period of adjustment after the birth. The bodies of the women they love have become biological factories capable of producing and supplying food for another human being! ("I remember my husband looking at my breasts one day and saying, 'I just don't look at them the same way anymore. They're too functional,'" recalls one mother of two.)

It may take time for you and your partner to become sexually active again, but with any luck, the mood and the opportunity will strike at the same time and you'll be able to squeeze in some lovemaking before your baby wakes up looking for food. Here are some tips to help make your first post-baby rendezvous as stress-free as possible for both yourself and your partner.

- **Take things slowly.** There may be some tenderness the first time you make love, particularly if you had a bad tear or your episiotomy site hasn't had the chance to heal over completely (it's best to wait until your episiotomy heals before going for it). And even if your stitches have long since healed, it can take months for soreness in the area to disappear.

- **Experiment with different positions.** Since the traditional missionary position tends to put pressure right on the very area where you're most likely to be sore—your perineum—you might prefer to make love in other positions (for example, side-lying or woman-on-top).

- **Keep in mind that Mother Nature may need a little help.** Even if lubrication isn't normally a problem for you, it could be after the delivery. This is because breastfeeding hormones tend to dry up your vaginal secretions, reducing the amount of lubrication that's available when you want to make love. (And even if you're not breastfeeding, vaginal lubrication levels can be altered for six months following the birth as a result of decreased estrogen levels following the delivery of the placenta.) While an over-the-counter water-soluble lubricant will do the trick for most couples, don't be afraid to ask your doctor for a prescription for estrogen cream if vaginal dryness is a particular problem for you.

- **Don't expect sex to feel quite the same right away.** If you gave birth vaginally, your vagina may feel a little looser than it did prior to the delivery. Of course, you'll regain much of your vaginal muscle tone over time if you make a point of doing your Kegel exercises on a regular basis. And don't be horrified if the big O is a little o at first. Orgasms may be shorter and less intense during the first few months after the birth, the result of decreased blood flow to the labia majora and minora and reduced perineal tone. This is just a temporary blip. You will return to your usual sexy self once your body has a chance to finish up the necessary repair work. Keep the faith, Mama (and the sizzling hot fantasies, too).

- **Be prepared for a bit of a milk bath if you're a breastfeeding mom.** Don't be surprised if you end up leaking milk during intercourse (stimulation of the vagina and the cervix increases oxytocin levels) or if your breasts feel very uncomfortable if your partner puts any weight on them. The solution to both problems, by the way, is to feed your baby right before your romantic tryst—and, as an added bonus, your baby might even sleep through the whole thing!

---

mother wisdom While breastfeeding offers some protection (it's considered to be a reliable method of birth control for women whose babies are under six months old, exclusively breastfed, and not given any bottles or pacifiers, and whose period has not returned), the Lactational Amenorrhoea Method (LAM) shouldn't be treated as a foolproof method of birth control once your baby starts solids. There are also some other caveats, so you'll want to do your homework on this method if you intend to treat it as your one-and-only form of birth control.

You probably won't want to count on breastfeeding as a method of birth control if you're holding down a full-time job, for example. A study published in the medical journal *Contraception* indicates that more than 5 per cent of breastfeeding women who return to work can expect to become pregnant within six months of the birth of their child. Previous research had indicated that less than 2 per cent of women who breastfeed exclusively will conceive within a six-month period provided that they have not yet started menstruating again, their baby is exclusively breastfed (no formula or solid foods), and there are no more than four hours between feedings. The researchers concluded that women who are away from their babies while they are at work may miss out on olfactory (scent-based) or physical stimuli that affect their hormones in a manner that protects against pregnancy.

- **Give some serious thought to birth control.** There's a very good chance that you'll ovulate *before* you get your first period—something you might want to bear in mind if you're not exactly eager to see the pregnancy test come back positive again just yet. Fifty per cent of new mothers who aren't breastfeeding and not using birth control will be pregnant again within six to seven months of the birth of their babies, while 50 per cent of new mothers who are breastfeeding and not using birth control will be pregnant again within nine months of the birth of their babies. It's a good idea to give your body a bit of a break between pregnancies, even if you are totally enchanted with your little one. Your body needs time to replenish the vitamins, minerals, and amino acids that are depleted during pregnancy.

Understand that having sex less often is the norm for most couples who have just had a baby. The frequency of lovemaking typically drops by 40 per cent during the year after childbirth. Those who have researched the impact of having a baby on a couple's relationship have concluded that frank and open communication, regular sex (even if it's just a quickie), and couple time are the keys to remaining emotionally and sexually connected during the early months and years of parenthood.

mother wisdom   Am I Pregnant? That's a question you can ask an online and mobile application launched by the Society of Obstetricians and Gynaecologists of Canada. The app—which was launched in early June 2010—is designed to help Canadian women better understand the signs and symptoms of pregnancy, and to assess their odds of having conceived. The *Am I Pregnant?* app can be found on the SOGC's www.sexualityandu.ca website alongside two contraception-related apps that were launched in 2009: the *Choosing Wisely* application, which is designed to help you choose the contraception method that is best for you right now, and the *S.O.S.—Stay on Schedule* application that is designed to help you to decide what to do if you miss a birth control pill, forget to get your Depo-Provera shot, or commit another type of birth control faux pas.

As you can see, you have plenty of important health issues to grapple with during the postpartum period. In the next chapter, we tackle life after baby.

chapter 3
THE POSTPARTUM SURVIVAL GUIDE

> "I remember driving home with our new son and marvelling at how much everything looked the same. It felt so different, but it was the same. We got home and the house was quiet, almost eerie. I felt there should have been something special, like in the movies—huge crowds of cheering people, balloons, jugglers—something."
>
> —JENNIFER, 32, MOTHER OF ONE

No matter how much time you spent babysitting as a teenager or how many baby-care books you've devoured since the pregnancy test came back positive, nothing can ever fully prepare you for the experience of becoming a mother. Many new mothers describe the early weeks after the birth as the best of times and the worst of times all wrapped up into one exhilarating and yet exhausting package: a time in which you celebrate your newfound status as a mother while simultaneously mourning the loss of your pre-baby freedom. Add to this the fact that your body is busy morphing back to its pre-pregnant state and the fact you haven't had a good night's sleep since the second trimester (if then!), and you can see why the postpartum period tends to be a bit of a rocky ride.

In this chapter, we'll cover some of the emotional aspects of life after baby: how you may feel about becoming a mother and what you need to know in order to spot the warning signs of postpartum depression.

LIFE AFTER BABY

In years to come, when you look back on this time, you will envision a giant dividing line. On the one side, life before baby; on the other, life after baby. The line marks the point at which everything changed.

Right now, you're so close to the line that it's hard to have much perspective on the future, to imagine that there will ever be a time when you're not exhausted, baby-obsessed, and struggling to find your new-mom equilibrium. What you need is for the community of mothers (mothers who have survived this crazy time and lived to tell) to reach out their hands and help you find your balance. That's what this section of the chapter is all about—helping you to find your feet without stumbling too hard or too often.

Here are some tips on making the most of this new-mother time.

- **Be prepared to feel unprepared.** It takes time to grow into the role of parent. At first you may feel shaky, like a 6-year-old trying to ride a two-wheeler without training wheels for the first time. But your confidence will grow day by day.

- **Accept the realities of parenting a newborn.** You may not be thrilled that you haven't had an uninterrupted meal or a decent night's sleep since your baby was born, but you'll do yourself and your baby a favour if you simply accept the fact that your life is going to be topsy-turvy for the foreseeable future.

mom's the word

"Everyone tells you their labour stories and neglects to mention that the truly trying times are ahead! Until I spoke to other women about it, I thought I was a failure because I found the first two months of my baby's life to be exhausting, frustrating, and emotionally draining."

—CAROLE, 33, MOTHER OF TWO

- **Learn to go with the flow.** Newborns are notoriously unpredictable. Just when you think you've figured out your baby's eating and sleeping patterns, she'll change her schedule dramatically. Rather than trying to force your new baby into adopting patterns she's not yet ready for—which will only serve to frustrate the two of you—focus your energies on trying to follow her lead and enjoy this special time in your lives.

- **Don't worry about spoiling your baby.** Ignore any well-meaning or not-so-well-meaning relatives who warn you about the evils of indulging your infant. It isn't possible to spoil a newborn. Responding quickly to his cries teaches him to trust the world around him—something that will ultimately lead to a much happier baby. (A now-classic study conducted at Johns Hopkins University during the early 1970s revealed that babies whose cries were responded to quickly cried less at 1 year of age than those babies whose cries were not responded to quite so quickly.)

- **Clear your calendar of all but the essentials, and limit your number of visitors for at least the first few weeks.** Pace yourself until you know what you can handle, and gravitate toward activities that are energy enhancing, not energy draining. You want to conserve your energy for yourself and your new baby.

- **Rather than trying to catch up on the housework each and every time your baby takes a nap, hit the couch yourself.** Your rest is more important than trying to live up to impossibly high housekeeping standards. On the other hand, if living in chaos is making you crazy, ask for help or hire someone to help out for a few weeks. Think of the money you spend as an investment in your health and your baby's (which it is).

- **Figure out how to deal with unhelpful advice, particularly unhelpful advice of the random, unsolicited variety.** You know your baby best, so it's important to allow your rapidly emerging parenting instincts to guide you when you're trying to decide which bits of parenting advice and information are useful and which bits are best ignored. If you're struggling with a particular parenting problem, it's a good idea to talk to other parents who have faced a similar challenge and to do some research on your own (read books; consult some trusted websites; put in a call to your local health unit and ask to speak to a public health nurse). Then spend a bit of time mulling over the different approaches you've learned about. Ask yourself which approach seems like the best fit for your baby, given his temperament, his stage of development, your parenting philosophies, and anything else that seems relevant to your situation. Reserve the right to go back to the drawing board if your initial solution doesn't work out. Parenting is a mix of both art and science. Expect to spend a lot of time in the parenting lab.

mother wisdom Learn about infant development so you'll know what types of developmental milestones are typical for each age and stage. That way, you'll be able to filter out a lot of advice that is clearly off the mark. (At the same time, don't get so obsessed with developmental milestones that you forget to enjoy who your baby is today. Babyhood zooms by quickly enough. You don't want to wish it away any more quickly by forever anticipating the next milestone.)

- **Accept any and all offers of help, and be prepared to ask for help, too.** Don't deprive others of the joy of helping you, or make life harder for yourself by refusing to accept these offers of assistance. There is a long-standing tradition of mothering the mother (and the father, too) in many cultures. Don't mess with tradition!

- **Keep a running list of jobs that can be delegated to others who have offered to help.** For example, picking up fresh fruit and vegetables at the grocery store and creating a fruit-and-veggie platter for you, folding a load or two of baby laundry, loading the dishwasher or washing whatever dishes happen to be stacked up on the kitchen counter. "A girlfriend of mine picked up groceries for us," recalls Tina, a 32-year-old mother of one. "Some other friends brought over supper. These things mean so much during the first few weeks."

- **Get out of the house.** Nothing can add to your stress level more than being housebound day after day with a newborn—especially if she is trying out for the position of Town Crier. (See the section on dealing with crying further on in this chapter.) Whether you decide to take the baby for a walk or to hit the local parent resource centre, it's important to do whatever you can to avoid getting cabin fever. "Go for walks with the baby as soon as you can," suggests Janet, 32, who recently gave birth to her first baby. "You'll feel much better physically and the baby's cries will seem that much quieter in the great outdoors!"

- **Connect with other parents.** Keep in touch with the other new parents you met at prenatal class and compare notes on your babies' sleeping, eating, and crying patterns. Or connect online with other women who gave birth the same month as you did. (You'll find groups like these at every major parenting website.)

- **Resist the temptation to compare your baby to other babies.** No two babies are alike, so there's no need to hit the panic button just because your baby's spitting up a bit more than the babies of the other couples in your prenatal class.

- **Accept the fact that there can be a few potholes on the road to breastfeeding success.** Don't feel inadequate if breastfeeding doesn't come easily to you at first; it doesn't for everyone. "Breastfeeding is more difficult than giving birth," says Carrie, 34, who is currently pregnant with her second child. "My body did what it was made to do during the birth. Breastfeeding required some thought and learning on my part." If you run into breastfeeding difficulties, get support from an experienced nursing mother or a lactation consultant. The benefits of breastfeeding are tremendous, so it's worth persevering. Most mothers will be able to enjoy a successful breastfeeding relationship with their babies if they receive adequate information and support.

- **Recognize that it may take your older child time to warm up to the new baby.** Even if you do all the right things, you can expect to experience the odd rough spot as your child learns how to share you and your partner with the newborn. Jane recalls how frustrated she felt when her older child refused to accept the new baby: "We talked about the baby, we read books, we made a special 'I'm a Big Brother T-shirt,' and we brought suckers for him to distribute at daycare. We even brought a present from the baby home from the hospital for him. It didn't really help, though. He was nearly 3 at the time and had had lots of attention before Emma's arrival. It was an event that really, truly rocked his world. He was very jealous of her and tried to hit, poke, bite, and so on. The only thing that seemed to help was when I finally clued in that he needed some time alone with me."

- **Expect your worry-o-meter to go into overdrive.** Now that you're responsible for ensuring the health and well-being of another human, you'll suddenly find a million and one things to worry about. "I worried about finding a good daycare for her when I returned to work, especially after reading a lot of horror stories in the news," recalls Bevin, a 27-year-old mother of one. "I worried about getting into an accident, dropping the baby, all kinds of silly things."

- **Don't expect to feel Madonna-like 24 hours a day.** (I'm talking about the classic type of Madonna here, not the pop diva.) If you're expecting to feel totally euphoric all the time, you could be in for a major disappointment. Hey, even the women I'd personally consider nominating for the Motherhood Hall of Fame have days when they feel like running away from home! "I had many guilty feelings about not bonding instantly with my first baby," recalls Jane, a 33-year-old mother of two. "I expected overwhelming feelings of love, and I didn't have them. I didn't dislike him, but I just didn't feel the gushiness I expected. When I was finally brave enough to talk about these feelings with other moms, I was so relieved to find out how common this is. I wish I'd read about that beforehand! It could have saved me so much grief. Eventually, probably several months down the road, I did feel overwhelming love for him." And if you do fall head-over-heels in love with your baby right away, don't let other people rain on your happy parade by telling you that you're too attached to your baby (not possible, by the way). Simply soak up those amazing feelings and enjoy your baby.

- **Savour every moment (well, as many as you can!) of this very special time in your life.** "This is a strange and magical time, but it's so very fleeting," says Maria, a 35-year-old mother of two. "Take a million photos and write everything down—every feeling, every thought. Time really does pass so quickly, and you can't remember everything."

---

learn how to manage the stress that goes along with being a parent Parenting can be stressful, even when you're caring for an impossibly cute baby. That's why it's important to learn how to manage stress, right from day one.

- √ **Figure out which stress-management techniques work best for you.** Then make those techniques part of your regular routine.

    Exercise. It helps to reduce stress, boost your mood, increase your energy, and improve your overall health and wellness.

    Meditation. It can help to reduce stress, relieve pain, lower both your blood pressure and your heart rate, and improve the quality of your sleep.

Breathing. Focusing on your breathing helps to relax you. Place one hand on your abdomen, and breathe in air all the way into your abdomen so that your hand rises and falls while you breathe. Continue for five to ten minutes.

Massage. It soothes and relaxes the nervous system by releasing endorphins.

- √ **Set the parenting bar high, but not too high.** Parents who try to be perfect are at risk of burnout. Besides, there's no such thing as perfection when it comes to the art and science of child rearing, so cut yourself some slack and you'll find parenting a whole lot more enjoyable, and you'll be less likely to burn out. As your child grows, you'll both learn together.

- √ **Don't let multi-tasking make you crazy.** Living life at hyper-speed can leave you feeling five times as stressed at the end of the day—and only one-fifth as happy. Slow your life down to a saner pace. It's okay to breastfeed your baby without trying to balance the chequebook at the same time.

- √ **Put your parenting support team in place.** Connect with other moms and dads who can offer you support and encouragement as you tackle the mother—and father—of all challenges: raising kids. You can meet these parents at the playground, in parenting classes, and on online message boards—anywhere that moms and dads hang out.

- √ **Trust yourself to make good parenting decisions.** There's no one-size-fits-all parenting solution, and trying a parenting technique that doesn't feel right to you will only add to your parenting stress. (If the technique is out of sync with your parenting philosophies or doesn't mesh with what you know about your child, your heart and your head will rebel.) You'll find that you make better parenting decisions if you do your research, talk to other parents, and allow your intuition to guide you. You know what's right for your family.

On your mind after baby

Don't be surprised if you find yourself walking around like a zombie, putting your car keys in the refrigerator and the milk—well, who knows where the milk might end up. This is perfectly normal. It's not just sleep deprivation messing with your head. You've got a lot on your mind.

How you may feel about becoming a mother

After months of looking forward to having her baby, Maria, a 35-year-old mother of two, was hit with a bad case of stage fright when the moment of truth finally arrived. "I said to the nurse when we left the hospital, 'How can you send this tiny baby home with us? We don't know how to be parents.'"

The feelings of insecurity that Maria experienced are very common among first-time mothers. Janet, a 32-year-old first-time mother, remembers feeling more than a little shell-shocked after her daughter arrived: "I felt completely ready for the baby before the birth," she confides. "Once she was born, however, I felt less ready. I guess reality set in and I realized I had to spend 24 hours a day with a real live baby."

Jennifer remembers feeling awestruck that she was actually capable of giving birth to such a perfect human being: "I think through it all we both had doubts as to whether we were capable of such a miraculous act," the 32-year-old mother of one recalls. "Even now, we're still in awe of the whole process of conception, gestation, and birth, and find it hard to believe that our bodies are actually made to do that." Her confidence in her mothering abilities was badly shaken, however, in the weeks that followed, as the result of a difficult breastfeeding experience. She persevered and managed to partially breastfeed her son until he was six months old, but she still remembers the anger and frustration she experienced during those early weeks of motherhood: "There can be no greater pain than knowing that your child is hungry and feeling powerless to feed him. It still angers me that I had to defend my actions to those who argued that breast is best. I agree wholeheartedly. But breast milk is only best if it's actually in the baby. No one told me that a baby might not breastfeed. None of the stack of books and pamphlets I was given in prenatal class even mentioned the possibility that a baby might

---

mom's the word

"Giving birth gave my life a whole new meaning. Raising children is the most difficult thing a person can ever do. I've never been happier in my entire life since I became a 'Mommy.' I've also never been so busy, tired, drained, and fulfilled."

—SUSAN, 34, MOTHER OF FIVE

---

refuse the breast. As a result, I was unprepared emotionally for being unable to feed my child in this 'oh-so-natural' way."

Joyce, a 41-year-old mother of two, found that becoming a mother changed her priorities and her view of the world. "Having the girls has made me look at life in such a different way—much less selfishly. I'm no longer the most important person in my world. They are! It's also made me much more conscious of my own mortality, partly because their growing up makes you more aware of the passing of time, but also because life is so much more precious to me. I worry about dying young because I want to be their mother for a long time—to be here for them as they grow up."

Chris, a 36-year-old mother of three, believes that becoming a mother has opened her up to a whole new world of love, but a whole world of heartache as well. "A good friend once warned me that once you become a mother, you become a mother to the whole world. That is so true. Any kind of news that has to do with children suddenly becomes personalized and the child in question is compared to your own child. The pain this can bring is excruciating when the news is bad. Famine. Murder. The loss of a child through illness."

Lori, a 29-year-old mother of four, feels that becoming a mother is the best thing that ever happened to her: "It's amazing. In some ways, it's changed my life in negative ways—there's not a lot of quiet time for me, I'm not able to be as spontaneous as I once was, there's more cleaning and cooking to do. But that doesn't even compare to the positive ways my life has changed. I feel a bond—a love that nothing can compare to. I have a pride that comes from knowing I created this wonderful life and that I'm responsible for it. I'm learning as much as I'm teaching. Not a day goes by that I don't laugh at something they say or do. I look forward to the future so that I can see their science experiments, their graduations, their weddings, their children. But I'm also desperately holding onto the past so that I don't forget that innocent look of theirs when they look right into your eyes and deep into your heart; that hearty laugh they give when they're playing hide-and-seek and have just been found; the look of amazement when they see something new or the look of pure happiness and delight when they open a birthday present or blow out their candles. I can't even begin to explain how having a baby has changed my life. It's the most rewarding experience I'll ever have."

mom's the word "The first month of Anya's life, we used to sit and hold her, breathing in her smells and marveling at this 'madly, deeply' love we felt for her. What an amazing feeling. That is something you are never really prepared for—the feeling of being so hopelessly in love with this little creature."

—KAREN, 28, MOTHER OF ONE

Worrying about being a good mother

One of the toughest things about becoming a mother is figuring out what you need to know (and what you don't need to bother obsessing about 24/7), as well as where and how to access the need-to-know information. What you don't know about mothering can leave you feeling like a bit of an imposter during the early weeks of motherhood—like you're not a real mother yet.

Fortunately, our hard-wired tendency to turn to other women for support during times of stress helps to ease our learning curve when it comes to mastering the art and science of mothering. We quickly learn that there's no easy solution to any issue we'll ever face with our children, starting with something as seemingly simple as which style or brand of diaper to use. (Your baby's bum is a slightly different size and shape than all the bums of all your friends' babies, so the diaper that fits their babies perfectly could leave your baby sopping wet.)

And as for the sense that the experts have all the answers—you quickly learn to ditch that theory, too. Even your baby's doctor doesn't know your baby as well as you do. While she may know everything you could ever want to know about strange and obscure pediatric illnesses (and probably a whole lot more!), you're the one who knows which types of sounds soothe your baby to sleep, how he likes to be held, and whether he loves—or loathes—the stroller.

Expert advice certainly has a valuable role to play in your education as a mother, but you need to carefully balance the mother learning with the mother knowing. You don't want to undercut your mothering self-confidence by exposing yourself to so much conflicting advice that you end up feeling totally overwhelmed.

Sometimes it makes more sense to

- talk to other moms;
- develop a sense of your emerging parenting philosophy; and
- zero in on those parenting resources that are in sync with your sense of who you are as a mother.

You'll be less likely to feel like there's a constant battle raging in your head between the various experts and advice-mongers, a battle that has the potential to drown out the voices that you really should be listening to: your own and your baby's.

---

mother wisdom A study conducted at the Sleep Research Centre at the Hôpital du Sacré-Cœur de Montréal has confirmed what many of us moms have discovered for ourselves: pregnancy and postpartum dreams can be the stuff of which nightmares are made.

The study's lead researcher, Tore Nielsen, Ph.D., found that 59 per cent of pregnant women and 73 per cent of new mothers experienced dreams in which a baby was in danger. New mothers found these dreams so disturbing that they continued to feel anxious even after they were wide awake (41 per cent), experienced confusion (51 per cent) and felt a need to go and check on their babies to make sure that their babies were safe (60 per cent). The results of this study were published in the September 1, 2007, edition of the journal *Sleep*.

These nightmares are believed to be triggered by a combination of physical, hormonal, and emotional factors. Long-term sleep deprivation (the result of pregnancy-related discomforts followed by round-the-clock parenting responsibilities); the hormonal changes associated with pregnancy, birth, and postpartum; and the many conflicting and powerful feelings that accompany the transition to motherhood play out in the world of dreams in unexpected ways.

While these dreams can be frightening and upsetting, they tend to become less frequent as you get more sleep, your body morphs back into something resembling its pre-pregnant state, and you begin to feel more comfortable in your new role of "mom."

---

mother wisdom — Mothering is easier the second time around. A study published in the *Journal of Nurse Midwifery* found that mothers having their second or subsequent child function better, experience fewer sleep disturbances, feel less tired, and feel more energetic than first-time mothers. First-time mothers may be more exhausted and less functional than experienced moms because they have to devote a lot of their energy to figuring out what it means to be a mom.

Thinking about the birth

Odds are motherhood isn't the only thing on your mind. Most new moms find that they also spend a lot of time thinking about how the birth went. They are particularly likely to be preoccupied with the birth if their birth experience was traumatic, if they felt that they were unable to control the way that events played out, or if what happened was significantly different from their hopes and dreams for the birth. (See the appendices for leads on resources you may find helpful.)

Most women find that they want to share their birth experiences with other women—to talk about how the events played out and how they were affected by the birth. Some of the points that you might want to think about when you reflect upon your birth include how involved you were able to be in making decisions throughout your labour and birth, and whether you felt that you were well-informed of your choices and treated with respect.

If you have questions about your birth (you were working hard and focusing intensely on the events that were taking place inside your body, so you might not have noticed everything that was happening around you), be sure to ask your caregivers and labour support people to help fill in any blanks for you. If you have a midwife, ask for a copy of your records (if the midwife hasn't already given a copy to you). Likewise, if you had a doula, ask what information she can share. Note: It is common for doulas to write up a copy of the birth story for the families they work with.

You may want to involve your partner in this conversation. He or she may have questions or concerns about the birth that need to be resolved as well. It's important that you are clear about what happened and why, so that you can feel at peace with your baby's birth. You may also want to write down your birth story while the memory is still fresh.

Hopefully your baby's birth was blissfully uneventful (other than resulting in the birth of a baby, of course). The advantage of coming to a full understanding of the birth is that you won't be left with nagging questions about your baby's birth months or years after the fact.

---

mom's the word "I feel a bond with any woman who has ever given birth. When I see a woman with a baby, I feel as if I should become her friend: after all, we went through the same things and have so much in common."

—LORI, 29, MOTHER OF FOUR

Until now, we've been talking big-picture survival strategy. Now it's time to get down to specifics. The final section of this chapter is designed to tell you the need-to-know information about postpartum depression. Note: Even if you don't think you're going to need this section on postpartum depression, read it anyway. And have a family member or friend read it, too. It's important that someone else in addition to you is alert to the warning signs of postpartum depression.

---

mother wisdom Just over half (54 per cent) of Canadian women who responded to the Maternity Experiences Survey reported that their overall experience of labour and birth was "very positive." Another 26 per cent considered their experience to be "somewhat positive," while the remaining 20 per cent chose a neutral or negative rating. Women who received maternity care services from a midwife were more likely to report having a positive birth experience than those who were cared for by obstetrician/gynecologists, family doctors, or nurses, and nurse practitioners 53 per cent.

COMING THROUGH POSTPARTUM DEPRESSION

As wonderful as motherhood can be, it's not unusual to be hit with the "postpartum blues"—that hormone-driven wave of emotion that tends to come crashing over you one to three days after the birth. In fact, studies have shown that 50 to 80 per cent of women suffer a brief episode of mild depression at some point during the first week as their hormones return to their pre-pregnancy levels. If you find, however, that you continue to feel exhausted, anxious, and depressed for weeks after the birth, you could be suffering from postpartum depression—a much more severe case of the blues that won't go away on its own.

Postpartum depression occurs in approximately one in four women who have recently given birth. It generally appears during the first six to eight weeks after the delivery, but can show up at any time during the year after birth. (By the time they celebrate their babies' first birthdays, one in five new moms will have experienced postpartum depression.) Postpartum depression can last anywhere from several weeks to several months, with 4 per cent of cases lasting for a full year.

In one out of every thousand births, a woman will develop a more serious form of postpartum depression known as postpartum psychosis. It's characterized by extreme confusion, fatigue, agitation, alterations in mood, feelings of hopelessness and shame, hallucinations, and rapid speech or mania, and can cause the affected woman to become a threat to both herself and her baby. Note: In a study published in the August 2008 issue of the *American Journal of Obstetrics & Gynecology,* researchers compared two groups of mothers and found that a history of psychiatric disorders or substance abuse was a strong predictor of postpartum suicide attempts.

Prenatal depression is the strongest predictor of postpartum depression, and postpartum depression is the strongest predictor for parenting stress. That's why it's so important to diagnose and treat perinatal mood disorders (mood disorders during or after pregnancy) promptly. Other risk factors for postpartum depression include a history of depression and other psychiatric disorders (both personal history and family history), prenatal depression, prenatal anxiety, stressful life events, a pessimistic life view, low self-esteem, low income, and not having a lot of support (which can lead to feelings of isolation and fatigue, and a sense of being overwhelmed).

Postpartum depression is much more than the "blues." You may be suffering from postpartum depression if you experience one or more of the following symptoms on an ongoing basis: despondency, tearfulness, feelings of inadequacy, guilt, anxiety, irritability, and fatigue. Physical symptoms include headaches, numbness, chest pain, and hyperventilation.

Note: Please share this information with family members and friends. It is important that they know how to spot the warning signs of postpartum depression. You may not be able to detect the symptoms in yourself. And the sooner someone can alert you to the fact that you might be struggling, the sooner you can seek treatment. Untreated postpartum depression can be harmful—even deadly—to mother and baby. The longer postpartum depression remains untreated, the greater the mother's risk of lifelong and recurrent depression and the greater her risk of suicide. Untreated postpartum depression can also interfere with the relationship between mother and baby, and result in intellectual, emotional, and behavioural problems in the baby.

---

mother wisdom While many people are tuned in to the warning signs of postpartum depression in new mothers, friends and family members are far less likely to make the connection between a mom's overwhelming feelings of anxiety about her new role as a mother (after all, isn't it normal for new moms to be a little anxious?) and the possibility that she is struggling with postpartum anxiety (another type of perinatal mood disorder).

If you suspect you're struggling with postpartum depression or anxiety, let your health-care provider and/or some other trusted person know how you are feeling. Motherhood doesn't have to be this hard.

Note: Some new moms delay seeking treatment because they are worried about the possible effects of anti-depressants and other medications on their babies. If this is what is stopping you from seeking treatment, it is important to know that medication isn't the only treatment for postpartum depression or anxiety. Interpersonal therapy, cognitive-behavioural therapy, and group therapy have all proven to be beneficial in the treatment of perinatal mood disorders. Depending on your situation, your health-care provider may recommend therapy and/or a breastfeeding-friendly medication.

What has helped other moms

Wondering what you can do to start feeling better—or even to give yourself the hope that you might someday start feeling better? Here are some strategies that have proven to be helpful for other moms who have struggled with postpartum depression and anxiety.

- **Make sleep a priority.** Practise relaxation techniques so that you can fall asleep quickly when your baby does. (You want to maximize your opportunities for sleep.) Other things that can help your body to unwind and your mind to relax before bedtime: taking a bath, reading a book, meditating, or repeating a calming word or phrase to yourself (try "calm" and "relax").

If you can arrange for your partner or a trusted friend or relative to care for your baby for a two-hour block of time, go to bed with ear plugs in your ears (so you won't be put on mother alert each time your baby makes the slightest sound.) A two-hour nap every now and then could be all you need to keep you going.

Note: It's important to let your health-care provider know if you're too stressed out to get the sleep you so desperately crave and that your body and mind require to refuel.

---

mother wisdom Symptoms of depression can worsen in mothers with perinatal mood disorders if they start to become sleep deprived. Sleep deprivation can interfere with the mother's ability to care for her baby as her judgment and concentration decline, and the mother's sleep difficulties begin to impact the baby's sleep quality as well. The net result? Mom and baby can quickly find themselves in a downward spiral.

Ironically, sleep deprivation, taken to the extreme, may have the opposite effect. A study involving critically timed sleep deprivation interventions helped to reduce symptoms of depression in some new mothers. For now, this is something best left for the sleep lab. In other words, don't try this at home.

- **Eat for energy.** Eat foods that will boost your energy naturally. Including protein and high-fibre foods in every meal or snack will help a lot. And make a point of staying well hydrated. (Remember, you need extra fluids while you're breastfeeding.)

- **Move your body.** Find fun ways to be physically active. Exercise will help you to feel better both physically and emotionally. And it reduces your risk of lapsing back into depression once you're recovered. So stick with that workout over the long-term. And try to take advantage of the mood-boosting benefits of being active outdoors. (Research has shown that spending time outdoors on a daily basis helps to reduce the severity of postpartum depression.)

- **Take time for yourself.** Mothers as martyrs is so 1950s. It's important to take care of yourself and to take breaks from motherhood when you're busy caring for a new baby.

- **Seek out the support you need in order to start feeling better.** Talk to friends and family members about how you are feeling and let them know what kind of support and hands-on help you need. Consider hiring a postpartum doula for a few days or a few weeks to help with baby care and household tasks. (If you or your partner have an extended health benefits package at work, the doula's services may be covered under one of your plans.) Tap into online or face-to-face support groups for women coping with perinatal mood disorders so that you can share your feelings with others who truly understand.

- **Start keeping a journal so that you can work through your feelings and monitor your progress.** It can be reassuring to look back and see that you are making progress, even if that progress isn't always quite as speedy as you'd like.

- **Remind yourself that you're not alone, that what you're experiencing is not your fault, and that you won't feel this way forever.** It's easy to lose sight of that at times, so write this out and post it where you can see it. One in every five moms will go through this. You didn't do anything to cause this. And you will feel better again.

- **Practise good sleep hygiene.** Go to bed at the same time every night. Avoid caffeine, nicotine, and alcohol. And don't nap or exercise within four hours of bedtime.

- **Stick with breastfeeding.** Breastfeeding will help you to get the sleep you need. (Mothers who breastfeed exclusively get more sleep than mothers who bottle-feed on a part-time or full-time basis.) And breastfeeding helps to offset the effects of postpartum depression on infant development. (Baby's brain gets an added boost.)

mother wisdom   Elevated levels of a brain protein known to deplete the body of feel-good hormones like serotonin may be responsible for triggering powerful feelings of sadness in new mothers. That's the key finding to emerge from a study conducted at the Centre for Addiction and Mental Health in Toronto and published in *Archives of General Psychiatry*.

The researchers discovered that, four to six days after a new mom gives birth, levels of the brain protein monoamine oxidase A (MAO-A) are elevated by 43 per cent in her brain (as compared to levels of the protein in the brains of women who have not recently been pregnant). MAO-A levels reach their peak on Day 5, the day when the postpartum blues tend to be at their worst.

The researchers involved in the study hope that their findings will lead to the development of nutritional supplements that could compensate for the nutrients that become depleted by high MAO-A levels, thereby reducing the risk that a woman will develop postpartum depression.

mother wisdom   Unresolved trauma can boomerang back into the lives of new moms, making the transition to motherhood more difficult. Researchers at the University of Missouri–Columbia and the University of Texas–Austin found that mothers who have experienced an unresolved trauma were more likely to be frightened of their infants and to exhibit behaviours that were frightening to their infants: for example, sudden voice changes or movements. This pattern of behaviour (which the researchers described as "frightened/frightening" behaviours) has been linked to attachment problems in children (difficulty forming friendships, increased aggression, and anxiety or depression). The good news is that, in situations where one or both parents have a history of unresolved trauma, therapy combined with parenting classes may help to ease the transition to parenthood and help the parents to feel more at peace with the events of the past.

dear mom with postpartum depression . . .

Dear Mom,

It takes time to get used to that name, no matter how desperately you've longed to be someone's mother. It's one thing, after all, to have the idea of a baby dancing around inside your head; it's quite another to have the reality of a baby nestled in your arms.

That tug of war between the dream and the reality of motherhood can mess with a mother's head. Toss in sleep deprivation, postpartum hormones, and the responsibilities of caring for a tiny, helpless human being, and the experience of early motherhood can feel a lot like a hurricane.

So how do you care for yourself and your baby if you find yourself caught up in the postpartum storm, struggling with a perinatal mood disorder such as postpartum depression, postpartum anxiety, or postpartum psychosis (the postpartum storm at its most severe)? Here's what I suggest:

√ Seek the shelter of friends and family.

√ Let others nurture you so that you can focus on caring for yourself and your baby.

√ Don't feel guilty about what you are or aren't feeling: a groundswell of positive, healthy emotions will surround you and your baby as soon as you start to feel better.

√ Understand that the world is impatient with mood disorders. Have a friend or family member advocate for you so that you are given the time and space you need to recover until you are strong enough to advocate for yourself.

√ Recognize that what you are experiencing is a brief stopover on your motherhood journey, not a permanent detour.

When you emerge from your cocoon, you will be a stronger and wiser woman who is capable of advocating for herself, her child, and the other mothers and children of the world. That is the silver lining of the gift you never asked for—a gift you will seize as you emerge from the darkness, following in the well-worn footsteps of other mothers who have walked this path before you.

chapter 4

CARING FOR YOUR NEWBORN

> "The time immediately following birth is precious . . . A child is born, and for a moment the wheeling planets stop in their tracks, as past, present, and future meet."
>
> —SHEILA KITZINGER, *HOMEBIRTH*

It's common knowledge that it's a good idea to get plenty of sleep when you're trying to master a new skill. Unfortunately, parents of newborns don't have that luxury: the crash course in parenting that they've signed up for follows a punishing around-the-clock schedule.

Good thing we come hard-wired with powerful instincts that are designed to help us get through the early days and nights of parenting. We're programmed to find our newborns utterly enchanting and to want to respond to their cries.

In this chapter, we zero in on these exhausting but exhilarating early weeks: getting off to the best possible start with breastfeeding, coping with sleep deprivation, and tried-and-true techniques for soothing a crying baby.

BREASTFEEDING: WHAT EVERY NEW MOM NEEDS TO KNOW

Entire books are written on the subject of breastfeeding. While I can't summarize all the fascinating information that you'll find in one of those big, thick, juicy guides (I hope you'll load up on an armful of them, too, by the way), what I can do is provide you with a quick intro that addresses two key questions: How do I get started? And, what do I do if I run into difficulty? Here goes.

mom's the word "Sometimes breastfeeding can be a drag. It prevents you from getting very much else done and it deprives you of sleep—particularly when Baby has a growth spurt and feeds every two hours for several days. However, most of the time it's a thoroughly enjoyable experience. Your baby will never be as happy as when she's on your breast. Sometimes she looks into your eyes with so much love. The feeling is just incredible."

—JANET, 32, MOTHER OF ONE

Getting started

So you're ready to put your baby to your breast. You'll be relieved to know that you don't have to master any IKEA-like assembly instructions (insert breast part A into baby mouth part B). I'm not the least bit mechanically inclined or coordinated and I managed to pull it off four times. Here's my best advice to you as you prepare to get started. Note: Step one is really important. Repeat as many times as necessary.

- **Find a position that will work well for you and your baby.** What most experts recommend now, for the first few days and weeks at least, is to get in a semi-reclining position in bed or on the couch, with pillows to support you so you're not flat on your back. Then lay your baby, tummy down, on your tummy so that your breasts are available to her. She may head for the breast and latch on without much help from you, or you may find you need to help a bit in supporting her or supporting your breast. Because she's lying on top of you, you don't have to support her weight, so your hands will be more available to provide any help she needs.

- **Offer the breast at a time when your baby is likely to be receptive: when she's alert, calm, and sending out signals that she's ready to eat.** Babies may not be able to talk, but they have ways of communicating their desire to breastfeed: rooting (turning the head to one side when something touches the cheek), making sucking movements with their lips, breathing rapidly, clicking their tongues, and sucking on their fingers or their hands. If held against your chest (especially if you are skin-to-skin), a hungry baby will move toward your breast—sometimes so enthusiastically that he practically throws himself toward it! A baby can also tell you when he's had enough to eat. He may stop nursing and turn his head away, relax in your arms, and stretch out his arms and legs and his fingers. That's the body language of a satisfied baby.

- **Help your baby to achieve a good latch.** Most of the time, letting your baby latch on while you are semi-reclined will work well. If that is not working for some reason, or if you need to sit up to feed your baby, you may need to help with the latch. Aim for what breastfeeding experts Nancy Mohrbacher and Kathleen Kendall-Tackett describe as "the comfort zone"—a deep latch that is comfortable for Mom and that provides a steady milk flow for Baby. Position your baby's nose in line with your nipple and at the level of your breast, and turn her body in to yours—think "nose to nipple, tummy to Mummy." Avoid placing your hand behind your baby's head. Most babies dislike this. To encourage a good latch, lightly stroke your nipple against Baby's lips. When she opens her mouth very wide (like a yawn), pull her toward the breast so your nipple and areola find their way deep into her mouth. Aiming your nipple toward the roof of her mouth helps. (Note: You don't want her to latch on to just your nipple. Not only is that painful, it's ineffective at removing milk from your breast.) Her chin should be buried in the breast, and her nose should be clear of the breast. If it isn't, try tucking her bottom in more closely—this should ensure that her head tips back a bit more, thereby improving the latch.

- **Understand that your milk supply is more abundant in the morning than it is at night.** There are also peaks and valleys in your energy cycle. (These are tied to your sleep-wake cycle, the last time you ate, and your baby's sleep-wake-feeding cycle.) You can be caught off guard by leaks, squirts, and spurts. Breast pads and a sense of humour are a breastfeeding mother's best friends.

- **Trust your body and your baby to get this thing right.** Yes, it's helpful to have some basic knowledge of breastfeeding, but you'll learn most of what you need to know by working with your breastfeeding partner: your baby. Just as you can only learn so much from a dance manual, most of your true learning will occur once you start putting your breastfeeding theory into action.

---

mother wisdom Breastfeeding mothers and babies were the original inventors of supply-demand economics and just-in-time manufacturing. The quantity and the specific composition of breast milk changes in order to meet Baby's need at any given time. A baby may breastfeed more frequently in hot weather or during a growth spurt. Growth spurts typically occur at around 2 to 3 weeks, 6 weeks, 3 months, and 6 months of age, although each baby is unique.

- **If you run into breastfeeding problems, seek help sooner rather than later.** More than breastfeeding is at stake, suggests breastfeeding expert Kathleen Kendall-Tackett in the *International Breastfeeding Journal* (in an article entitled "A new paradigm for depression in new mothers: The central role of inflammation and how breastfeeding and anti-inflammatory treatments protect maternal mental health," March 30, 2007): "When breastfeeding is going well, it protects mothers from stress, thereby protecting maternal mood … Breastfeeding not only reduces stress for mothers; it also lowers stress that babies experience when their mothers are depressed … When breastfeeding is not going well, particularly if there is pain, it becomes a trigger to depression rather than something that lessens the risk [of depression]. Mothers' mental health is yet another reason to intervene quickly when breastfeeding difficulties arise." It's normal to feel disappointed or angry if you're having trouble breastfeeding. If you're upset, talk to someone you trust and who you know will support your feelings. And be sure to find out where and how to access breastfeeding support in your community so you can get help right away.

Note: See Table 4.1 (Top Worries and Concerns about Breastfeeding) and Table 4.2 (Troubleshooting Common Breastfeeding Problems) for additional information on getting started with breastfeeding. You will also find more information about breastfeeding your baby in Chapter 6.

CHAPTER 4 — CARING FOR YOUR NEWBORN

TABLE 4.1

Top Worries and Concerns about Breastfeeding

What you may be worried about	What you need to know
"Which position should I use to breastfeed my baby?"	The position that works best for you and your baby. What usually works best to start with is the semi-reclining position where your baby's inborn breastfeeding skills can "kick in." Note: As you begin to breastfeed in other positions, you may notice that your baby doesn't breastfeed well if • her body is twisted; • her feet are pushing against the arm of a chair or other surface, which makes it easy for her to push herself off the breast; or • her chin is not pressed into the breast, because she can't remove milk from the breast effectively that way.
"I can't tell how much milk my baby is getting."	Your baby is getting enough milk if she is making swallowing signs (a distinct pause during each suck at the point where the baby's mouth is open wide), producing a couple of bowel movements every 24 hours after the first few days of life (although some babies may go a week or longer without a bowel movement starting at around week six), and gaining weight (after the initial post-birth weight loss of 5 to 8 per cent of birth weight, which is normal).
"My milk hasn't come in yet. I'm worried my baby is starving."	Newborns only need tiny quantities of colostrum—the nutrient-rich first food—when they first start to nurse. By the time your transitional milk comes in (around day four) he'll be getting about 59 millilitres (2 ounces) of milk per feeding. That will be up to about 59 to 74 millilitres (2 to 2.5 ounces) of breast milk by the time your actual breast milk comes in the following day (around day five). Your health-care provider will want to see your baby regain his birth weight by age 2 weeks and to continue to gain 113 to 227 grams (4 to 8 ounces) per week during the first three months of life.

(continued)

What you may be worried about	What you need to know
"Is breast milk supposed to look like that?"	Breast milk is supposed to look like a whitish-bluish to whitish-yellowish version of the most watered-down skim milk you've ever seen. That's normal. Don't expect your breast milk to look like whipped cream. And realize that your breast milk may look different than the breast milk of another mother.
"How often should my newborn be nursing?"	*Up to 3 months of age:* At least eight times a day (but it may be many more times than that each day). What is more important than how *often* the baby feeds is how *effectively* the baby feeds. You'll probably notice that your baby "cluster feeds" (has a couple of feedings that are closely spaced together). This is normal. Resist the temptation to schedule feedings, to time feedings, or to limit time at the breast. Your baby will let you know when he's hungry and when he's had enough to eat. Of course, there's a difference between a baby who's actively nursing and a baby who wants to keep a nipple in his mouth all day—whether he's asleep or awake!
"My baby just spit up half his feeding."	Don't be concerned if your baby regurgitates small amounts (or what looks like large amounts) of breast milk after his feeding. Breastfed babies have less acid in their stomachs, so they don't experience any painful burning in their tissues when they spit up. There is even evidence that spitting up may be beneficial to breastfed babies. A small amount of regurgitated breast milk may end up reaching the respiratory tract, conveying immunological benefits. This may help to explain why breastfed babies develop fewer respiratory infections than formula-fed babies. Note: Spitting up is different from projectile vomiting and reflux. See Appendix A.

"What foods should I eliminate from my diet in order to reduce my baby's fussiness?"	If you eliminate every possible food that has been linked to fussiness in breastfeeding babies, you'll be on a very bland diet. A better approach is to try to figure out what food might have triggered your baby's fussiness and then try to eliminate that food or food group for two weeks. Then gradually reintroduce the food and see if you notice a difference in your baby's symptoms. Note: Foods that have been blamed for making babies edgy, cranky, or colicky include caffeine, dairy products, eggs, gluten, corn, garlic, fish, nuts, soy, gassy vegetables, and spicy foods.
"What's the earliest that I should introduce a bottle or a pacifier?"	The first thing you should know is that many mothers never give their babies bottles or pacifiers. Don't feel you need to introduce them, ever, if you'd prefer to breastfeed exclusively. The next thing you need to know is that you'll hear various answers to this question. That's because the most honest answer is, "It depends on how well your baby is doing with breastfeeding." You are less likely to run into problems (but still may) if you wait until your baby is breastfeeding well and your milk supply is well established before introducing a bottle or a pacifier. That might be at four weeks with one baby, but it could be at eight weeks with another who got off to a rough start. Despite the advertising, no nipple is really similar to a human nipple. And be aware that time spent sucking on an artificial nipple is time that isn't spent at the breast stimulating milk production. (On the other hand, if you're feeling like you've turned into a human pacifier 24/7, it may be worthwhile weighing the pros/cons of pacifier use. In addition, there is an association between pacifier use while sleeping and reduced incidence of SIDS.)
"Is it okay to offer a breastfed baby the occasional bottle of formula?"	Exclusive breastfeeding for at least six months is preferred (and is what the World Health Organization recommends).

(continued)

What you may be worried about	What you need to know
"Is it okay to drink alcohol while you're nursing?"	Most health authorities advise avoiding alcohol while you are breastfeeding, but note that limiting yourself to one alcoholic beverage and timing that drink so that you have it right after a feeding will limit the amount of alcohol your baby receives.
"Is it okay to smoke while you're nursing?"	Smoking decreases milk production, interferes with milk ejection, lowers prolactin levels and fat levels in milk, and increases the incidence of infant colic. What's more, exposure to second-hand smoke increases a baby's risk for SIDS, respiratory infections, and cancer. *Nutrition for Healthy Term Infants* states that breastfeeding mothers should be encouraged to stop or reduce smoking, but adds, "Even if smoking is continued, breastfeeding is still the best choice." The baby of a mother who smokes will be healthier if he is breastfed than if he is fed formula. La Leche League International offers some sensible advice: smoke away from the baby (outdoors, or in a separate room); and change your clothes before picking up the baby again); smoke right after nursing sessions; and smoke as few cigarettes as possible. Note: If you decide you're ready to quit or you'd like to cut down on the number of cigarettes you smoke, talk to your doctor about the best ways to go about quitting.
"Is it safe to take this medication or herbal product while I'm breastfeeding?"	Medications and herbal products pass through breast milk to babies. While many medications can be taken by breastfeeding moms, some products are known to be harmful to babies. Contact your doctor, pharmacist, or the Motherisk Clinic (www.motherisk.org or 1-877-439-2744) for information.

TABLE 4.2

Troubleshooting Common Breastfeeding Problems

Type of problem	What causes it	Possible solutions
Your nipples are sore.	A poor latch, breast infection, or initial tenderness that many women experience when they first start to breastfeed.	• Get help from a breastfeeding expert (lactation consultant) to see if Baby's latch can be improved. • Expose your nipples to the air as much as possible (leave the flaps of your nursing bra undone or go braless and wear a loose-fitting shirt). • Express some milk and drip it on your nipples. Then allow your nipples to air dry. • Get the milk flowing before you put your baby to the breast (hand-express or use a breast pump). • Avoid washing your breasts with soap. • Use breast pads made from natural fibres and change them regularly to keep your breasts dry. • Work with a breastfeeding expert to rule out or get treatment for other causes of sore nipples.
Baby is too sleepy to nurse.	Following a period of initial alertness, most newborns become quite sleepy. Babies with jaundice are extra sleepy.	• Keep Baby skin-to-skin as much as possible. This is the most effective way to help a sleepy baby wake. • Watch for signs that Baby has fallen asleep (Baby's eyes are moving behind his eyelids and he's "nursing" in his sleep). • If necessary, try giving Baby a little bit of expressed milk (with an eyedropper or syringe in the corner of his mouth) to help wake him up.

(continued)

Type of problem	What causes it	Possible solutions
Baby doesn't want to nurse. (If a newborn refuses the breast, it's called "breast refusal"; when an older baby refuses the breast, it's called a "nursing strike.")	Often the problem in a newborn is that he has been given bottles. You can overcome this, but it's a good idea to ask for help.	• Keeping up milk production is crucial, so you will want to pump or hand-express. • Keep the baby skin to skin, bathe with Baby, and give Baby lots of opportunities to self-attach. • Try offering the breast when Baby is sleepy, or while walking around with Baby in a sling. • Offer pumped breast milk with a cup or spoon. Avoid bottles!
Your breasts are engorged.	Your baby can't extract milk from your overly firm breasts, and Baby's poor latch leaves you susceptible to sore nipples.	• Apply warm compresses right before feedings to encourage milk flow, and apply cold compresses (frozen peas or cabbage leaves) in between feedings to reduce swelling. • Assess the latch, nurse frequently (at least eight times a day), and watch for signs of a breast infection (fever, redness, breast soreness). • Hand-express a little milk before feeding. Use your fingers to press in a circle around the nipple to create a "moat" where you have pushed the fluid back. Then latch Baby on right away.
You're afraid that your baby isn't getting enough milk.	Most women produce enough milk for their babies. In general, if your baby is producing one wet diaper on Day 1, two wet diapers on Day 2, and so on until Day 5 (at which point you want to see five to six wet diapers per day and a couple of yellowish stools), you should feel reassured. If you are still worried, have your health-care provider check your baby's weight, latch, and overall health.	To build up your milk supply • have someone knowledgeable about breastfeeding check your baby's latch; • ensure your baby nurses actively for at least 10 minutes at each breast (you want to see slow sucks with a noticeable pause at the point where Baby's mouth is open wide); • breastfeed your baby as often as he seems interested, which should be at least eight times per day but is usually much more frequently, offering each breast at each feeding and expressing milk (or pumping) after each feeding to further stimulate milk production; • use breast compression while the baby is sucking to help him get more milk; • ensure you get adequate fluids; and • ask your health-care provider if a prescription or herbal product to build up your milk supply would be advisable in your situation.

Your baby chokes, gulps, or pulls away from the breast because he can't manage the flow of milk. Some babies simply refuse to nurse.	You have an overabundant milk supply.	- Offer one breast per feeding. - Pump or hand-express some milk before you offer the breast to your baby so that the milk flow won't be quite so overpowering. - Nurse in the side-lying position so that Baby can let any extra milk dribble out of his mouth. - Lie on your back once your baby is latched so gravity is on your side rather than your baby's. - Be cautious with this approach and be sure to monitor your baby's bowel movements via the number of soiled diapers: it is easy to decrease your milk production too much.
Your nipples are flat or inverted.	Provided that you access good breastfeeding support, this is rarely a problem. Babies breastfeed, they don't nipple-feed. The key is getting a really good latch so that a good portion of the areola is in Baby's mouth.	Use a breast pump immediately prior to each nursing session. This will encourage the nipple to protrude long enough for Baby to get a good latch. Or use a nipple everter (a syringe with the end cut off) to help an inverted nipple to protrude.
Baby has positioning problems.	Baby is latching on to the nipple itself rather than the areola (shallow latch). This leads to sore nipples, poor letdown, poor milk flow, and reduced milk production.	Check Baby's position. See "Which position should I use to breastfeed my baby?" in Table 4.1.
You are suffering nipple trauma.	This is most often the result of a poor latch, an improperly fitting pump, or infection in a damaged nipple.	If your breast pump is causing you pain or discomfort, stop pumping and consider getting a different-sized flange or pump, or hand-expressing. Get help with your baby's latch and seek treatment for the infection right away.

(continued)

Type of problem	What causes it	Possible solutions
You have a thrush (candida) infection on your nipples.	You can catch thrush from your baby, or thrush can be the result of other unrelated health conditions. Thrush causes shooting or burning pain in the nipple and breast that can persist during and after feeding.	Several anti-fungal medications can be used; you will probably need to treat your baby as well.
You have mastitis.	If a plugged milk duct becomes infected, you can develop a fever that is accompanied by symptoms of a breast infection (red streaks on your breast, a swollen and tender lump in the breast, and possibly pus or blood in your milk).	Keep nursing to avoid making the infection worse. There is no risk to the baby: he can't catch the infection. Apply warm water (hot wet washcloths, a hot water bottle) and massage your breasts in the area where the lump is to encourage the milk to flow.) If Baby refuses to nurse on the affected side, pump from that side and continue to offer the other breast. Note: Most babies will continue to nurse on the affected side. Other tips: • Avoid tight clothing, particularly tight bras, and take pain medication as needed. • Get plenty of rest. • Consult your caregiver if you don't see any signs of improvement within 24 hours. You may need an antibiotic.
Baby has reflux.	Gastroesophageal reflux disease (GERD) occurs when stomach acids back up into the esophagus, causing extreme distress to the baby during and after feedings and when she is lying down after a feeding.	Positions that keep your baby's head elevated during a feeding work best for babies with GERD. Keep Baby upright for at least half an hour after each feeding. (A baby carrier works well for this.) And talk to your health-care provider.

Baby has special feeding issues.	Babies who are premature may not be capable of feeding at the breast or staying awake for a full feeding at the breast initially. Babies who are tongue-tied (whose frenulum—the string-like membrane under the tongue—is unusually short), or who have a physical condition or structural problem that makes breastfeeding more difficult (such as Down syndrome, cleft lip, or cleft palate) may require modified breastfeeding holds or surgery in order to breastfeed, and, in some cases, partial breastfeeding may be a more realistic goal.	Speak with a lactation consultant to find out how to make breastfeeding and breast pumping work for your baby. There are special feeding devices that can be helpful to babies with cleft palate; for example, a palatal obdurator (a mouth appliance that provides a firm surface at the roof of the mouth) and a Haberman feeder (a bottle that can be adjusted for slower or faster flow and that is compression-driven rather than sucking-driven).
Baby is having latch difficulties or is too premature to feed at the breast, and/or you are having milk supply problems as a result of breast reduction surgery or other issues.	If you and your baby are experiencing breastfeeding challenges, a lactation consultant may be able to suggest alternate methods of delivering your breast milk (or breast milk from a breast milk bank: see Chapter 6) to your baby on a short-term or long-term basis.	A feeding tube can be taped to your breast or to your finger so that your baby can be fed expressed breast milk. Other alternative feeding methods include syringe-feeding, spoon-feeding, dropper-feeding, and cup-feeding.

mom's the word

"Nothing prepared me for the baby who wouldn't wake up to nurse and who would scream in protest at the late afternoon feeding, for breasts that didn't ever seem to live up to my expectations, or for the emotional turmoil I went through—feeling as though I was failing my baby because I couldn't seem to feed her adequately. It took a while for my husband to realize how emotionally involved I was in the process. To him, at first, it was just a matter of breast milk versus formula. As time progressed, he began to understand that it was so much more than that, and he was very supportive of my decision to persevere, even though he occasionally wondered if it was worth the emotional toll it took on me."

—JOYCE, 41, MOTHER OF TWO BREASTFED BABIES

mother wisdom

Breastfeeding doesn't come naturally or easily to every mother and baby. There can be a learning curve for one or both, and the problems to be overcome during the early weeks can range from the easy-to-troubleshoot to the much more challenging to resolve.

The pressure to breastfeed can be considerable—something that can be either motivating or overwhelming, depending on both the amount of pressure and the individual mother's reaction to the pressure that is being exerted.

Learning about breastfeeding before your baby is born (by sitting in on a La Leche League meeting: see www.lllc.ca), setting a breastfeeding goal for yourself, and connecting with sources of breastfeeding support and information after the birth can increase your odds of being able to breastfeed over the long term.

Once you reach the reward period of breastfeeding, you'll be so happy you persevered. Breastfeeding is a wonderful way to snuggle up to your baby, a source of feel-good mothering hormones, and a powerful mothering tool.

COPING WITH SLEEP DEPRIVATION

Sleep may feel more like fantasy than reality if you're a sleep-deprived new parent. Here are some tips on coping with sleep shortage while you wait for Baby to start sleeping a little longer at night. (Five and a half hours at a stretch is what you're holding out for, by the way. That's the medical definition of "sleeping through the night" when you're a baby—and your newborn likely won't be doing that for quite some time.)

mom's the word "I was severely sleep deprived. I can only appreciate how badly my abilities were impaired in retrospect. My friend used the expression 'stupid tired,' which I think is very apt. Sleep deprivation left my postpartum emotions very raw. I couldn't problem solve, organize my day, or think ahead. I felt drained, unimaginative, and as if my brain had turned to mush. I had trouble learning and coping with anything unexpected. All told, the sleep deprivation greatly magnified my feelings of being an incompetent mother. It was rather frightening at times and, unfortunately, I was so tired that it was hard at times to enjoy my baby."

—JENNIFER, 25, MOTHER OF ONE

- **Have realistic expectations of your baby when it comes to sleep.** Most newborns sleep for just a few hours at a stretch (three hours or less), repeating this sleep-wake pattern around the clock so that they can fill their tiny tummies on a regular basis. (A newborn's stomach can only hold 10 to 20 millilitres (2 to 4 teaspoons) as compared to a 12-month-old's, which can hold 200 millilitres (40.5 teaspoons). Don't forget that every baby is unique. Some newborns sleep for five-hour stretches while others wake up every hour on the hour all night long.

mother wisdom What you ate during pregnancy can affect how well your baby sleeps after the birth—and that, in turn, may affect your risk of developing postpartum depression. Mothers who consume high levels of DHA (an Omega-3 fatty acid) during pregnancy tend to give birth to babies who exhibit more mature sleep patterns during the first days of life. Having a baby who sleeps well during the early days should lead to a better-rested and happier mom. Or at least that's the theory.

- **Learn to spot and respond to your baby's sleep cues.** You'll have more luck getting your baby to settle down to sleep if you can get her to bed when she's tired rather than overtired. (When babies get overtired, they get wired—the way you feel when you've had too much caffeine. They desperately need sleep, but their bodies won't let them relax and wind down.) That's why it's important to learn how to spot the warning signs that your baby is getting sleepy before she reaches the point of no return and heads into the overtired zone. Your baby is probably winding down and getting ready for sleep if she becomes calmer and less active, she is less tuned in to her surroundings, she is quieter, she is nursing more slowly and less vigorously, and she starts yawning. You can assume your baby has gone from tired to overtired if you notice that she's becoming fussy, irritable, or rubbing her eyes. (That's bad news for you.)

- **Set the stage for sleep—for yourself and your baby.** The ideal sleeping environment is cool, dark, quiet, and well ventilated, and a place that you associate only with sleep and sex. (If your bedroom doubles as a workspace and a home entertainment zone, you'll find it tough to wind down when you get the chance.) It's also a good idea to limit your consumption of caffeine and alcohol (you're probably doing this anyway, if you're breastfeeding), both of which can interfere with a good night's sleep. And if you're smoking (or you recently started again), you've got another good reason to quit (again): smoking interferes with sleeping as well. (Being exposed to second-hand smoke also increases your baby's risk of SIDS, an even better reason to butt out.)

- **Help your baby to learn to distinguish between night and day.** Exposing your baby to sunlight in the morning will help to set your baby's natural circadian rhythm (the body's built-in sleep/wake clock). You also want your baby to learn that daytime is for playing and nighttime is for sleeping. You can help her to learn this important lesson by keeping the lighting low and keeping conversation and activity to a minimum in the wee hours of the morning, and ensuring that Baby benefits from plenty of activity and stimulation during the day.

- **Learn to differentiate between the half-awake noises your baby sometimes makes in his sleep and the more urgent pick-me-up sounds.** (Until you learn how to tell the difference, you may find yourself picking up a baby who is still asleep and trying to comfort a baby who wasn't in distress at all.) Of course, you'll want to trust your instincts on this. If the sound makes you want to reach for your baby, then that's what you should do.

- **Recognize that sleep deprivation makes parenting harder.** When you are missing out on sleep on a consistent basis, your brain and your body rebel. You become forgetful, your communication and problem-solving skills decrease, you become impatient and edgy, and you feel sapped of your usual energy and drive. You may find yourself experiencing some of the physical symptoms of sleep deprivation, such as cravings for high-carbohydrate or high-fat foods and an increased susceptibility to illness.

- **Understand that even very young babies are able to pick up on their parents' stress levels.** One of the best ways to help your baby wind down and fall asleep is to stay calm yourself. With any luck, you'll both enjoy the payoff: a good night's sleep.

- **Ask for what you need from other people.** Trusted friends or relatives can take care of Baby right after a feeding so that you can nap until it's time to nurse again. Friends or relatives can also assist with other household chores, cook meals, and run errands so that you won't be tempted to tackle these tasks during Baby's naps, when you could be sleeping.

Note: For tips on dealing with sleep issues in older babies, please see Chapter 9.

---

baby talk A Yale University study involving 2,299 mothers found that just 61 per cent of mothers consistently placed their babies to sleep lying on their backs (the position that has been proven to reduce the odds of a baby succumbing to sudden infant death syndrome (SIDS)). Mothers who believe that their babies find this sleeping position uncomfortable or who worry that the position increases their babies' risk of choking are less likely to use the recommended position. The study was reported in the April 2010 issue of the *Archives of Pediatrics and Adolescent Medicine*.

---

mother wisdom If your baby tends to wake up each time you try to lay her down, try warming her bed with a hot water bottle. She is less likely to protest the transition from being cuddled in your arms if she's placed on a warm (not freezing cold) sheet. (Important: Remove the hot water bottle before you place her in bed. Overheating is a risk factor for SIDS.)

COMFORTING YOUR CRYING BABY

Who's crying now? If you've got a baby who spends a lot of time crying, you might be ready to cry along with her. You might also be wondering if your baby is colicky, what that means, and what to do if she is. Here's what you need to know.

So what is colic? Medically speaking, colic (also known as purple crying) is defined as crying that begins and ends for no obvious reason, lasts at least three hours a day, happens at least three days a week, and continues for three weeks to three months.

So what do you do if you think it might be colic?

- **Talk to your baby's doctor.** The doctor may want to give your baby a checkup to rule out any physical causes for your baby's discomfort (such as gastroesophageal reflux, when stomach acids are regurgitated, causing extreme discomfort after eating and when your baby is sleeping). Be sure to let your baby's doctor know if you feel angry at or resentful toward your baby, you are worried that you may hurt or harm your child or yourself, your baby isn't nursing as well as he was or he has lost weight, your baby reacts negatively to new situations, or your baby has a strong reaction to sensory stimuli.
- **Play parent detective.** See what you can learn about your baby by observing his behaviour:
  - Does your baby cry at certain times of the day?
  - Do certain situations tend to trigger episodes of crying?
- **Offer your baby the breast.** Most babies enjoy nursing for comfort. Breastfeeding is soothing for you, too, thanks to the release of bliss-out breastfeeding hormones oxytocin, prolactin, and cholecystokinin.

mother wisdom — Some babies are colicky because they are sensitive to cow's milk protein. If you think your baby could be reacting to cow's milk protein in your diet, try avoiding all dairy products for two to three weeks to see if this improves your baby's symptoms. Then try reintroducing dairy to your diet. If your baby is only mildly sensitive to cow's milk protein, you may be able to consume small quantities of dairy products. If your baby is severely sensitive, however, you will need to read food labels carefully and choose only dairy-free products. Note: Choosing lactose-free products won't solve the problem because your baby is reacting to cow's milk protein, not lactose.

- **Experiment until you figure out what else soothes your baby (or at least what soothes your baby today).** You may have to go back to the drawing board tomorrow. Colicky babies are notoriously fickle! The more techniques you have at your disposal, the better. Your baby might be comforted by some skin-to-skin time (strip Baby down to her diaper and place her between your breasts), being snuggled against your chest (she will find the sound and feel of your heartbeat soothing), being carried over your shoulder (so she can see what's going on) or in a colic hold (hold your baby so she is lying across your forearm with her tummy down, with your hand supporting her chest), or being carried in a sling or a wrap while the two of you go for a walk (the motion will soothe her), and/or listening to the sound of your voice (she finds that soothing because she knows your voice so well).

mother wisdom — Wrap one of the bottom sheets from your baby's crib around you when you go to sleep at night so that it can pick up your scent. Then use it to make up your baby's bed. Your baby finds your scent very soothing.

baby talk A University of Miami study found that babies who are massaged are calmer and less fussy, and wake in the night less often. Massage also aids in digestion, makes it easier for babies to relax and fall sleep, and promotes healthy growth. Massaging your baby is also beneficial to you. It's soothing and it helps to promote a healthy parent-child bond.

- **Too much stimulation (sound, light, touch, and activity) can be overwhelming for very young babies.** They have not yet developed the ability to tune out or self-soothe. They need you to help them take a break from all the hustle and bustle. Watch for the following signs that your baby may have had too much excitement for now and may need your help winding down: Baby is looking away, covering her face with her hands, wrinkling up her entire forehead, arching her back, tensing her body, fussing, or crying. Note: Using a sling-type baby carrier can be very helpful if your baby is sensitive to stimulation and you need to go out with her. It reassures her by keeping her close and blocks out some of the outside world.

- **Pay attention to how your baby's crying is affecting you.** Some parents find their babies' crying very distressing and need to work at calming themselves. You may find it helpful to talk to other parents who are coping with a crying baby or who have been there and made it through. If it's really upsetting you, put your baby in a safe spot, like the crib, and take a break.

- **Accept all offers of help.** This is no time to play the martyr. You need all the help you can get when you're caring for a colicky baby. Oh, and by the way, don't put off waving the white flag for very long: if you have a baby who cries a lot, you are more likely to be arguing with your partner about parenting issues by the time your baby is 2 weeks of age, reporting decreased satisfaction with the amount of support you are receiving from your partner and other family members by the time your baby is 2 weeks of age, and experiencing feelings of self-doubt about your effectiveness as a parent by the time your baby is 6 weeks of age.

mother wisdom — Some babies cry more than others because they have extra-sensitive temperaments: they are easily upset. Even being held by a number of different people (excited grandparents, aunts, and uncles) may be all that it takes to throw an extra-sensitive baby out of whack. A baby like this craves consistency: when things smell the same (like Mom or Dad or other familiar things), this easily upset baby knows that all is right with the world.

If you have a baby with a challenging temperament, you are going to need people to take care of you (to ensure that your basic needs for food and rest are met, and to remind you to take breaks from the physically and emotionally demanding job of caring for an infant 24/7). You'll also want someone to reassure you that you're doing just fine. (Studies have shown that parents of colicky babies tend to feel incompetent, something that can make it more difficult for them to enjoy and connect with their babies.)

- **Don't blame yourself because your baby is colicky.** Colic happens. Remind yourself that you are making a difference for your baby, even if he is still spending a lot of his time crying.
- **Remind yourself that it won't be like this forever.** Crying in newborns typically begins a few weeks after birth and reaches its peak at around 6 weeks of age. Colicky babies generally morph into much happier babies by the time they are 3 to 4 months old. In the meantime, the following tips will help to keep you sane:
  - Work with—not against—your baby's needs.
  - Respect your baby's individual likes and dislikes.
  - Get as much rest as you can so that you can cope with your baby's demands.
  - Try to recreate the uterine environment for your baby (think motion, warmth, and white noise).
  - Provide skin-to-skin contact.
  - Use soothing tones and handle your baby calmly.

- Practise infant massage.
- Remind yourself that things will get easier as Baby becomes more settled and more tuned in to the world around him.

---

mother wisdom Research has shown that mothers of colicky babies tend to find it difficult to take breaks from mothering and that they tend to feel very anxious when they are away from their babies. This continues to be the case even after the crying diminishes. So if you have a baby who cries a lot, you may need extra encouragement from others to take a break from your baby (even if that "break" means taking a nap in another part of your house), and you may be so worried about how your baby is doing without you that you may find it difficult or even impossible to actually fall asleep during the time that you blocked off for this desperately needed nap. Accept that this is normal and use the time to relax and rest, even if you can't actually fall asleep. Listen to a meditation tape or other extremely soothing music while you lie down and breathe deeply. Who knows? You may surprise yourself by drifting in and out of dreamland after all.

---

major first-year firsts The moment your baby is born, the two of you head off on a journey of discovery together. Here's some mom-proven advice on coping with seven of the major first-year "firsts."

1. THE FIRST TIME YOU HOLD YOUR BABY
Your doctor or midwife places a wet and naked baby in your arms and covers the two of you with a toasty-warm blanket (to help keep you both warm).

- √ **What other moms want you to know:** Just relax, gaze into your baby's eyes, talk to her, and stroke her. She'll be surprisingly alert and checking you out, too. (Your face is the perfect distance away for her newborn eyes to focus on when you're holding her in your arms.)

2. THE FIRST FEEDING

Begin breastfeeding as soon as possible after the birth. That way, you can take advantage of that initial period of wide-eyed alertness. (If you or your baby require extra care after the birth and you can't offer your baby the breast as soon as you would have liked, don't worry. Simply offer the breast at the first possible opportunity in whatever position works best for both of you.)

- √ **What other moms want you to know:** It's a good idea to take a breastfeeding class, to do some reading about breastfeeding ahead of time, or to have some hands-on help lined up from an experienced nursing mother. Breastfeeding is perfectly natural, but there can be a bit of a learning curve involved for both you and Baby.

3. THE FIRST DIAPER CHANGE

You're going to change a lot of diapers by the time your baby learns how to use the toilet: something in the neighbourhood of 4,000 diapers.

- √ **What other moms want you to know:** First, gather up all the necessary supplies (diaper, change pad, wet wash cloths, and a baby towel or receiving blanket) before you start the diaper change so that you won't have to carry around a naked baby while you try to find the one thing you forgot. Secondly, if your newborn cries, it's likely because he doesn't like the sensation of being naked. Minimizing the amount of skin that's exposed at any given time (or covering these exposed areas with a baby towel or receiving blanket as you change him) can help to keep him comfortable while he's *au naturel*.

4. THE FIRST BATH

There are few things as nerve-racking as bathing a baby for the very first time.

- √ **What other moms want you to know:** If you're worried that your baby is going to go slip-sliding away, thanks to all the soap and the water, slip on a thin pair of cotton gloves (use them like built-in washcloths) and wash Baby in a plastic baby bathtub or in the kitchen sink (well-scrubbed and rinsed, of course). Wash the cleanest parts of Baby first, starting with his head. Use a small amount of soap or stick to plain water to avoid over-drying Baby's skin. Rinse Baby thoroughly and then wrap him in a towel and pat him dry.

Note: Once you start feeling comfortable bathing Baby, you can take an entirely different (and much simpler) approach: simply bring Baby into the bathtub with you. You might need to hand him off to your partner when he's been washed so that you can spend a few moments bathing yourself.

5. THE FIRST SLEEPLESS NIGHT

After those first few hours of wakefulness right after the birth, your baby is likely to experience a few extra-sleepy days before settling into a normal newborn rhythm of eating, sleeping, and waking around the clock. This means you'll likely find yourself keeping the same kind of hours—getting up a number of times in the night.

- √ **What other moms want you to know:** Keep the baby as close to you as possible at night. You'll sleep better knowing that baby is close by—and you won't have to fully wake up when you're up in the night caring for your baby. To help your baby start to learn the difference between night and day in the months to come, keep the house dimly lit and the noise level as low as possible when you're up feeding the baby in the night. Learn some other basic facts about infant sleep—including how it's likely to affect your life during the early months of parenthood. And if friends and family members offer to pitch in and help with housework and laundry so that you can remain as rested as possible, accept all offers of help.

6. THE FIRST TIME BABY GETS SICK

Whether it's a cough, a sniffle, or something more serious that has you poring over the baby-care books, hitting the Internet, or dashing off to Emergency with your baby, coping with your baby's first illness can be really worrisome. It's hard not to panic when someone so little seems so sick.

- √ **What other moms want you to know:** There's no need to worry about "looking silly" if your baby's symptoms prove to be something minor: your baby's doctor will be pleased that you decided to trust your gut feelings and check out those worrisome signs. After all, that's part of the job description of being someone's parent.

7. THE FIRST CRYING JAG

Baby's wailing away, and you feel like you should be able to pinpoint the cause of his misery and make the tears disappear. You run through a checklist of all the usual causes—Baby's hungry, overtired, uncomfortable, wet, ill—but he continues to sing the blues.

- √ **What other moms want you to know:** This is a situation when you may find you need just as much comfort as Baby. It's distressing to hear your baby this upset. Call a friend who has had first-hand experience in coping with a crying baby of her own and who can offer both moral support and hands-on help. If you find yourself getting frustrated, put your baby in a safe spot, such as the crib, and take a few minutes for yourself until you regain your cool.

chapter 5

BECOMING PARENTS

"I'm probably the poster child for women who were shocked with parenthood, in spite of the fact that I had always wanted children. The 24-hour-a-day nature of the job really hit me hard. I had intense feelings of guilt about feeling this way, and figured that I must be a terrible mother because I didn't have those mushy, lovey feelings about my son. To this day, I still feel badly that his first few weeks were so rocky, and I often wish I could do it over again."

—JANE, 33, MOTHER OF TWO

"The first month of Anya's life, we used to sit and hold her, breathing in her smells and marvelling at this 'madly, deeply' love we felt for her. What an amazing feeling. That is something you are never really prepared for—the feeling of being so hopelessly in love with this little creature."

—KAREN, 28, MOTHER OF ONE

The early weeks of parenthood are the best of times and the worst of times all wrapped up in one exhausting yet exhilarating package. One moment you're feeling head-over-heels in love with your new baby; the next, you're wondering if you actually have the patience and the stamina required to cope with the round-the-clock demands of parenthood.

This chapter focuses on the early weeks of parenthood (why they're challenging and how to get through them) and what parenting a newborn is all about.

WHY THE EARLY WEEKS OF PARENTHOOD CAN BE SUCH A CHALLENGE

Feeling a little overwhelmed by the realities of caring for a newborn? You're certainly in good company. Most new parents feel this way. Fortunately, as you get to know your baby and you become more confident in your ability to meet her needs, your enjoyment of parenting will increase. But, until that happens, it can be reassuring to understand why the early weeks of parenthood tend to be such a challenge—and what you can do to make life easier for yourself and your new baby.

Nothing you can do ahead of time can fully prepare you for life after baby.

Even if you do everything your prenatal instructor suggests in order to prepare yourself for the rigours of parenthood (you load up on baby-care books, sign up for pre-baby breastfeeding classes, and spend your Saturday nights forgoing the latest romantic comedies or action flicks in favour of child safety and birth videos), chances are you'll still feel decidedly unprepared for the challenges of parenthood once your baby actually arrives. Most parents find out the hard way that there's a world of difference between their expectations of parenthood and the realities of life after baby.

---

mother wisdom "My children cause me the most exquisite suffering of which I have any experience. It is the suffering of ambivalence: the murderous alternation between bitter resentment and raw-edged nerves, and blissful gratification and tenderness."

—ADRIENNE RICH, *OF WOMAN BORN: MOTHERHOOD AS EXPERIENCE AND INSTITUTION*

Dawn, a 38-year-old mother of four, remembers feeling shocked by just how unprepared she was for the challenges of early parenthood. "I am a highly educated person, as is my husband," she explains. "With all our education, we felt that parenthood would be a piece of cake. What a surprise it was when the first baby came and we were at a total loss as to how to make this little child fit neatly into our world! Our orderly, planned life was turned upside down. Ian just didn't seem to get it: when we were ready to go somewhere, a dirty diaper or a hungry baby didn't fit into the 'plan.' We soon learned to plan in 15-minute intervals and to accept it if we were late arriving because of Ian, but many times we felt as if we were flying by the seats of our pants. And then, 21 months later, baby number two came along."

Part of the problem, of course, is the fact that it's almost impossible to explain to those who've never been in the parenting trenches themselves just how much hard work is involved in caring for a new baby. It's a point that Lisa, a 36-year-old mother of three, is quick to make: "You have to be emotionally mature enough to realize that parenthood isn't all about cute babies all dressed up. It's also about spit-up, poopy diapers at 3 a.m., and evenings when you don't get to eat your dinner in peace because the baby is being fussy. It's tons of hard work, and I don't think a lot of people out there realize that."

That's not to say that every first-time parent makes the mistake of assuming that the early weeks of parenthood will be like a scene from a baby product commercial: a drop-dead gorgeous mom and an incredibly hot dad frolicking with their picture-perfect offspring. Some parents have heard so many horror stories about life after baby that they go into parenthood expecting the worst. That was certainly the case for Cindy, a 31-year-old mother of one: "Life with a newborn turned out to be even better than I had expected," she recalls. "So many people scared me with comments like, 'Oh, your life is really going to change—you'll lose all your freedom.' Or they'd warn me about the fatigue, the anxieties, and so on. In the end, I was blessed with a happy, contented baby who slept well, took to breastfeeding immediately, and who rarely cried. I do have my moments of fatigue and frustration, but having a baby has been the most fulfilling thing I have ever done."

If you're not quite as lucky as Cindy and you find that you're experiencing a bit of disconnect between your romantic fantasies about parenthood and the day-to-day reality, you might find it helpful to share your feelings with other new parents. "Knowing that some of the joys and fears you're experiencing are 'normal' can be very reassuring," insists Joyce, a 41-year-old mother of two. Allyson, a 32-year-old mother of two, agrees: "I was very lucky to have made friends with two women in our Lamaze class. They had their babies within three days of when I had Joey, and we have been having play dates weekly ever since. I credit Leanne and Stasey for helping me to keep my sanity during the early months of Joey's life. We were really able to support one another."

mom's the word "Life with a newborn was even more gratifying than I had expected. The nights were long, and breastfeeding and changing diapers in the moonlight at 2 a.m. was draining, but never once did I ever second-guess my decision to have children. There can be no feeling in heaven or on earth that compares to lying beside your newborn as he latches on and feeds, dozing on and off and looking into your eyes with trust, love, and comfort. It was amazing."

—CHONEE, 35, MOTHER OF TWO

You have no idea what the term "sleep deprivation" actually means until you've had a baby.
You've no doubt missed out on the odd night of sleep at some point in your life—perhaps during your senior year when you were cramming for final exams. While you no doubt felt like hell after pulling such an all-nighter, what kept you going was the fact that you knew you could crawl back into bed the moment the exam was finished and sleep for the next 12 hours or so.

The type of sleep deprivation you face as a new parent is, however, an entirely different ball game: you have no way of telling when or if you'll ever have a solid night's sleep again. And even if you do head off to bed an hour or two earlier than usual in a naive attempt to try to catch up on some of the sleep you have missed since Junior made his grand entrance, chances are you'll be called to your baby's side at least once or twice in the night. Parenting a newborn is, after all, a round-the-clock job.

Like many first-time mothers, Andrea, 32, found herself feeling overwhelmed with fatigue during the early weeks of her baby's life. "I knew it was going to be hard work, but I didn't realize how tired I would feel. It was exhausting," she recalls.

Alyson, a 32-year-old mother of two, was surprised to discover the extent to which the chronic sleep deprivation took its toll on her emotions: "I never thought I could be so frustrated by such a little person. And even though I never let my babies know just how upset I was, I always felt badly afterwards for getting so angry."

As exhausting as the early months of parenthood can be, it's important to remind yourself that there's light at the end of the tunnel. Unfortunately, it's impossible to predict ahead of time just how long that tunnel may be! According to Lisa, a 35-year-old mother of two, the payoffs to parenting become increasingly apparent over time: "That first six weeks is the hardest period—and it seems to be the longest, too. But before you know it, your baby will be smiling, then sitting up, then crawling, standing, and taking his or her first steps. Don't let the crying, up-all-night, how-can-I-continue-to-function feeling take over. Try to appreciate those early days of your baby's life: watch your baby sleep and memorize that beautiful newborn face."

Other things you can do to stay sane until you finally get a solid night's sleep include taking catnaps during the day so that you're better able to cope with the sleep disruptions at night, sharing nighttime parenting duties with your partner, and knocking as many items off your to-do list as possible during this stage of your life. (Remember, you don't have the luxury of catching up on your sleep if you happen to overdo things right now, so this is no time to go totally crazy with housework.)

---

mother wisdom "Parenthood may be the most natural task in the world, but considered objectively, the job description matches that of, say, a serf."
—NEW YORK TIMES WRITER NATALIE ANGIERS, QUOTED IN *LAUGHTER AND TEARS: THE EMOTIONAL LIVES OF NEW MOTHERS* BY ELISABETH BING AND LIBBY COLMAN

Your body is in the midst of morphing back to its pre-pregnancy state.

Rome wasn't built in a day—and your body won't return to its pre-pregnancy state overnight. But that certainly doesn't stop it from trying. Your body is in major repair mode right now as it works at reversing all the remarkable physical changes that occurred during pregnancy and birth.

And even if you're one of those lucky women who have few physical complaints during the early days and weeks postpartum, you're bound to find yourself riding an emotional roller coaster as your estrogen and progesterone levels come crashing down after the birth. So if you find yourself freaking out about things that wouldn't normally affect you (like the fact that your incredibly self-centred partner just got a drink from the kitchen but didn't even *think* to ask whether the poor exhausted breastfeeding mother might want one too—or, worse, muttered something about going to bed early tonight because he/she "hasn't been getting much sleep"), don't assume that you've completely lost it. What you're experiencing is perfectly normal and, in most cases, blessedly short-lived. Unless you are unfortunate enough to develop full-blown postpartum depression (a subject we talked about back in Chapter 3), you can expect to be feeling more like your old self relatively soon.

Your birth experience may have been less than picture-perfect.

After months of preparation and buildup, the birth is now behind you. And now that it's over, you may find yourself spending a lot of time thinking about this momentous day in your life.

If things didn't go quite as you had planned, you may find yourself feeling angry or disappointed—and perhaps even a little ripped off. If, for example, you had hoped for a completely unmedicated and intervention-free birth but ended up being induced and then having a Caesarean, you might have questions about the choices that were offered to you. Similarly, if your baby's birth was scary or otherwise traumatic for you—your baby arrived three months early by emergency Caesarean, for example—you may need to take some time (or talk to a therapist) in order to come to terms with the fact that your birth wasn't the one you had envisioned.

---

baby talk A 2003 study conducted by researchers in Sweden found that 66 per cent of first-time mothers and 74 per cent of mothers giving birth for the second or subsequent time felt a strong need to talk about their birth experience with the health-care provider who was present at their baby's birth. The researchers found that 58 per cent of first-time fathers and 30 per cent of fathers of subsequent babies also felt a strong need to participate in such a conversation. Issues the parents wanted to discuss with the health-care provider included how the birth went, what led to any complications, how pain and pain relief were managed, and feelings about the birth.

Sandi, a 30-year-old mother of two, remembers feeling completely shell-shocked in the aftermath of her youngest child's birth. "During the delivery, my baby's shoulder got stuck," she explains. "When he came out, there was a lot of commotion, and he was whisked away from me very quickly because he was not pinking up the way they like, although he did cry. It was an hour before he was brought back to me. The whole time I just lay on the delivery table crying. In the end, he was fine and there was no explanation for his rough start in life; it was just one of those things. It did bother me for some time afterward and still occasionally does even now."

You might also find that you need some time to get used to the fact that you are no longer pregnant. If this is likely to be your last pregnancy, you may feel particularly wistful about letting go of this special time in your life. Here's how Marie, a 37-year-old mother of four, explains her feelings: "It's been almost four years since my son was born, and yet I still get teary-eyed at times when I stop to consider the fact that I'll probably never be pregnant again. I can say without a doubt that the happiest times in my life were the times when I was pregnant with one of my children. It makes me sad to think that I'll never experience the magic of being pregnant again: the excitement of watching the pregnancy test turn positive, the quiet joy of feeling the baby's flutters and kicks, and the unparalleled high of giving birth. I will always feel sad that this very special chapter in my life has finally come to a close."

You may not have gotten the baby you "ordered."

It's not just your birth experience that you have to come to terms with, of course. You also need to come to terms with that tiny little bundle in your arms.

As strange as this may sound—after all, you've just spent nine months eagerly awaiting the arrival of this new baby, so what could there possibly be to "come to terms" with?—there can be a period of adjustment involved if the baby you gave birth to wasn't quite the baby you were "expecting." Perhaps you were positive that you were carrying a baby girl, but ended up giving birth to a baby boy instead. You had pictured yourself easing into the early days of motherhood while your newborn slept—only to find yourself caring for a baby who survives on catnaps and demands all your attention and energy. Or you were hoping to give birth to a healthy full-term baby, only to find yourself giving birth to a premature infant with a serious—perhaps even life-threatening—birth defect.

mother wisdom "If you've thoroughly considered parenthood before your baby arrives, then loving your child won't be a problem. The main problems you'll face are the same ones all new parents face: anxiety over taking care of a tiny person and fear you might do something wrong."

—CHRISTINE ADAMEC, *IS ADOPTION FOR YOU?*

While you may feel tremendously guilty about feeling disappointed that your baby wasn't "perfect" or "your dream baby" or "the right sex," the best way to come to terms with your feelings is to simply accept them. Only then will you be able to give up "the dream baby" you carried around in your head for nine months and fall head-over-heels in love with the baby in your arms.

If you are really struggling with your feelings, you may find it helpful to connect with a counsellor or to join a support group (either a new parent support group or a support group that is designed to meet the needs of parents in your situation: parents who have given birth to a baby who has special needs, parents of premature babies, and so on). Your health unit or your family doctor can refer you to such supports in your community.

Of course, some women who've experienced infertility; who've been through a high-risk pregnancy; who have previously experienced miscarriage, stillbirth, or infant death; or who have adopted a baby or previously given a baby up for adoption may find it difficult to accept that they've actually ended up with a baby at all.

That was certainly the case for Shauna, a 36-year-old mother of one, whose daughter was diagnosed with a potentially fatal heart condition prior to birth: "I realized after Deirdre was born just how unprepared for parenthood I really was. I had spent so much of my energy coping with the issues surrounding her heart defect, running back and forth to doctors for prenatal monitoring, and preparing myself for a myriad of possible worst outcomes that I suppose a part of me was afraid to actually visualize myself coming home with a baby. When we finally arrived home with Deirdre, I felt completely lost."

Marie, a 37-year-old mother of four who also lost a baby through stillbirth, had a similar experience: "My goal throughout most of my pregnancy was simply to get through the pregnancy and give birth to a living baby. I hadn't allowed myself the luxury of thinking about what life would be like after my baby was born."

Parents like Marie who have previously experienced the death of a baby often find that their feelings of joy about the safe arrival of their new baby are accompanied by renewed feelings of grief about the baby they lost. According to Deborah Davis, Ph.D., author of *Empty Cradle, Broken Heart*, parents can be quite disconcerted to discover that the grief they thought they had worked through months or years earlier may suddenly surface again: "Your grief may intensify as you realize that this new baby in your arms doesn't fill the longing you still harbor for your baby who died. Your babies aren't interchangeable. Each one is precious and deserves his or her own special place in your heart. And believe it or not, by letting your feelings of grief flow, you will also be able to reclaim the joy that comes with having a healthy baby—a joy that is your right and which you certainly deserve to feel."

Whether your reproductive history has been complicated or not, it may take a little while for your maternal feelings to kick in. But once they do, watch out: you may be blown away by their sheer intensity. "I experienced extreme love and attachment and this overwhelming 'mother bear' feeling that I would willingly take a bullet for this kid," recalls Jennifer, 35, a mother of one. "These feelings brought me to my knees in a way I never, ever imagined. They continue to this day."

Your worry-o-meter is working overtime.

If there were a million and one things to worry about back when you were pregnant, there are easily 10 million and one things to worry about now that your baby is here. Is the baby too warm or too cold? Is that rash baby acne or something more serious? The list just goes on and on. The best way to cope with garden-variety new-parent fears such as these is to arm yourself with the facts: pull out your baby books, talk with an experienced friend or family member, or make a call to your doctor's office to get the information you need. More often than not, all you really want is a bit of reassurance—to have someone else who has been there and lived through that confirm that your parental instincts are working just fine.

> **baby talk** A 2002 study of more than 8,000 mothers in Switzerland found that the fear of something happening to the baby was even greater than the fear of labour pain (expressed by 50 per cent versus 40 per cent of pregnant women).

Of course, some new parents have been through experiences in the past that make it easy for them to hit the panic button the moment anything out of the ordinary occurs—something that Heather, a 34-year-old mother of two, discovered shortly after her second child was born: "We lost our first baby 15 minutes after delivery, so we were afraid of everything with our next baby. We even called the hospital once when she was four days old because we thought she was sleeping too much and we were having trouble waking her up. The nurse at the hospital told us to undress her slowly and put cold compresses on her. Once she woke up and the nurse heard her screaming, she advised us not to tell any other new parents that we were upset because our baby was sleeping too soundly and too long: we wouldn't win many friends that way!"

It's not unusual for parents in Heather's situation to experience heightened anxiety, given their history, notes Deborah Davis: "One of the most vivid and prominent experiences that bereaved parents encounter after the birth of a subsequent baby is anxiety. After all, if you've already experienced the death of a baby, you *know* that bad things can happen to you, your children, your family. You also see how little control you can have over the things that are important to you. Your vulnerability to tragedy is a frightening realization, and can add fuel to normal parental worries."

If the bereaved parent's anxiety continues to thwart her attempts to "let go," interfering with her emotional or physical health or functioning, or affecting her relationships with others, some professional help may be in order. "Counselling with someone who understands parental grief can help you move beyond crippling anxiety so that you can enjoy your surviving children," says Davis. "You do deserve to enjoy parenthood and the precious gifts that your children are to you."

You and your partner may be out of sync at the very time in your life when you need his support most.
Feel as though there's something coming between you and your partner? You're right! It's a tiny, 8-pound (3.5-kilogram) human who needs to be fed and changed every two to three hours!

There's no denying it. The postpartum period can be a time of incredible adjustment for couples. Not only are both partners trying to wrap their heads around the whole idea of becoming a parent, they're also trying to work out new ways of relating to one another. And given that they're trying to accomplish these tasks in a sleep-deprived, zombie-like state, it's no wonder that so many couples end up experiencing a bit of a relationship meltdown during the weeks after the birth. Here are some tips on surviving the postpartum period as a couple.

- **Accept the fact that there may be some difficult times ahead.** The postpartum period is a time of tremendous adjustment for both of you. It's easy for tempers to flare and for feelings to get hurt when you're both exhausted and overwhelmed by the responsibilities of parenthood. "Be nice to your husband," advises Janet, a 32-year-old mother of one. "Remember that he's also overwhelmed by the baby's arrival and is suffering from sleep deprivation, even if you're the only one who's suffering from the physical after-effects of the birth."

- **Recognize that your partner may also end up being hit with the baby blues.** Studies have shown that up to 3 per cent of fathers exhibit signs of depression after their babies are born and that men whose partners experience postpartum depression are at particular risk of experiencing some sort of depression themselves.

- **Make a conscious effort to invest in your relationship.** It's easy to start feeling resentful and out of touch if you haven't had so much as a stolen kiss in weeks. "Take time for your marriage," recommends Nicole, a 29-year-old mother of one. "It's hard to do when the little one is consuming all your time, but it's important to still find ways to connect as a couple. We were told in prenatal class to set a date for two months after the baby's birth and go out for coffee, a drive, or even for dinner—to do something. As a new mom, this really gives you a feeling of freedom, even if all you do is talk about the baby!"

mother wisdom Couples who are good friends before they start their families are better able to adjust to the stresses of early parenthood than couples who are less satisfied with their relationships. According to University of Washington marital researcher John Gottman, if a new father is genuinely kind and affectionate toward the new mother, he understands how she's feeling about becoming a mother (what she loves and what she is finding most difficult), and both partners take a problem-solving approach to dealing with the challenges in their new life together as parents, the relationship is likely to thrive.

However, a couple is more likely to experience relationship difficulties following the birth of a baby if the decision to start a family was not mutual, one or both partners suffers from poor self-esteem or has pre-existing problems with depression, the couple was experiencing sexual problems prior to or during the pregnancy, and/or the father was irritable or uninvolved during pregnancy.

the birth of a family Families are born out of "messy processes" during which new ways of relating to one another are created. That's the theory of a group of researchers from the Université de Sherbrooke in Quebec—and it makes a lot of sense. After all, it's not as if you can assign parental roles and responsibilities ahead of time. You don't even have a handle on the job description of parent until you're at least a few weeks into the job. So be prepared to talk things through with your partner, try things out, renegotiate responsibilities, and then talk things through again. It's okay to make this up as you go along. You're inventing your own one-of-a-kind family.

You'll find it easier to learn the steps in this new dance called parenting (without stepping on your partner's toes too often) if you remember the following advice.

- √ **Accept the fact that you're each going to have your own unique parenting styles.** Not only were you raised in different households: you're entirely different people. Remember, there's no such thing as a one-size-fits-all parenting style.

- ✓ **Be generous with your praise when you think your partner has done an amazing job.** Everyone benefits from a pep talk every now and again, and there's nothing sweeter than hearing your parenting style being raved about by your partner.

- ✓ **Commit to an ongoing program of parental development, and encourage your partner to come along for the ride.** If you find a parenting book or video that's particularly helpful to you, share your favourite parts with your partner. It's easier to talk through issues like how to handle biting during play dates (whether your child is the biter or the bitee) if you have a bit of a game plan figured out in advance. Ask parents whose parenting styles you admire what books, websites, and other resources they found helpful in learning about parenting. Your local health unit and your local family resource centre (if you're lucky enough to have one in your community) are excellent places to turn to for leads on parenting-related programs and services in your area.

- ✓ **Realize that it may take time to get your sexual relationship back on track.** You may be too exhausted or too sore to think of anything but sleep during the early weeks and months after the birth. And if you're not exactly feeling terrific about your postpartum body, you may find that your libido nosedives for a while—one of the side effects of the hormone prolactin, which is produced while you're breastfeeding. You may also be reluctant to have sex for fear that you might become pregnant again. "We had sex for the first time about three weeks after giving birth," recalls one new mother. "It was kind of awkward as I was a little leery about doing the very thing that had caused me to go through such pain. And as for my sexual desire, it was like a switch had been turned off completely." Not everyone feels this way about sex, however. One first-time mom found that she felt so good about her body after giving birth that she couldn't wait to become intimate with her partner. "My hormones must have been raging after my son was born because I was interested in sex almost immediately after the delivery," she recalls. "I think I was high on the thrill of giving birth to this amazing baby. I felt almost omnipotent and was so pleased that my body was doing everything it was designed to do—get pregnant, grow a healthy baby, give birth, and breastfeed this perfect baby. I felt an overwhelming desire to make love with my husband."

- ✓ **Maintain the intimacy and affection in your relationship (and celebrate them as something separate and distinct from sex).** A hug may be just what you need to ease some of the stress of parenting. Researchers at the University of Zurich in Switzerland have discovered that daily intimacy between partners—even something as simple as a heart-felt hug or a few minutes holding hands—helps to bring down blood cortisol levels (a biological measure of just how stressed we are).

- ✓ **Make time for one another on a regular basis, even if that means keeping your eyes open for an extra 15 minutes after your baby falls asleep.** Staying connected is an important investment in your well-being as a family. With any luck, the time and energy you invest in your relationship will reap tremendous dividends for you and your partner, both inside and outside of the bedroom.

- ✓ **Keep your sense of humour.** A shared laugh at the end of a particularly rough day can work wonders by cementing the ties between you and your partner and relieving some of the stress of parenthood.

- ✓ **Allow your shared love for your baby to bring you closer together.** "Having a baby made my relationship with my partner even stronger," says Carrie, 34, who is currently pregnant with her second child. "Watching him take care of our son and seeing what a great dad he is made me love him even more, if that's possible." Christina agrees that having a baby can enrich your relationship tremendously. "Birth is one of the most life-altering experiences you'll ever have and share as a couple," the 25-year-old mother of two explains. "Enjoy every moment and let it bring you closer together as a couple and as a family."

baby talk University of Illinois child development researcher Sarah Schoppe-Sullivan has discovered that the ability of two parents to function as a team when their child is 6 months of age can accurately predict how well that couple's relationship will be doing by the time that child reaches 3 years of age.

mom's the word "When you see a man you love with tears in his eyes as he thanks you for giving birth to his baby, when you see him up at night comforting a crying infant, or cleaning up vomit without even mentioning it, or sitting with your child reading his favourite book again, your feelings for him change in so many ways and it's wonderful."

—LORI, 29, MOTHER OF FOUR

baby talk Becoming a father doesn't just affect a new dad's sex life and sleep patterns: it also affects his biochemistry in far-reaching ways. Researchers at Bar-Ilan University in Ramat Gan, Israel, studied 80 couples and found that oxytocin levels rise in both mothers and fathers following the birth of a baby. While oxytocin encourages moms to gaze at their babies, touch their babies, and talk to their babies in a singsong voice, it encourages dads to play with their babies.

This latest study builds on two earlier studies (conducted in 2000 and 2002 by researchers at Memorial University in Newfoundland and Queen's University in Kingston, Ontario).

The 2000 study revealed that levels of prolactin (the hormone responsible for breast milk production in women) in an expectant father's blood rise by about 20 per cent during the three weeks before his partner gives birth, and that blood levels of the stress hormone cortisol rise to double what they were earlier in the pregnancy. At the same time, levels of testosterone—the hormone that underlies competitive, aggressive behaviour—dip during the three weeks following the birth.

The 2002 study concluded that the estrogen levels in a father-to-be rise 30 days prior to the birth. (Estrogen increases the brain's sensitivity to oxytocin, boosting nurturing behaviours.) Contact between partners allows for this biochemical meeting of minds, in which pheromones (chemical substances) given off by the woman's body as birth approaches signal to the father-to-be that it's time to start switching into daddy mode.

mom's the word "We had more arguments in the first year of Kayleigh's life than we did in the previous five years! We disagree more about child rearing than anything else. We also don't have sex as much as we used to. That said, having children together brings you closer together. In some ways, it strengthens your partnership. Your relationship changes because the kids are so much a part of your life. It isn't just the two of you anymore: you are part of something bigger."

—KATE, A 36-YEAR-OLD MOTHER OF TWO

How your partner is adjusting to becoming a parent
You've known your partner for a long time (or at least long enough to have a baby together). But seeing your partner as someone's parent may require a bit of a mind shift—for you and for him.

There may be times when you swear you're living on two different planets—and that conditions are a lot tougher on your planet than on his. (I'm saying "his" because the research about the impact of the transition to parenthood on partners focuses almost exclusively on new dads.) You'll find it easier to carry on a civil conversation if you try to see things from your partner's point of view.

Here are a few things that every new mom should know about new dads.

- **It's not a lot of fun being the invisible man.** A new dad can feel all but invisible: visitors make a huge fuss over you and the new baby, but he may barely be noticed or acknowledged. If you want him to provide you with the emotional support you need to survive the postpartum roller-coaster ride, be prepared to return the favour by making time to listen to his worries and concerns (finances, your health and the baby's health, and whether the two of you will ever get your sex life back on track), and by acknowledging all the extra work he's doing so that you can invest your time and energy in caring for the baby.

mother wisdom

Think it's tough being the mom? Try being the dad. Many new dads are surprised by the extent of their partner's preoccupation with the baby. Sure, they knew she would be busy with the baby, but head-over-heels in love? In Rhonda Kruse Nordin's book *After the Baby: Making Sense of Marriage after Childbirth,* marriage counsellor Daniel Norby explains the struggle many new fathers go through as they try to make sense of their relationships after baby: "Women typically take all nine months to get ready for a new baby. During this time, they make room for it in their hearts and lives. They make plans to care for it. The process is quiet and gradual, yet it makes a tremendous impact on a woman and consequently on her marriage. A father usually needs some time after the baby is born to catch up. Most women aren't ready to refocus on their husband until they are willing to let go of the baby. This could be when a woman goes back to work or feels comfortable with a baby—or it may not be until the child enters school! This change in focus or behavior can be mystifying to a husband and terribly upsetting to his marriage."

- **Dad's way may not be Mom's way, but that doesn't necessarily mean it's the wrong way.** Researchers at Ohio State University found that a new mom plays a major role in determining how hands-on or hands-off her partner ends up being with their baby, and that even the most committed new father can lose his motivation to be actively involved with baby-care tasks if he receives repeated messages of disapproval from his partner. The feedback doesn't have to be verbal for fathers to become discouraged: a mom's body language can tell a new dad everything he needs to know about her feelings about his fathering abilities—and then some. Fathers are more likely to choose to be actively involved in baby care if they receive encouraging feedback about their fathering skills from their partners—and if new mothers don't hover too much. Everyone fares better when new moms give new dads the time and space needed to figure out their own ways of soothing babies and mastering all the other need-to-know skills of early parenting. Dad's way won't be Mom's way, but that doesn't mean it's the wrong way. It's just different. That's all.

- **Fathers' support networks aren't as fully developed as mothers' support networks.** A University of Bristol study examining how women and men make the transition to parenthood found that while moms tend to have a wide range of sources of support (their mothers, their partners, friends, colleagues at work, health-care professionals, and other mothers they've met at prenatal or postnatal groups), dads primarily have just three sources of support (their partner, colleagues at work, and/or health-care professionals). Because they have fewer sources of support, many new dads find it difficult to find someone other than their partner to talk to about sensitive issues that are really bothering them. It's important for fathers to form close relationships with other fathers so that they can act as one another's sounding board on fatherhood-related issues. (No matter how close partners are to one another, they shouldn't be one another's sole confidante. That's a pretty big burden to place on one relationship. It is also terribly limiting. You want to benefit from the experiences of others when you're trying to make sense of a life-changing experience like becoming a parent.)

---

mother wisdom According to a study reported in the medical journal *Health Education Research,* a mom-to-be is most likely to turn to her health-care provider, her pregnancy confidante (typically her mother or a close female friend or relative), or her partner for advice—in that order. A new dad, on the other hand, is overwhelmingly likely to turn to his partner for advice. The *Journal of Perinatal Education* found that 91.8 per cent of expectant fathers seek advice from their partners, 37.1 per cent from their mothers or mothers-in-law, 34.6 per cent from other fathers, 24.4 per cent from coworkers, 23.9 per cent from nurses, 21.0 per cent from doctors, and 15.6 per cent from their fathers or fathers-in-law.

Sleep deprivation makes everything harder. "Going through this first year, and all the sleep problems we've had, has really made me understand why some marriages fall apart when a baby is added into the mix," says Jen, a 30-year-old mother of one. "There are so many new stresses, and sometimes it's almost like getting to know and understand a whole new partner—something that it's hard to find the energy for when you are already exhausted."

You have to ask for what you need from your partner. Kelly, a 35-year-old mother of two, found that her marriage came close to reaching the breaking point after she gave birth to two children in just a little over two years. "We were overwhelmed with joy in both cases, but eventually reality set in and the responsibilities all fell on me," she recalls. "My husband wasn't willing or able to change his routine. We fought a lot, mostly because I was angry that he wasn't helping more: he didn't rush home every day to relieve me and he slept in another room because he 'needed his sleep.' When I look back on the situation, I can see that I was my own worst enemy. I allowed him not to help during those early years and I accepted 100 per cent responsibility for the baby."

Having a baby leaves you open to unwanted and often conflicting advice.

Having a baby also changes your relationship with other people in your life, most notably older relatives and other people in your life who already have children. Overnight, these usually mild-mannered people may feel empowered or even obligated to offer you advice on any number of parenting topics.

If you're lucky, your nearest-and-dearest will instinctively understand that it's not a good idea to weigh in with an opinion unless their advice has been specifically solicited. But if they don't seem to understand that basic fact of relationship harmony, you may need to learn how to ignore any advice that doesn't mesh with your own parenting philosophies. Karen, a 28-year-old mother of one, quickly learned to tune out her mother's breastfeeding advice. "My mother is from the generation of mothers who didn't breastfeed because it wasn't fashionable," she explains. "She is the biggest anti-breastfeeder I know! She is always making remarks about someone or other whose breastfed baby isn't growing quickly enough, or a mother who has 'bad' milk, or a baby who 'eats all the time.' I found this very frustrating, and had I not known as much as I do about breastfeeding, I might have been deterred by her comments."

Regardless of the actual cause of the conflict, it can be helpful to remind yourself that the advice-giver usually has your well-being or the best interests of the baby at heart, even if the advice that they're offering is a generation or two out of date. So the next time your mother suggests that you start weaning your four-month-old, just smile sweetly and say that you'll be sure to raise the issue with your baby's doctor at the next checkup. (Hint: All but the most rabid advice-givers will back off once they find out that a doctor's going to be weighing in on a particular issue, so feel free to play this particular trump card as often as necessary. It's sure to save your life on at least one occasion.)

Here are a few other tips:

- Listen to what the person offering the advice has to say and politely thank them for sharing their words of wisdom with you. Then quietly decide whether this particular piece of advice is a keeper or whether you can mentally hit the delete key.
- Trust your instincts and have faith in your ability to make the best possible decisions for your baby. You're less likely to be hurt or offended by unsolicited advice if you feel confident in your mothering abilities.
- Finally, don't be afraid to ask for advice when you need it. Tap into the knowledge and experience of others. Being a parent is tough enough. Why make it tougher?

It's difficult to find time to take care of your own needs.

One of the biggest challenges that new mothers face is finding time to ensure that their own needs are met. It can be hard to find time to have a shower or sit down and eat a sandwich, let alone fit in time to spend on your favourite hobby during this challenging stage of your life. But, as Elisabeth Bing and Libby Colman point out in their book, *Laughter and Tears: The Emotional Lives of New Mothers,* mothers who go into martyr mode and ignore their own needs aren't doing their babies any favours: "Just as the fetus cannot get a nutrient the mother does not consume, so an infant cannot receive emotional nutrition that the caregiver does not receive. To be able to feed your baby the emotional calories of love, you must consume 'nutritious' love yourself. If you don't get enough love and attention and pleasure yourself, you will have trouble providing these things for your baby."

So if a friend offers to watch your baby for an hour so you can enjoy an hour-long soak in the tub or hit your favourite bookstore by yourself, take her up on the offer (or, if you don't want to be away from your baby, make her a counter offer that will work for you: "How about you come to the bookstore with Baby and me?"). You'll feel a lot better for it.

mother wisdom

"The how-to-parent books make family sound like a problem with a solution, a skill that can be mastered... But family is a work in progress, a never-ending renovation job that begins with tidy, visionary blueprints and ends in plaster dust and daily chaos."

—MARNI JACKSON, "BRINGING UP BABY,"
SATURDAY NIGHT, DECEMBER 1989

You could find yourself facing the Mother of All Identity Crises.

It takes time to adjust to any new role—and you've just stepped into the Mother of All Roles. So don't be surprised to find yourself having a bit of an identity crisis. The very landscape of your life has, after all, shifted overnight.

The transformation tends to be particularly dramatic if you were working outside the home until shortly before your baby's birth. In that case, your concept of what you can reasonably hope to accomplish in a day will have to be completely reworked. "Getting anything done is a challenge," insists Molly, a 36-year-old first-time mother. "For a mother who has been used to working and being in control of her life, staying home and having difficulty even squeezing in a shower can be very frustrating at first!"

And then there's the sense of isolation that many women experience when they're first "home alone" with their babies. "I remember it feeling so strange when John walked out the door and left me and Joey alone for the first time," recalls Alyson, a 32-year-old mother of two. "It was as if Joey and I were the only people on earth."

Althea, a 30-year-old mother of one, found herself experiencing total culture shock during the early weeks of motherhood. "The early days were more difficult than I had anticipated. No matter how much you read or how many times your friends and family members warn you about the sleepless nights and the incessant crying, nothing can really prepare you for how you'll feel during that time. Not only was I exhausted, frustrated, and emotionally upside down, I was really mourning my old life! I loved my baby, but I would walk by people on the streets who were 'babyless' and carefree, and I'd actually cry."

Just as it takes time for you to fit back into your pre-pregnancy jeans, it takes time to grow into the role of mother. But, with any luck, you'll soon discover that the role feels comfortable and familiar. Connecting with other mothers who can share their stories while encouraging you to find your own way to mother your baby can help to ease the transition for you.

As you can see, there are a number of reasons why the early weeks and months of parenthood tend to be a tremendous challenge for first-time parents. Fortunately, the boot camp initiation rites tend to get a little easier with each subsequent baby—something that you'll no doubt be relieved to hear if there's likely to be another baby in your future.

FIRST COMES LOVE

The early weeks of parenthood are hard work, for sure, but there's an upside. And that upside is love. Baby love, to be specific.

Babies are designed to elicit a powerful response from the adults around them. You are hard-wired to want to respond to your baby's needs.

If you go with the flow—if you respond to that biologically based urge to nurture your baby—parenting is less stressful for you.

What's more, your baby learns to trust in you and her world. The happiest, most confident babies are those whose early needs are met by loving parents who understand that you can't spoil a baby or make a baby too dependent simply by meeting his needs.

Forming such a bond—or attachment—to a parent or other primary caregiver is an important step to forming healthy relationships later in life because having their needs met consistently and lovingly teaches babies about the give-and-take of relationships. "Early relationships and attachments to a primary caregiver are the most consistent and enduring influence on social and emotional development for young children," according to *From Neurons to Neighborhoods*, a report published by the U.S.-based National Research Council and Institute of Medicine.

Bonding with your baby gives you a biological boost, too, triggering the release of energizing, feel-good endorphins that make it easier for you to cope with the sleep deprivation of early motherhood. Fortunately, the things that help to promote a healthy attachment with your baby are things you are naturally inclined to do: spending time gazing at this amazing new person in your life, trying to figure out what your baby is thinking and feeling so that you can anticipate and meet his needs; breast-feeding your baby and otherwise engaging in skin-to-skin contact (which your baby finds very calming and reassuring); and providing reassurance when your baby is upset. A young baby doesn't have the skills to soothe himself. You lay the groundwork for important self-regulation (emotional control) skills down the road by providing him with comfort and reassurance when he is very young. Rather than spoiling the baby, you're helping to ensure that your baby will become an emotionally healthy toddler, child, teenager, and adult. A healthy attachment lays the foundation for everything else that is to come.

It's a win-win.

---

mother wisdom Bonding can be a bit more challenging for some parents and babies. You may want to talk to your health-care provider about the best ways to maximize the opportunities for bonding and encouraging a healthy attachment if your baby was born prematurely or with health problems; you are struggling with postpartum depression or anxiety; you are dealing with a lot of stress; you experienced abuse or neglect when you were a child and/or you have mainly negative memories of your growing up years; you are living in an unsafe environment; or you are otherwise having difficulty connecting with your baby.

INTUITIVE PARENTING: READING YOUR BABY'S CUES

While your baby is a newborn, she has a limited number of ways of making her needs known. She's counting on you to decode her signals by learning how to read her body language and to make sense of her various cries (Table 5.1).

As you get to know your baby, you'll find it easier to meet her needs. This will reduce the amount of time your baby spends fussing and crying, leading to a much happier baby and a much more confident you.

Every baby is unique, so you're likely to find that she uses some signals that are uniquely her own in addition to some of the more common baby body language signals listed in Table 5.1.

TABLE 5.1
What Your Newborn Is Trying to Say

What your baby is trying to tell you	Watch for these types of baby body language
I'm hungry	Turning head from side to side; putting his hands near his mouth; sucking on other objects near his mouth; rooting (trying to nurse when placed in the nursing position); fussing or crying; and breathing rapidly. Your baby may also make efforts to move toward the breast. Note: As the American Academy of Pediatrics points out, "crying is a late sign of hunger." Your baby will find it easier to settle down to breastfeed if you are able to offer the breast before your baby gets all worked up from crying. The earlier signs are your cues that feeding time has arrived.
I'm in pain	A high-pitched shriek that is unrelenting; Baby is red in the face.
I'm sleepy	Redness or pinkness around the eyes, eyebrows, and nose; rubbing eyes; pulling on her ear; acting fussier than usual. Some babies cry until you retreat to quieter surroundings and help them wind down and fall asleep. Note: Don't worry if your newborn needs help falling asleep. This is normal for young babies, although it can be exhausting for you. Most babies fall asleep breastfeeding. You can teach your baby other self-soothing skills as she grows older.
I need a break	Looking away, covering face with hands, wrinkling up entire forehead, arching back, tensing body, fussing, crying.
I'm ready to play	Wide-eyed and excited. Breathing may speed up. May move her arms and legs—a whole-body greeting.

Here are a few key points to keep in mind as you begin to experiment with this intuitive style of parenting, something that will add to your confidence as a new parent.

- **Understand that parenting a newborn inevitably involves some trial-and-error.** Figuring out what your baby needs requires a bit of experimentation. Don't expect perfection of yourself. No one expects that of you. That said, you can reduce your new parent learning curve by learning some basic facts about infant development so that you'll have a rough idea of what to expect from your baby and when. See Chapter 10 for an introduction to this important (and fascinating) topic.

- **Give in to your desire to reach out to other mothers for support.** Stress causes women's oxytocin levels to rise, triggering what researchers have described as a "tend-and-befriend" response (as opposed to the "fight-or-flight" response which is more typical in men). This encourages two behaviours that help us with mothering: an urge to tend to our babies and to befriend other women who can, in turn, support our mothering efforts.

- **Be honest about what types of support you need right now—and communicate those needs to other people.** Martyrs don't make for good mothers. Perpetual self-sacrifice leads to resentment—resentment that could too easily end up being directed toward your baby. A healthier alternative is to recognize your limits as a parent and to know when to ask for help.

- **Find your community.** It takes a village to raise a child; and wise parents quickly realize that connecting with and investing in that community will reap tremendous dividends for their growing family. Your child will benefit by knowing that he is loved by people other than just his parents; and you will benefit from knowing that there are people you can turn to for wisdom and support on the extra-challenging days of parenthood—people who also know and love your child.

- **Think about the kind of parent you want to be.** Here are some questions you may want to consider now and revisit from time to time:
    - What do you admire most/least in other parents?
    - What does a happy childhood look like to you?

- How would you like your children to be able to describe you to their friends—or when they reflect upon the type of parent you were to them in years to come?

- What types of wisdom or life lessons do you want to pass along to your children? How will you do this through your actions and your words? Does the way you live your life right now reflect the lessons you want to convey?

- What kind of family do you want to be? What kinds of relationships do you need to build or actions do you need to take to become that family?

- How will you continue to prepare yourself for the challenges of parenting (both the challenges that accompany each developmental stage and the ongoing emotional challenges of being a parent)?

- What do you want for yourself (both as a mother and outside your role as mother)? What passions do you want to nurture? What dreams do you want to pursue?

- How well do your dreams mesh with those of your partner (if you are raising your children with a partner)? Are you on a similar path? Do you have the same types of hopes and dreams for your child and your family?

chapter 6

BOSOM BUDDIES

"Breastfeeding is much more than a form of nutrition. It is a special way to bond with your child—to learn how to be a mother."

—ELISA, 27, MOTHER OF TWO

"Breastfeeding is the most natural way of nourishing your baby, and it makes mothering easier."

—JENNIFER, 26, CURRENTLY PREGNANT WITH HER SECOND CHILD

Breastfeeding can be a powerful, life-altering experience for both mother and baby. In addition to the tremendous health advantages that may be enjoyed by both a breastfeeding mother and her baby, there are also tremendous emotional benefits associated with breastfeeding—a subject that Michele Landsberg touches upon in her book *Women and Children First*. She writes: "Between . . . the early nurturing and the weaning lay . . . a time of enfolding intensity that I have never known in any other kind of love or work. I'm quite sure that this mother time was the making of me as a person, and the making of my three children."

Like Landsberg, Laura, a 37-year-old mother of two, believes that it's the bond that develops between a breastfeeding mother and her baby that makes breastfeeding such a memorable experience. It's the logical continuation of the bond that began long before your baby was born. "Sometimes after your baby is born it can be hard to accept that your pregnancy is over and your baby is no longer moving around inside of you," Laura explains. "Nursing gives you that connection as well as the knowledge that your body is still producing nourishment for your child."

> **mom's the word** "I love to watch my 18-month-old fall sleepily off my breast, his wee mouth curved in a contented smile, his lips full from the effort of nursing. For me, it's a moment of peace in a hectic day. It's a time for us—a chance for him to have 'mommy time' in an otherwise busy household."
> —LAURA, 37, MOTHER OF TWO

That's not to say that breastfeeding is automatically problem-free for every nursing couple. Karen, a 29-year-old mother of two, compares breastfeeding a new baby to hitting the dance floor with a brand-new partner: "Breastfeeding is like dancing with someone for the first time. You have to learn from each other."

In most cases, the learning curve is blessedly short: within a few days or weeks, you and your baby will be into a well-established breastfeeding rhythm. What you need during that time of transition is support from other people who understand the importance of breastfeeding and who are committed to helping you and your baby trouble-shoot any problems you are experiencing.

"A lot of breastfeeding obstacles can be overcome with support," adds Elisa, a 27-year-old mother of two. "Support is the key to success. If you can persevere and make it through, you will be rewarded with the most incredible experience of your life, that of nursing your child. The relationship and memories that are created by breastfeeding are unbelievable, irreplaceable, and more incredible than you could even imagine."

> **mom's the word** "Enter into breastfeeding with an open mind. You may feel now that you only want to breastfeed for six weeks or so, but you may be shocked by your pull to keep going."
> — JENNIFER, 26, CURRENTLY PREGNANT WITH HER SECOND CHILD

It also helps to be fiercely determined, adds Karen, a 36-year-old mother of two whose nursing experiences as a first-time mother were anything but picture-perfect. "I simply did not anticipate the types of problems I had with breastfeeding," she confesses. "I had read enough to know that things don't always go smoothly at first, and that it might take a month to six weeks to really establish a good nursing pattern. However, I never produced enough breast milk and had to use a lactation aid in order to supplement my baby's feedings with formula. It was very stressful in the beginning: I was crying, the baby was screaming, and I couldn't get the lactation aid into the baby's mouth. Fortunately, I was very committed to breastfeeding and I persevered, but there were times when I just wanted to give up and offer her a bottle."

If a mother experiences breastfeeding difficulties, she deserves support and reassurance, not blame. In a March 30, 2007, article in the *International Breastfeeding Journal*, Kathleen Kendall-Tackett notes: "Breastfeeding has a protective effect on maternal mental health because it attenuates stress and modulates the inflammatory response. However, breastfeeding difficulties, such as nipple pain, can increase the risk of depression and must be addressed promptly." If you and your baby need a little extra help with breastfeeding, ask friends and family members to help you find and access the help you deserve.

THE SCIENCE OF BREASTFEEDING

Just as it can be helpful to understand what's going on inside your body when you're pregnant, it can be useful to have at least a rudimentary understanding of the science behind lactation.

You might be surprised to discover how much of the prep work for breastfeeding is done during pregnancy. Breastfeeding is serious business for Mother Nature—so serious, in fact, that she starts constructing the milk factory long before your baby is ready to be born. Your breasts began developing when you first entered puberty—when you first needed a training bra. Additional growth and development occurred during your pregnancy. (Most of the time, breast growth is completed by 22 weeks of pregnancy, but sometimes a woman's breasts continue to grow throughout her entire pregnancy and even after her baby has been born.)

Preparing your breasts for lactation is truly a team effort between you and your baby: the result of the interaction between three maternal hormones—estrogen, progesterone, and prolactin—as well as lactogen, a little-understood hormone produced by the baby's placenta. These hormonal changes during pregnancy trigger the milk glands to develop the extensive system of milk ducts (they look like a network of tangled roots) that will be required for the manufacture and transport of colostrum and then milk.

The milk factory "on switch" doesn't get flipped on, however, until after the placenta has been delivered. At that point, your progesterone and estrogen levels crash, sending a clear signal to your breasts that it's time to start making milk.

During the first few days after the birth, your breasts produce a type of milk called colostrum. Despite the name, it's still milk, just milk in a concentrated form with high levels of the protein, carbohydrates, and (perhaps most importantly) immune factors that give your baby's immune system a valuable jump-start. Colostrum lays down the bacterial foundation for the gut to begin processing nutrients. The combination of probiotic and antibiotic properties contained in colostrum protects the gut from diarrhea—a powerful defence for a tiny newborn to have.

Within two to three days of the birth, your breasts start producing transitional milk. Because of the increased volume, the antibodies and protein are less concentrated, but this milk has more lactose (milk sugar) and fat to help your baby grow.

Within two weeks, your breasts will be producing what is known as "mature milk," milk that is lower in protein but higher in lactose. The exact composition of your milk changes from feeding to feeding, from day to day, and from month to month, depending on your baby's age, the time of day, how often your baby feeds, what you are eating, and many other important factors that Mother Nature is wise enough to factor in.

---

baby talk Colostrum is the clear, yellowish fluid that your breasts produce during the second half of pregnancy. It is high in protein and low in fat and carbohydrates; it's easy to digest; and it has a laxative effect that helps to clear the meconium out of your baby's bowels. It promotes good digestive health by encouraging the growth of bifidus flora (a healthy type of bacteria) in your baby's digestive system.

Colostrum is also rich in immunological factors that help to protect the baby against illness until his own immune system is firing on all cylinders, something that can take many months or as long as a year to occur. (The World Health Organization refers to colostrum as "baby's first immunization.")

Your baby won't get a lot of colostrum during each feeding—2 to 10 millilitres (1/4 teaspoons to 2 teaspoons) on average—but he'll certainly get a lot of benefit out of each drop of colostrum he ingests.

---

baby talk — Wondering what gives colostrum its yellowish colour? An abundance of carotenoids, the same compounds that are found in carrots and squash. Colostrum is 10 times richer in carotenoids than the mature milk that your body will start producing within a few days of the birth.

Your breasts make milk continuously, but they make more milk, more quickly, when your breasts are relatively empty, and slow down milk production when your breasts are full. It's the ultimate supply-demand economics system. Your milk ejection reflex (let-down reflex) is triggered by the hormone oxytocin—the very same hormone that brought you those delightful labour contractions and that is likely to be serving up some equally delightful afterpains as well. Oxytocin causes the band-like muscles around the milk-production cells to contract, forcing the milk through your internal canal system and into your nipples, where it can be obtained by your baby through an average of seven to twelve tiny openings.

Oxytocin isn't the only hormone involved in breastfeeding, of course. Prolactin plays an equally important role. As your baby nurses at the breast, she stimulates the nerve endings in your areolae, sending a message to your pituitary gland that triggers the release of more prolactin. Your rising prolactin level then triggers your breasts to produce more milk. Prolactin levels are nudged higher during night feedings than daytime feedings, so those middle-of-the-night feedings may play an important role in maintaining a good milk supply.

The best description I've seen of the remarkable interplay between oxytocin and prolactin in successful breastfeeding is this quote from reproductive physiologist R.V. Short in Meredith Small's book *Our Babies, Ourselves*: "Oxytocin serves today's meal while prolactin prepares tomorrow's."

Prolactin, not Prozac

You've no doubt heard about the so-called breastfeeding high that many women get while they're breastfeeding—a peaceful feeling that all is right with the world. What you might not realize is that the hormone responsible for triggering this beneficial by-product of breastfeeding is none other than prolactin—the so-called mothering hormone.

Your prolactin levels increase 20-fold during pregnancy and lactation, reaching their highest levels during the first 10 days of breastfeeding. (I don't know about you, but I think it was very wise of Mother Nature to ensure that new mothers have an ample supply of "natural sedatives" on tap right when the stresses of caring for a newborn are at their greatest.) While women who don't breastfeed lose this beneficial jolt of prolactin by the time their babies are 2 weeks old, the prolactin levels of breastfeeding women remain elevated until after their babies are weaned. (One study showed that prolactin levels can be as much as 10 times higher in breastfeeding mothers than non-breastfeeding mothers during the first three months of a baby's life. Talk about getting hooked on motherhood.)

---

mother wisdom Mothers who breastfeed their babies exclusively get more and better quality sleep than mothers who supplement with formula or who bottle feed. Partners of women who breast feed their babies exclusively also report getting more sleep. While offering a baby a nighttime bottle might seem like the perfect solution over the short-term, it actually results in less sleep for you, your partner, and your baby over the long-term. Bottom line? Nursing Baby at the breast is the secret to a well-rested family.

The breastfeeding high has an added advantage. It encourages you to relax and let your body do what it is designed to do. It's possible to overthink breastfeeding (applying too much left-brain attention to what is essentially a right-brain task, according to breastfeeding expert Nancy Mohrbacher), and that's when mothers tend to run into trouble. While it's important to understand a few basics about breastfeeding, your best teacher is your baby. Being flooded with too much information at the wrong time can take your focus off your baby and leave you feeling overwhelmed. If that starts to happen, retreat to a quiet place and find your own way by learning from your baby.

---

mother wisdom The brains of breastfeeding mothers respond differently to the sounds of their own babies in distress than the brains of mothers who are not breastfeeding. MRI scans reveal that the areas of the brain associated with nurturing and empathy light up with activity when a mother who is breastfeeding hears the sounds of her own baby crying.

THE ART OF THE LATCH

Location is everything, realtors tells us. This bit of wisdom also applies to breastfeeding. If your baby takes only your nipple into his mouth, breastfeeding will be painful and ineffective. She'll be hungry, and you'll be miserable! What she needs to do is get the nipple to the back of her mouth, and to do that she needs to take in a good portion of the breast as well. How do you help her get a good, deep latch? Getting in position helps.

You can assume that your baby is probably positioned properly at the breast if

- her tummy is against your stomach, and she doesn't have to turn her head sideways to reach the breast;
- you wait for her to open her mouth wide and latch on, and then use your hand or arm behind her shoulders to bring her in closer;
- her chin is pressed into your breast, and her nose is clear of the breast;
- she sucks with noticeable pauses when her mouth is open wide (she may start off with a series of quick, fluttering sucks, then shift to this slower sucking as the milk lets down);
- her head is tipped slightly back, with more of the breast covered by the baby's bottom lip as compared to the amount covered by her top lip; and
- you can see and hear your baby sucking and swallowing regularly as milk is released into her mouth.

mother wisdom Your areola may change colour while you're pregnant and retain its darker pigment thereafter. While the areola of a woman who has never been pregnant will tend to be pink, the areola of a woman who has had a baby tends to be reddish-brown. Note: This doesn't always happen in the first pregnancy for fair-skinned women; it may take two or three babies before a change in pigment is noticeable.

While some babies seem to know intuitively what to do, other babies need a little help figuring out how to latch on. You can help your baby by ensuring that you're both in a comfortable position (babies and mothers come in all shapes and sizes, so you'll want to experiment until you find a position that works best for you). Tip: Work with, not against, gravity. Get into a comfortable, semi-reclining position, using pillows if needed so you feel supported and relaxed. Pick up your baby and lay her on her chest, tummy to tummy with you, and let her find your breast. She will instinctively know how to find the nipple, and gravity will help her latch on well.

Skin-to-skin contact between mother and baby makes breastfeeding easier. Your breasts help to regulate Baby's temperature, so you don't have to worry about keeping Baby warm when you're snuggled up, skin-to-skin. Skin-to-skin contact acts as a stress-reliever for you, releasing oxytocin and bringing your blood pressure down. It reminds Baby what she needs to do in order to find the breast and latch on.

---

baby talk Rather than the miracle cure it was once touted as being, swaddling has been receiving a lot of critical attention lately—and for good reason. Over-reliance on swaddling as a baby-soothing technique can actually impede your baby's development. The reason? Swaddling tends to encourage babies to shut down and to tune out rather than to tune into and respond to their environment. Swaddling is associated with lower infant temperature, less competent early sucking, later establishment of breastfeeding, greater weight loss after the birth, and shorter duration of breastfeeding. Babies who are swaddled tend to sleep longer and to wake less frequently, something that can interfere with breastfeeding. Regular swaddling during the early months is also associated with some serious health issues: an increased risk of overheating (a key risk factor for SIDS), respiratory infections, and hip dysplasia. Instead of swaddling your baby, soothe your baby by practising kangaroo care (placing your baby skin-to-skin against your chest). He will be soothed by the sound of your heartbeat as well as the contact with your skin. See **Chapter 4** for more suggestions on ways to soothe your baby.

WHAT BREASTFEEDING FEELS LIKE

You may experience some initial discomfort when your baby first latches on—a noticeable tightening in your breast tissue that feels as if someone is pumping up a blood pressure cuff around your breast. This is your "let-down" reflex in action. The feeling tends to go away quickly (within 30 seconds or less) and becomes much less noticeable over time. You can expect to experience several let-downs during a typical feeding, but you will probably only be aware of the first one or two.

You may also notice that your breasts are a little tender during the first few days of breastfeeding as they get used to your baby's round-the-clock feeding schedule. And you may find that your breasts feel warm and heavy around the time that your milk is increasing in volume (approximately the second to fourth day postpartum), but that should be the extent of your discomfort.

If you experience pain in your nipples or breasts, it's important to get help quickly from a lactation consultant or other breastfeeding expert. Most often, nipple pain is caused by a baby who isn't latching well, but there are other possible causes, so you should get things checked out right away. The sooner you catch a breastfeeding problem, the easier it is to correct.

To reduce your chances of developing sore nipples, keep these tips in mind:

- **Get comfortable before you start nursing.** If you're sitting down in a chair or couch with arms, make sure the arms don't get in your way when you're feeding the baby. Pillows can help you get comfortable if you sit on the floor or if you nurse in a semi-reclining position. If you're lying down, make sure that you've got enough pillows under your head to prevent your neck from getting sore and that you've tucked a pillow between your knees if lower back pain tends to be a problem for you. Remember that you want to choose a situation that will allow your baby to find the breast (possibly with a little help from you). You don't want to have to contort your body in an effort to try to bring the breast to your baby. That can lead to sore nipples (and a tired and achy mother) very quickly.

- **Don't underestimate the strength of your newborn baby's latch.** If you need to remove your baby from the breast, slip your finger into the corner of your baby's mouth, gently breaking the suction. The alternative—trying to wrestle your breast out of your baby's mouth without breaking the suction—can hurt. A lot.

YOUR TOP BREASTFEEDING QUESTIONS ANSWERED

Here are answers to the questions that are likely to be on your mind once you start breastfeeding your baby.

How can you tell if a baby is interested in nursing?

Look for these signs of hunger:

- rapid eye movements and/or rapid breathing followed by stretching, stirring, and waking;
- hand-to-mouth activity (for example, your baby seems determined to stuff one or both fists into her mouth);
- plenty of mouth activity (your baby starts smacking her lips, sucking or licking her lips or her fingers, or frantically rooting around in search of a passing nipple); and
- attempts to move down (some will practically throw themselves sideways) toward the breast if you are holding your baby.

Of course, if you don't manage to pick up on these preliminary cues, your baby will soon resort to fussing and crying. Whenever possible, you should try to feed your baby before she starts to cry. Otherwise, she may become so upset that she may have a hard time settling down to nurse—something that can lead to a very unhappy baby and a very stressed mother.

That's why it makes sense to offer the breast if you think your baby might be hungry. If your baby isn't hungry, she'll either turn her head away or nurse for a few minutes and let you know (by letting the nipple slip out of her mouth and looking around) that she's ready to move on with her day.

How often should I feed my baby?

The answer to this question is simple: as often as your baby wants to eat. You don't have to worry about overfeeding an exclusively breastfed baby. She'll regulate her own food intake.

While babies normally wake as needed to breastfeed, some babies are a little sleepy for a day or two after the delivery. While you might be tempted to "let sleeping babies lie," you won't be doing yourself or your baby a favour by allowing her to sleep through a feeding or two. Your baby needs to nurse frequently in order to learn how to breastfeed and to help build up your milk supply. Otherwise, when she becomes a little less sleepy and realizes how hungry she is, there won't be enough milk on hand to satisfy her ravenous appetite. Therefore, instead of letting your resident Rip Van Winkle doze for hours at a time, you should encourage your newborn to nurse at least every three hours during the day and at least once or twice during the night. (Your goal should be to fit in at least eight to twelve feedings during a 24-hour period in order to stimulate adequate milk production, prevent your breasts from becoming overly engorged, and ensure that your newborn is gaining enough weight.)

---

mother wisdom Wondering how to go about waking a sleeping baby who seems determined to doze through her next feeding (a common problem in newborns—particularly newborns with jaundice)?

The best way to rouse a baby is to strip her down to her diaper, remove your own shirt, and put her skin-to-skin with you. If she still doesn't want to wake up

- watch for signs that your baby is moving into a period of active sleep. (You'll notice that her eyes are moving under her eyelids, her legs and arms may be twitching, and she may appear to be nursing in her sleep.)
- start stroking and talking to your baby.
- express a bit of colostrum and rub your nipple along the baby's lips and tongue to give her a taste of what's to come.

These techniques usually do the trick, but you may be astounded to find that after all your hard work, your baby starts dozing off at the breast. You may find that the only way to keep her awake is to continue to stimulate her by rubbing her head, her feet, her palms, and the underside of her chin while she is nursing. Compressing the breast as she sucks will also increase the flow of colostrum.

How long should I feed my baby on each side? How will I know when it's time to change breasts?

You should allow your baby to nurse on the first breast until she stops sucking, falls asleep, or releases the breast. When she pauses to take a break, simply burp her (pat or rub her on the back gently to see if she needs to burp), and then offer her the second breast. Don't be surprised if your baby isn't as interested in nursing on the second side as she was on the first: her appetite is already partially satisfied. She may, in fact, decide to pass on the second side entirely, leaving you with one breast that feels like a cantaloupe and another that feels like a pancake. If you happen to offer the same breast for a couple of feedings, your other breast will be quick to remind you that it's time to switch sides. You'll either wake up in a puddle of milk after putting pressure on an overly full breast or you'll end up with a tender, engorged breast that's practically crying out to be emptied. (If your baby's not quite ready to nurse again, you may need to express or pump a bit of milk in order to relieve your discomfort.) Note: In order to maximize milk production, you want to offer your baby both breasts at each feeding as often as possible.

There's a simple remedy for this lopsidedness, by the way: simply alternate which breast you offer first at each feeding (and a simple hand on the chest is all that it takes to figure out which breast is scheduled to receive star billing at the next feeding). Another option, if you find she is often just taking one breast, is to stop nursing after a few minutes and switch to the second breast. You can then switch back to the first breast again if she is still hungry.

My baby barely finishes one feeding before it's time to gear up for the next. Is this normal?

Every breastfed baby's feeding pattern is unique. There can be significant variations when it comes to the length of a typical feeding and the duration between feedings. If your newborn is a slow nurser who likes to eat every two hours, you could find yourself breastfeeding practically non-stop during the early days of your baby's life. Fortunately, it won't be like this forever. Your breasts will become more efficient at making and releasing milk, your baby's breastfeeding technique will improve, and her tummy will grow and become capable of holding more food so she won't need to nurse quite so often. But all this takes time.

While a typical nursing session lasts between 20 and 30 minutes, not all babies like to settle for being average. Just as some adults like to linger over coffee and dessert for hours at a time, perhaps even ordering a round of liqueurs to top off dessert, some babies prefer to stretch out each meal as long as possible, clearly reluctant to see the feeding draw to a close until they've enjoyed the breastfeeding world's equivalent of a nine-course meal. These babies tend to alternate sucking periods with periods of resting that may last for several minutes at a time, resulting in longer-than-average nursing sessions. Other babies prefer to take a much more business-like approach to their feedings, barely taking time to breathe as they work at extracting maximum milk in minimum time.

There are also significant variations when it comes to the frequency of feedings (the length of time between the start of one feeding and the start of the next). Some newborns like to nurse every two to three hours around the clock, while others prefer to nurse more often during the day (daytime "cluster feeding") and less frequently at night. (Some babies adopt the opposite pattern: nursing frequently at night and sleeping a lot during the day—a schedule that can require exceptional parental endurance if there are toddlers and preschoolers to care for during the day.) And, of course, while some babies follow a predictable pattern, most eat at different times every day.

While almost all women can make plenty of milk for their babies, women do vary in their milk storage capacity. This means that some women have more milk available at each feeding than others and that mothers with a smaller milk storage capacity need to feed their babies more often.

What can I do to build up my milk supply?

The best technique for building up your milk supply also happens to be the one that comes most naturally—putting your baby to the breast whenever she's interested. The more often (and more effectively) your baby nurses, the greater your milk supply. If a newborn starts nursing shortly after the birth and is offered the breast whenever she is interested (at least eight to twelve times during the first 24 hours of life), the transition from colostrum to mature milk will be made within about 48 hours. This is because frequent feeding ensures that milk production keeps chugging along.

The vast majority of women have little trouble manufacturing milk for their babies. However, problems are more likely to arise if.

- the mother received synthetic oxytocin to speed up her labour (A study published in the April 2012 edition of a Spanish pediatric journal indicated that babies born to mothers who received synthetic oxytocin during labour may have a poorer sucking reflex and may breastfeed for shorter durations.);
- the baby was delivered via Caesarean section;
- there is a delay in putting the baby to the breast after the birth;

- the length or frequency of feedings is restricted in the mistaken belief that it makes sense to put breastfed babies on a schedule;
- supplements are introduced;
- the baby isn't able to nurse effectively due to poor positioning and/or an ineffective latch or suck, or because of a congenital abnormality (such as cleft lip, cleft palate, or Down syndrome) or a health problem (such as prematurity or illness);
- a pacifier is introduced before breastfeeding is well established (early pacifier use may cause the mother's breasts to miss out on some critical early stimulation and may be confusing for some newborns);
- the mother has had breast reduction surgery;
- the mother is experiencing "primary lactation failure" (a rare medical condition); or
- some fragments of the placenta have been retained. (The placenta continues to produce hormones—including estrogens and progesterones—that can severely limit breast milk production. This problem can be diagnosed via a blood test and/or an ultrasound. Surgery may be required to remove the placental fragments. Provided that this condition is treated promptly, the mother's milk supply usually increases dramatically shortly after the surgery.) Note: If a mother is not at risk of hemorrhaging, increasing the frequency and duration of breastfeeding may be recommended as an alternative to surgery. In such a situation, the mother will need to be monitored carefully to ensure that the remaining placental fragments are expelled.

---

the baby department

Finding yourself with a million and one questions about breastfeeding? Fortunately, there are many excellent sources of breastfeeding support and information in most Canadian communities. Here are a few tips on tapping into the help you need.

√ Visit the La Leche League Canada website (www.lllc.ca) to find out the name of the closest La Leche League leader. La Leche League is a non-profit association run for and by nursing mothers. Meetings usually take place in members' homes, and both pregnant women and nursing mothers are welcome to attend. Some La Leche League leaders provide telephone support and/or make personal visits to breastfeeding women in need of support and information. There is also a free iPhone app that gives answers to common questions, plus information about the nearest LLLC Leader and meeting locations. Search iTunes for "La Leche" to find it.

✓ Ask your doctor or midwife and/or contact your public health department to find out what type of lactation consulting and breastfeeding support services are available in your community. You'll want to ask whether there is a mother-to-mother breastfeeding support program (through which experienced nursing mothers are hooked up with first-timers to provide support and information) or a help line (where women with breastfeeding questions can call to get answers) available to women in your community, and whether your local hospital or health unit operates a breastfeeding clinic and/or has a lactation consultant on staff to help nursing mothers troubleshoot any difficulties.

✓ Check the website of the International Lactation Consultant Association (www.ilca.org) to see if there are any lactation consultants in practice in your community. (Or ask your La Leche League leader.) When you're inquiring about their services, you'll want to find out whether their services are covered by your provincial or territorial health plan or by any extended health benefits plan you or your partner may have through work, and whether the lactation consultant in question is an International Board Certified Lactation Consultant (IBCLC)—the "gold standard" for the profession.

✓ Don't forget to look for support within your own circle of friends. Chances are you know at least one woman who is currently breastfeeding or who breastfed a baby recently. Sometimes all you need is a little reassurance from another nursing mother who has faced breastfeeding challenges of her own—and who can provide you with the encouragement you need to achieve the breastfeeding goals you have set for yourself.

Most mothers have little difficulty producing enough milk to feed their baby (or babies) once any underlying breastfeeding-related issues have been resolved. In rare cases, however, milk supply may continue to be a problem for a breastfeeding mother, in which case her doctor may decide to prescribe a drug (domperidone) that is designed to aid in milk production. Such treatment can typically bring the milk supply back up to its previous level and, in some cases, can even increase the amount of milk that is available for pumping. Mothers of adopted children can exclusively breastfeed their babies using a combination of this drug along with some additional hormonal support.

Note: In March 2012, Health Canada issued a warning about domperidone, advising that the drug has been associated with serious heart-related problems that could result in death. It added, however, that it had not received any reports of such problems "in relation to the use of domperidone used to stimulate milk production in breastfeeding women." Your health-care provider can help you to weigh the advantages of using domperidone to boost your milk supply against the potential risks.

My milk looks really thin and watery. Is this what breast milk is supposed to look like? Or could there be some sort of problem?

A lot of nursing moms are surprised to find out how thin and watery breast milk looks. After all, how can a baby be expected to thrive on a beverage that looks like watered-down skim milk? No worries. You are feeding a baby human, not a baby calf, and your milk is perfectly designed to meet your baby's needs.

How can I tell if breastfeeding is working?

Pay attention to your breasts and your baby. Breastfeeding is working if:

- your breasts feel fuller before a feeding and emptier afterwards. This is especially noticeable in small-breasted women. Large-breasted women may not notice this as much.

- your baby is nursing regularly (at least eight to twelve times per day during the newborn stage).

- your baby is gaining weight. It's normal for breastfed babies to lose weight during the first few days after the birth, but this initial weight loss should turn around quickly once breastfeeding becomes established. There's no need to panic in the meantime. Babies are born with more fluid in their tissues than they need—the result of being immersed in amniotic fluid prior to birth. Note: Babies who have been exposed to intravenous fluids and synthetic oxytocin during labour retain even more fluid. This can make the loss they experience the second time they are placed on the scale seem even more dramatic.

It can also jeopardize breastfeeding. A drop of what appears to be more than 7 per cent of Baby's bodyweight will put Baby at risk for supplementation (artificial feeding).

- your nipples are not sore.
- you know your baby is drinking at the breast because, after a short period of rapid sucking, she switches to a period of slower sucking that is alternated with pauses when her mouth is wide open.
- your baby seems sleepier and more satisfied toward the end of a feeding. Tip: Take a look at your baby's hands. At the beginning of a feeding, most babies have their hands bunched up into tight little fists. When they are satisfied after a feeding, their hands tend to relax and open up.
- your baby's diapers are wet and she's passing stools on a regular basis. (See below.)
- your baby is alert and responsive.

While most breastfed babies thrive, it's important to be on the lookout for signs that there could be a breastfeeding problem. You should get in touch with your baby's health-care provider to discuss the possibility that your newborn might not be getting enough to eat if

- your baby is having fewer than two substantial soft stools each day between Day 4 and 4 weeks of age;
- the baby's urine is becoming concentrated (darker yellow in colour);
- the baby is having fewer than one or two wet diapers daily during the first three days or fewer than six wet diapers daily by Day 6;
- your baby is sleepy and difficult to wake at feeding time;
- your baby is nursing fewer than eight times in a 24-hour period; or
- you have sore nipples.

---

mother wisdom By the end of the first week of breastfeeding, your breasts will be producing roughly 10 to 20 times as much breast milk as they were at the start of the week (from a little more than 37 millilitres per day (1 ounce) to between 280 and 576 millilitres per day (10 to 19 ounces). This does vary considerably among mothers, however.

My baby wants to nurse more frequently in the evening. Is this normal?

Your milk supply is likely to be at its lowest in the evening, so it makes sense that your baby wants to nurse more frequently. The more he nurses, the more your breasts are stimulated to produce more milk, and the more milk he gets. It's a win-win situation, ultimately (although it can be a bit challenging to figure out how to make dinner when your baby is in perpetual feeding mode). This is why take-out was invented, however, and why so many new parents are overjoyed when friends and neighbours drop off ready-made meals. There's also an upside to this all-evening grazing: many babies will "stock up" during the evening and then go for longer stretches at night—not a bad plan.

---

mother wisdom A breastfed baby's milk intake peaks at about 5 weeks of age. She will continue to consume about the same amount of breast milk (750 to 1,035 millilitres or 25 to 35 ounces) on a daily basis until age 6 months, at which point she will add solid foods to her diet. Here's another fascinating fact about breast milk that relates to the amount of breast milk babies consume: breast milk contains hormones that helps babies to regulate their appetite. Right from the start, breastfed babies learn to eat when they are hungry and to stop eating when they are full. What a brilliant design.

Should I give my baby a pacifier?

Even the Canadian Paediatric Society responds to this question with a definitive *it depends*. In their recommendations on pacifier use, updated in February 2011, the CPS writes: "The decision to use pacifiers in infants and children remains controversial and an individual choice for today's parents." So if you're feeling uncertain about whether or not to introduce a pacifier to your baby, at least you're in good company.

One thing that the experts do agree upon, however, is that if you're going to introduce a pacifier to a breastfed baby, you should wait until breastfeeding is well established. This is because pacifier use may reduce the amount of time an infant spends at the breast, a situation that may contribute to an inadequate milk supply and poor weight gain.

baby talk Pacifiers have been shown to have some very real benefits for very premature infants: babies who were given soothers gained more weight and stayed in hospital for less time than their soother-less peers. And they've also been proven to be an effective comfort measure for babies who are undergoing painful procedures such as heel sticks (pricking the heel to take a small sample of blood). All that said, kangaroo care (skin-to-skin care) and breastfeeding are even more effective when it comes to soothing and encouraging growth in premature babies. A pacifier may make a suitable stand-in, but the real thing is better.

That's not to say that every breastfed baby who's offered a pacifier is going to treat it as her new best friend. Some truly discriminating babies will refuse, in fact, to have anything to do with an artificial nipple—particularly one that's not even hooked up to a food supply. But if you do decide to offer your breastfed baby a pacifier, there's always the possibility that there could be some breastfeeding-related fallout. There is some evidence that babies who use pacifiers are more likely to bite at the breast, as well.

What else do you need to know about pacifiers? They're associated with an increased incidence of ear infections (the risk of developing an ear infection is twice as high in babies who use pacifiers) and, in children who rely on a pacifier after age 5, dental problems as well.

If you decide that the benefits of pacifier use (see sidebar about **SIDS and pacifiers**) outweigh the risks and you decide to offer your baby a soother, here are some important points to keep in mind.

- Choose the right size. Your newborn baby will barely be able to wrap her mouth around a toddler-sized pacifier, let alone suck on it.
- Be vigilant when it comes to safety. To reduce the risk of strangulation, use a pacifier holder rather than a string to attach your baby's pacifier to her clothing or her crib.
- Keep your baby's pacifier squeaky clean. Run it through the dishwasher on a regular basis (provided the product you have purchased is dishwasher safe) or scrub it with soap and water.
- Inspect your baby's pacifier regularly for signs of wear. Make sure that the nipple is firmly attached and be prepared to discard the pacifier if it starts feeling sticky (a sure sign that the pacifier is beginning to deteriorate).

- Never dip a pacifier in sugar, honey, or corn syrup. Exposure to such sweets can lead to tooth decay, and honey and corn syrup may contain botulism-causing bacteria that may pose a serious risk to a baby's immature digestive system.

- If your baby is dependent on her pacifier, keep plenty of spares around. It'll alleviate the need to turn your entire house upside down looking for a pacifier that's somehow gone astray. Regardless of how desperate you may be, don't even think of using a bottle nipple as a substitute for the missing pacifier. The risk of choking is simply too great.

- While a pacifier can be quite effective when it comes to soothing a crying baby, it's important to address the underlying cause of your baby's crying.

---

baby talk In 2005, the American Academy of Pediatrics updated its policy on Sudden Infant Death Syndrome. One of the new recommendations stated that infants should be offered a pacifier at bedtime and naptime. The AAP qualified this recommendation by noting that breastfed babies should not be offered the pacifier until age 1 month (in order to allow breastfeeding to become well established). The recommendation was made in response to research indicating that pacifiers may protect against SIDS by preventing babies from drifting into an overly deep sleep. It was also noted that pacifier use encourages a more forward position of the tongue, preventing blockage of the baby's airway, and that pacifier use tends to keep a baby on his back (the sleep position that has proven to be safest for babies). While breastfeeding advocates opposed to this recommendation have argued that breastfed babies do not need pacifiers to benefit from this type of protective effect because they receive the stimulation that comes from suckling during the night, more research needs to be conducted to be sure.

The Canadian Paediatric Society had this to say about pacifiers in its October 2011 *Joint Statement on Safe Sleep:* "Pacifiers appear to provide a protective effect for SIDS. No solid evidence demonstrates that pacifier use impairs breastfeeding; however, delaying the introduction of a pacifier is best left until breastfeeding is well established. Infants who accept a pacifier should have one consistently, for every sleep; however, a pacifier is not required to be reinserted if it is expelled during sleep."

How much extra food do I need to eat while I'm breastfeeding?

Milk production requires about 500 calories per day. Your body can obtain some of this energy from the extra calories it set aside while you were pregnant (one of the reasons you've retained a few pounds of your pregnancy weight gain). You can obtain any extra calories your body needs to support breastfeeding (about 300 calories per day) by eating according to hunger and ensuring that you have a variety of nutritious foods on hand.

If your diet is far from perfect, don't let that stop you from breastfeeding. Yes, good nutrition is important for everyone, but your milk will still contain the protein, carbohydrates, immune factors, and other essential elements your baby needs, in precisely the right proportions. (And now that you're doing a great job of feeding your baby, why not commit to taking the best possible care of yourself, too? Doesn't your baby's mom deserve the best?)

You're likely to be thirstier than usual while you're breastfeeding. Some moms find it works well to have a beverage handy whenever they sit down to nurse their baby. Water is always a good choice. (Add a slice of lemon, lime, or cucumber to give it a bit of zip.) Fruit and fruit juices, milk, and soups will also keep you well hydrated while delivering a variety of nutrients at the same time.

Here are some other nutrition tips to keep in mind while you're breastfeeding your baby.

- Eat a variety of foods. Certain foods may flavour your breast milk. This is a good thing: it prepares your baby for the various flavours he'll encounter when he makes the switch to solid foods. If your baby demonstrates a strong dislike for a particular flavour of breast milk (garlic-onion breast milk?), don't panic. Flavours pass through breast milk quickly. One of his preferred flavours should be back on tap within a feeding or two.

- Choose fibre-rich foods: fruits, vegetables, beans, and whole grain products.

- Zero in on foods that provide the nutrients that are most likely to be in short supply after the birth or during breastfeeding. Those nutrients (and recommended food sources) are as follows:

    - *Calcium*: milk; cheese; yogurt; fish with edible bones; tofu processed with calcium sulfate; bok choy; broccoli; kale; collard, mustard, and turnip greens; and breads made with milk.

- *Zinc*: meat, poultry, seafood, eggs, seeds, legumes, yogurt, and whole grains.
- *Magnesium*: nuts, seeds, legumes, whole grains, green vegetables, scallops, and oysters.
- *Vitamin B6*: bananas, poultry, meat, fish, potatoes, sweet potatoes, spinach, prunes, watermelon, some legumes, fortified cereals, and nuts.
- *Thiamin*: pork, fish, whole grains, organ meats, legumes, corn, peas, seeds, nuts, and fortified cereal grain.
- *Folate*: leafy vegetables, fruit, liver, green beans, fortified cereals, legumes, and whole-grain cereals.
- *Iron*: liver, meat, fish (halibut, haddock, perch, salmon, tuna), enriched breakfast cereal, cooked beans, seeds, and legumes.

- If you are vegan, be sure to supplement with vitamin B12. If you are deficient in your intake of this important nutrient, your milk will be, too, and your baby could suffer damage to his developing nervous system.
- If you're trying to lose weight, aim for slow, steady weight loss rather than rapid weight loss. Losing 1 to 2 pounds (1 to 1.5 kilograms) per month should not interfere with milk production.

---

mother wisdom Even though you use a lot of calcium while you're breastfeeding, there's no need to be concerned that breastfeeding will increase your chances of developing osteoporosis later in life. While you will lose some bone mass during lactation, within one year of weaning your baby your bone mass will have been completely restored. In fact, some research has even demonstrated that women who have breastfed their babies at some point in their lives face only half the risk of developing osteoporosis over their lifetimes of women who have never breastfed a baby. And, even better, your protection against osteoporosis increases with the length of time you spend breastfeeding.

TABLE 6.1

Canada's Food Guide

Canada's Food Guide to Healthy Eating is designed to provide you with an adequate number of servings from each of the four basic food groups: vegetables and fruit, grain products, milk or alternatives, and meat or alternatives.

Food Group	Why You Need This Type of Food	Number of Servings You Need in a Day	What Constitutes a Serving
Vegetables and fruit	Vegetables and fruit are good sources of fibre and excellent sources of vitamin C as well as hundreds of disease-fighting compounds called phytochemicals. Vegetables are also an excellent source of vitamin A.	7 to 8 servings	• 1 medium-sized vegetable or fruit • 125 mL (1/2 cup) fresh, frozen, or canned vegetables or fruit • 250 mL (1 cup) of tossed salad • 125 mL (1/2 cup) of fruit juice
Grain products	Grain products are critical for converting food to energy and for maintaining a healthy nervous system. They are also an excellent source of B vitamins.	6 to 7 servings	• 1 slice of bread or 1/2 bagel • 30 grams (1 ounce) of cold cereal • 175 mL (3/4 cup) of hot cereal • 25 mL (1/2 cup) of pasta or rice
Milk products	Milk products are an excellent source of calcium, the mineral that is responsible for keeping our bones healthy and strong and staving off osteoporosis, a debilitating bone-thinning disease.	2 servings	• 250 mL (1 cup) milk • 50 grams (1 1/2 ounces) of hard cheese • 175 mL (3/4 cup) of yogurt

(continued)

Food Group	Why You Need This Type of Food	Number of Servings You Need in a Day	What Constitutes a Serving
Meat and alternatives	Meat and alternatives are an excellent source of protein.	2 servings	• 75 grams (2 1/2 ounces of meat, poultry, or fish • 175 mL (3/4 cup) of cooked beans • 2 eggs • 30 mL (2 tbsp) of peanut butter

Women who are breastfeeding need an extra two to three Food Guide servings each day. Have fruit and yogurt for a snack or an extra slice of toast at breakfast and a piece of fruit at dinner.

You should also include a small amount of unsaturated fat (30 to 45 millilitres or 2 to 3 tablespoons) in your diet each day. Typical sources include salad dressings, margarine, mayonnaise, and oil for cooking.

For additional information about *Canada's Food Guide*, please visit www.myfoodguide.ca.

mother wisdom Health Canada recommends that Canadians eat at least two servings (of 75 grams or 2.5 ounces each) of fish a week. Your baby can benefit from the nutrients in fish, but because mercury in fish also poses a particular risk to young children, it is important that women who are breastfeeding understand which types of fish are a good choice for frequent consumption and which should be eaten less often.

Fish and shellfish that contain high levels of fatty acids but are also low in mercury include anchovy, capelin, char, hake, herring, Atlantic mackerel, mullet, pollock (Boston bluefish), salmon, smelt, rainbow trout, lake whitefish, blue crab, shrimp, clam, mussel, and oyster.

Predatory fish that eat lots of other fish for food tend to contain higher levels of mercury. These include fresh/frozen tuna, shark, swordfish, marlin, orange roughy, and escolar. Health Canada recommends that pregnant and breastfeeding women limit consumption of these fish to 150 grams (5 ounces) per month.

They also recommend a limit of 300 (10.5 ounces) grams per week for canned albacore (white) tuna. Note: This limit does not apply to canned light tuna. Canned skip jack tuna is low in methyl mercury too (compared to canned albacore tuna, which is higher in the methyl mercury toxins).

---

mother wisdom Keep your home well stocked with foods that are quick to prepare and can be enjoyed with a baby in your arms. These foods have been selected because they are ready-to-eat (or can be prepared ahead of time), they work equally well at mealtime and snack time, and you can mix-and-match them to come up with all kinds of interesting combos.

- √ Yogurt (especially Greek yogurt) mixed with cereal and fresh fruit
- √ Tzatiki with cut-up veggies such as celery and baby carrots
- √ Hard-boiled eggs
- √ Low-fat cheeses
- √ Sliced meat (cooked turkey, Black Forest ham)
- √ Hummus and other spreads/dips
- √ English muffins, bagels, pitas, rice crackers
- √ Whole-grain muffins
- √ Whole-grain crackers
- √ Dried fruits and nuts
- √ Fresh fruits and vegetables
- √ Pre-made salad (stuff the salad in a pita to make it easier to eat when you're holding a baby)

Can certain foods that I eat make my baby fussy?

A small percentage of babies are affected by the foods that their breastfeeding moms eat. (When this occurs, there is likely to be a family history of allergies.) Foods that can make babies edgy or unhappy include caffeine, citrus fruits, dairy products, eggs, gluten, fish, nuts, soy, and spicy foods.

If you're wondering about whether you need to give up your morning cup of coffee, you'll likely be reassured to hear that most mothers need to drink at least five cups of coffee before their babies are affected.

Certain types of herbs can affect breastfeeding. Sage, peppermint, and parsley can reduce breast milk production. If you're concerned about the possible effects of your favourite herbal tea, talk to your pharmacist or your health-care provider.

My baby spits up after every feeding. How can I be sure that she's getting enough to eat?

It's not unusual for a baby to spit up after a feeding. Babies spit up because they've swallowed air during a feeding or because they've eaten more than their stomach can hold. You can minimize the amount your baby spits up by

- feeding your baby before she is frantically hungry;
- keeping feeding times as calm, quiet, and leisurely as possible while minimizing both distractions and interruptions;
- burping your baby more often during feedings (to get rid of any trapped air);
- placing your baby in an upright position on your lap or in a sling, wrap, or soft baby carrier after a feeding; and
- if you're offering your baby breast milk in a bottle, making sure that the hole in the nipple is neither too large (causing the milk to flow too quickly) or too small (causing the baby to swallow a lot of air).

Some babies spit up more than others (most for no identifiable reason), but most babies stop spitting up by the end of the first year of life. There's rarely cause for concern unless your baby is experiencing projectile vomiting (a condition in which a large quantity of food is forcefully ejected from a baby's stomach with every feeding), in which case you'll want to discuss the problem with your baby's doctor. This condition is of particular concern if a baby isn't gaining weight.

My baby has reflux. What can I do to minimize his discomfort during and after feedings?

Gastroesophageal reflux disease (GERD) occurs when stomach acids back up into the esophagus, damaging the delicate tissues. This can lead to extreme distress in babies, both during and after feedings. Your baby may cry during and after feedings and experience bouts of extreme crying after he has fallen asleep because he is so uncomfortable when he is lying down.

Experiment with breastfeeding positions until you find one that works well for your baby. Generally, positions that keep the baby's head elevated higher than his bottom work best. Keep him in an upright position for at least half an hour following each feeding. And talk to your health-care provider to find out whether she recommends a modified sleeping position for babies with GERD.

---

mother wisdom If your baby gulps down large amounts of milk very quickly and then spits up a lot of milk when you go to burp her, consider sticking to one breast per feeding, as long as the baby is gaining weight well. This may help to reduce the amount of spitting up.

My two-week-old baby has been nursing about 12 times a day. Yesterday she nursed 18 times! What's going on?

Long-time La Leche League leader and author Teresa Pitman says: "We call these 'frequency days.' Most breastfed babies have these days when they nurse more frequently than usual. It can be to increase milk production because the baby is growing. It can also be because he's picked up a virus or germ and is wanting more of the antibodies and immune factors in your milk."

---

mom's the word "If you are planning to breastfeed, don't keep any formula in the house at all. There will be a day when things aren't going right or Baby won't latch on and your mind will focus on that can of formula sitting in the cupboard. At those weak moments, it is so easy to give in and say, 'Just this once.' Usually, it doesn't end up only being one time, and before you know it, your milk supply has dwindled and Baby is now being formula-fed. So if you are given any formula samples, donate them to a shelter or a food bank—just get them out of your house."

—LORI, 30, MOTHER OF FIVE

The best way to cope with a frequency day (or days) is to go with the flow. That means nursing as often as your baby wants to nurse, around the clock, drinking plenty of fluids, and ensuring that you're getting adequate rest. If you're going to be staying in one place, make it fun. Rent a movie, cuddle up on the couch with your baby and partner, and enjoy a relaxing evening with your baby at the breast.

My baby wants to nurse all the time, but fusses and squirms at the breast while she's nursing and then is gassy and hard to settle after a feeding. Could it be that I'm not producing enough milk?

It could be, but it is also possible that your problem is actually the opposite—too much of a good thing. These symptoms can sometimes indicate your baby is getting too much milk, too fast.

How do you know? It's likely that you have an overabundant milk supply (which often comes with an overactive let-down) if you see these signs:

- your baby is gaining weight rapidly;
- your milk sprays out whenever your baby lets go of the breast;
- your baby noticeably gulps and sputters when your milk lets down (you may see milk run out of the corners of her mouth);
- your baby has watery, green-tinged, mucous, explosive bowel movements and wets her diapers frequently (Sometimes green stools can be associated with poor milk intake, so you might want to check in with your baby's doctor if you're not sure what's going on.); and
- your baby may sometimes let go of the breast and suck her fingers instead.

There are a couple of ways to approach this problem. One research study found this method effective: feed the baby, then pump or hand-express both breasts until they are as empty as you can get them (they are never really empty, of course). Then, for the rest of the day, offer the baby just one breast at each feeding. Some women find it works better if they offer the same breast for a couple of feedings in a row, then the other breast for the next two feedings. Usually you only need to do this for a day or two before your milk production settles down again, and you can go back to offering both breasts at each feeding. Another approach used by some experts is to estimate how long the baby would typically feed. If the baby is usually nursing for fifteen minutes, for example (and these babies will generally only take one breast per feeding because they get full), the mother would switch the baby to the second breast after seven minutes. The goal is to get the baby to nurse for an equal time on each breast at every feeding, which should gradually reduce milk production. If these strategies don't seem to help, talk to a lactation consultant about other options.

My baby chokes and pulls away when he is trying to nurse. Then he starts crying. What's wrong?

This pattern is also common in babies whose mothers have an overabundance of milk. Hand-express or pump some milk before you put your baby to the breast so that your baby won't be overwhelmed by the volume of your milk flow. Lying on your back or semi-reclining, with Baby on top of you, can also help.

My baby is refusing to breastfeed at all! Is there anything I can do to solve the problem or should I cut my losses and switch to a bottle?

Babies usually have a good reason for refusing the breast, even if it's a mystery to the rest of us.

If your baby refuses the breast shortly after birth, it could be because she associates opening her mouth with a less than pleasant experience such as having her mouth vigorously suctioned after the birth. It's also possible that there's an underlying physical problem responsible for your baby's breast refusal: she may be "tongue-tied" (the thin membrane that connects the lower part of the tongue to the floor of the mouth may be too tight to allow the baby's tongue to extend far enough forward to take hold of the nipple) or your baby may have difficulty latching on (a lactation consultant should be able to provide you with some tips on solving this problem).

If your baby has been nursing for a period of weeks or months but then suddenly refuses to nurse (or nurses for a couple of minutes and then arches her back and cries), you're dealing with a frustrating occurrence known as a nursing strike. Some common reasons for a baby who has been nursing beautifully to suddenly refuse the breast are as follows:

- Your breast milk has developed a taste that your baby isn't exactly thrilled with and she's allowing her inner food critic to make her feelings known. Perhaps you've started eating a new food or taking a medication that has added an objectionable flavour to your breast milk, you're developing a breast infection, you've started a strenuous new exercise program, or you are pregnant. All of these situations can affect the flavour of your breast milk.

- Your baby is in physical pain or discomfort. If your baby's getting a new tooth, is developing thrush, has a bladder infection, is experiencing the symptoms of GERD (gastroesophageal reflux disease), or has an earache, it may hurt when she nurses. Likewise, if she has a bad cold, she may have trouble breathing through her nose while she's nursing—something that can cause her to pull back in frustration once the milk begins to flow.
- You smell different to your baby. You've started wearing a different brand of deodorant or you decided to slather some sort of body lotion all over your breasts. Baby is telling you, "I like my mom to smell like my mom."
- Your baby is stressed. Babies are highly intuitive and will react to changes in their routines (a family move, Mom's return to work, family travel, stress within the family, or prolonged separations between mom and baby). If your baby doesn't feel safe and secure, she may have a difficult time settling down to eat.
- Your milk supply has decreased. This can happen for a number of reasons, and a baby who is frustrated by not being able to get enough milk or who is annoyed because the milk is flowing more slowly than in the past will sometimes refuse to nurse.
- Your baby has been introduced to a bottle and has developed a preference for the fast flow and different type of sucking he does at the bottle. (He doesn't have to work as hard.)
- Your baby is afraid of biting you. If your baby bit you during her last feeding and you yelped in pain (understandably) and pulled her off the breast, she may not want to nurse for fear of biting you again.

Don't take the nursing strike personally. Your baby isn't rejecting *you*. She's trying to tell you that a breastfeeding problem has developed. She just doesn't have the words to spell out exactly what that problem is.

Express some breast milk and give it to your baby via an eyedropper, a teaspoon, or a sippy cup (to manage her hunger until she starts breastfeeding again).

Offer your baby the breast while she's in a relaxed, sleepy state. Use your baby's favourite breastfeeding position and make sure that there's milk waiting (hand-express so there's milk at the ready) when your baby latches on. Having a bath with your baby is often a good way to help her feel relaxed and provide some skin-to-skin contact as well. If your baby is still unsure, try walking or rocking your baby while you continue to offer the breast.

---

mother wisdom If your baby bites, pull her in close so that your breast covers her nose and she has to open her mouth to breathe (releasing the breast). Say "it hurts" to her (not that she'll understand). Biting tends to happen at the end of a feeding, because the baby has to pull her tongue back before she bites (otherwise, she'd bite her tongue). So keep a finger by the corner of her mouth, and if you feel that tongue move back, slip it into her mouth to protect your nipple. Usually you only need to do this a few times. Older babies who are teething and who have a powerful need to bite on something in order to relieve their discomfort may need to be provided with a teething ring or chew toy to chomp on as an alternative.

Continue to offer your baby the breast—ideally when she's asleep or very sleepy and least likely to become upset. Talk to your baby in a soothing voice and try varying your nursing position (for example, try nursing while you're walking around) to see if that makes a difference. Sometimes that's all it takes to settle the strike. Other times it isn't easily solved. Spending lots of time skin-to-skin or taking Baby to a group with other nursing babies are strategies that have worked for other mothers.

Under what circumstances is breastfeeding not recommended?

While breastfeeding is recommended for most babies, there are some situations when breastfeeding is not recommended. Your health-care provider is likely to recommend against breastfeeding if

- you are taking a medication that is not considered safe for use by breastfeeding mothers (such as radioactive isotopes, anti-metabolites, cancer chemotherapy agents). There are only a few medications in this category. If it is necessary for you to take a medication while you are breastfeeding, your health-care provider can help you to weigh the benefits of breastfeeding against any known risks of taking that particular medication while breastfeeding. In cases where there are known risks, your health-care provider may recommend an alternative medication. Note: The Motherisk Clinic (www.motherisk.org or 1-877-439-2744) is an excellent source of information on medication use while breastfeeding.

- you have herpes simplex, with active lesions on your breasts. (If there are lesions on only one breast, you can nurse from the other breast.) At first, both breasts will produce milk and you may experience some discomfort in your non-nursing breast, but, over time, your body will take note of the fact that you are only nursing from one breast and adjust milk production on the other side accordingly. If the non-nursing breast becomes extremely engorged in the meantime, express enough milk to relieve your discomfort (but not so much that you encourage more milk production).

- you develop chicken pox immediately prior to or after the birth.

- you have breast cancer. (The role of prolactin in advancing breast cancer is uncertain; chemotherapy and the use of radioactive compounds for diagnosis and/or treatment could also be harmful to the breastfed baby.)

- you have untreated, active tuberculosis.

- your baby is diagnosed with galactosemia (a rare genetic disorder in which babies are born without the liver enzyme required to process galactose, a simple sugar found in all kinds of milk, including breast milk). Note: Some babies with milder forms of this condition can be partially breastfed.

New research indicates that exclusive breastfeeding by mothers with human immunodeficiency virus (HIV) does not increase the baby's risk of infection.

While most breastfeeding mothers are able to produce enough milk to fully meet their baby's nutritional needs for the first six months of life and beyond, there are situations when it is necessary for a breastfed baby to receive some supplementary feedings. These are some examples of situations in which partial or total formula feeding might be recommended:

- if the baby is at risk of developing hypoglycemia or has hypoglycemia that is not improving with breastfeeding;

- if the baby is dehydrated and the degree of dehydration is not improving with increased breastfeeding;
- if the mother is severely ill and unable to breastfeed;
- if the baby has a metabolic problem that requires a special formula (for example, galactosemia, phenylketonuria). (Note: With careful monitoring, babies with phenylketonuria (PKU) can breastfeed provided that they are getting both Lofenalac—a special formula for babies with PKU—and breast milk);
- if the mother experiences primary lactation failure and isn't able to produce enough milk for her baby; or
- if an adoptive mother is breastfeeding (in most cases, some degree of supplementation will be necessary, although she will likely be able to breastfeed her baby on a part-time basis).

If breastfeeding is only interrupted temporarily, you or your partner might want to feed your baby using a cup (a shot glass works particularly well), a spoon, or a dropper, or by attaching a lactation device to your finger ("finger feeding") until you're able to put her back to the breast rather than introducing a bottle. Some babies are unwilling to resume breastfeeding once they've discovered that there's less work required in extracting food from a bottle than a breast. Because different sucking techniques are used for breastfeeding and bottle-feeding, some babies forget how to latch on to a breast after they've been exposed to a bottle.

---

baby talk Chicken pox can be harmful or even fatal to a newborn baby if it's contracted during the first week of life. Babies born to women who develop chicken pox five days before or two days after the delivery should be given varicella zoster immune globulin as soon as possible after the birth, and both the mother and the baby should be isolated. If the mother has lesions but the baby does not, the mother should not have any contact with the baby—including breastfeeding—until all the lesions are dry and/or the infant has received the immune globulin. Breast milk may be supplied to the baby as long as the milk does not come into contact with any active lesions.

If supplementation is required, your health-care provider will recommend that you supplement with breast milk from a human milk bank (if applicable to your baby's situation) or that you use one of the following types of formula:

- *Milk-based formula:* Milk-based formula is recommended for full-term and preterm infants who don't have any special nutritional needs. This type of infant formula is made from cow's milk, but much of the protein found in cow's milk is removed to make it easier for babies to digest. A new generation of partially hydrolyzed cow's milk infant formula products is also available for babies who have difficulty digesting the protein in cow's milk. In this case, the protein is partially pre-digested.

- *Soy protein formula:* Soy formula is derived from soy protein rather than cow's milk protein. Soy protein is not a suitable choice for all infants, however, as some babies are allergic to soy. A 2009 Canadian Paediatric Society nutrition committee position statement recommended that the use of soy-based formulas be limited to infants with galactosemia (a metabolic disorder in which people cannot digest the sugar in milk) and those who cannot consume dairy-based products for cultural or religious reasons.

- *Specialized formulas:* There are a variety of specialized formulas designed to meet the needs of preterm infants and infants with metabolic disorders and other medical conditions.

Most formulas are fortified with iron (critical for infant development) and many manufacturers are now adding DHA (docosahexaenoic acid) and ARA (arachidonic acid), also known as Omega-3 and Omega-6 fatty acids. These fatty acids are known to contribute to brain and eye development. DHA and ARA naturally occur in breast milk.

If your baby requires infant formula, be sure to follow the formula preparation instructions, pay careful attention to hygiene, and stick with the same formula unless there's a medical reason to change. Don't heat your baby's bottle in the microwave (hot spots in the liquid could burn your baby) and never prop a bottle to feed the baby (propping poses a choking hazard and deprives you and your baby of time that might otherwise be spent cuddling).

Do breastfed babies need to drink water?

You don't have to worry about giving your baby water until after she's started to eat a variety of solid foods. At that point (usually around age 9 months), you can introduce water in a sippy cup. This is more about sippy cup skill-building than her needing water. She'll still be getting plenty of liquid from breast milk and from fruits and vegetables in her diet.

Do I really need to give my breastfed baby vitamin D?

Vitamin D deficiency is common among children and adults in Canada. Not only does our northerly latitude contribute to the problem (sunlight is a source of vitamin D), until recently, public health authorities underestimated the amount of vitamin D our bodies need to function at their best. Vitamin D plays an important role in calcium absorption, bone health, cell growth, and neuromuscular and immune functioning.

So what does this mean for you and your baby?

- Health Canada recommends that all infants receive a vitamin D supplement of 400 IU/day.
- The Canadian Paediatric Society has chosen to make a series of more targeted recommendations as opposed to a single, across-the-board recommendation.
  - If a baby is living in a northern (above the the 55th parallel) or Native community, a dose of 800 IU/day is recommended, especially during the winter months.
  - If a baby is being fed an infant formula that has been fortified with vitamin D, the baby does not require a separate supplement because he is receiving adequate quantities of vitamin D through food sources.
  - If a breastfeeding mother consumes large amounts of vitamin D (at least 4,000 IU/day), her infant may not require additional vitamin D supplementation.
  - Breastfeeding moms may instead choose to take 2,000 IU/day to meet their own vitamin D needs *and* to supplement their baby with the standard 400 IU/day dose.

Your health-care provider can help you to make sense of these recommendations so you can make the best decision for your baby.

My breastfed baby isn't gaining weight as quickly as my sister's formula-fed baby. Should I be concerned?

All babies have their own individual patterns of weight gain. The difference in weight gain may have nothing to do with the fact that one baby is breastfed and the other is formula-fed. It could be simply that each baby had different sets of parents and therefore a different gene pool to draw upon. That said, breastfed babies do tend to gain weight differently than their formula-fed counterparts—the key reason why the World Health Organization (WHO) developed separate infant growth charts for breastfed babies (as opposed to formula-fed babies) in 2006. It doesn't make sense to compare apples to oranges—which is exactly what you're doing if you try to plot a breastfed baby's weight gain patterns on a growth chart based on data from formula-fed babies.

While many parents are concerned that the different growth patterns of breastfed babies may mean that those babies aren't thriving to the same degree as formula-fed babies, that's looking at the issue backwards. It may be that the formula-fed babies are overweight; not the other way around. While we may have been culturally conditioned to believe otherwise, breastfed babies are the norm. A now-classic article published in the medical journal *Pediatrics* in 1997 pointed out that formula-fed babies grow more rapidly than breastfed babies during some parts of their first year, but that "to mistakenly advise mothers to supplement unnecessarily or to stop breastfeeding altogether" is "a *misinterpretation* of the growth patterns of healthy breastfed infants" and an issue of "great public health significance."

Do I need to do anything special to care for my breasts when I'm breastfeeding?

Your breasts are finally getting a chance to do what they were designed to do, so they don't require an extraordinary amount of pampering. That said, there are a few important points to keep in mind.

- Soap can be very drying to your skin, so it's best to avoid using soap on your nipples when you're breastfeeding. Besides, your breastfed baby might object to the taste and scent of your favourite brand of soap: she much prefers you *au naturel*.

- Forget about that sexy black bra that's languishing at the back of your underwear drawer: stick to wearing bras that fit you properly and that provide adequate support. A bra that's too tight may cause your breasts to become engorged, while a bra that doesn't provide adequate support can be extremely uncomfortable. And avoid underwire bras like the plague: they can contribute to plugged ducts.

- Keep in mind that your breasts are pretty much able to take care of themselves. There's no need to resort to fancy creams and lotions if your nipples are feeling a little tender. (In fact, most lactation experts advise that you avoid such products entirely.) Your best bet is to simply express a few drops of colostrum or milk when you're finished nursing and then let your nipples dry naturally. Exposing your nipples to air and light can also be helpful. (See the discussion about **sore nipples** later in this chapter.)

Are there any substances I should be avoiding while I'm breastfeeding?

You should continue to lead a baby-healthy lifestyle while you're breastfeeding, but the rules for breastfeeding mothers aren't quite as stringent as the rules for pregnant women.

- **Prescription and over-the-counter medications:** Most prescription and over-the-counter medications are highly diluted and/or rendered inactive by the time they make their way into breast milk. In other words, it's safe to continue breastfeeding while taking them. That said, there are some noteworthy exceptions, including chemotherapy drugs and radioactive compounds used for diagnostic or therapeutic purposes. Since it can be difficult to keep up to date on which drugs are and are not suitable for breastfeeding mothers, your best bet is to check with your doctor, midwife, and/or pharmacist about the advisability of taking a particular medication while you're nursing, or to call the Motherisk Clinic at Toronto's Hospital for Sick Children (www.motherisk.org or 1-877-439-2744) to request this type of information. Of course, it goes without saying that street drugs should be avoided during lactation, and that you should also make an effort to prevent family members or friends from exposing your baby to the smoke from any drugs that are inhaled.

- **Alcohol:** While alcohol use isn't considered to be quite as taboo when you're breastfeeding as when you're pregnant, moderation is definitely the way to go. Most health authorities recommend that you limit yourself to one drink per day and that you have that drink right after a feeding, to minimize the amount of alcohol that your baby receives via your breast milk. Alcohol in breast milk can make a baby sleepy, which can interfere with breastfeeding. Alcohol use also increases the risk of SIDS when babies and parents are co-sleeping because an inebriated parent may not be as responsive as usual to the presence of the baby.

- **Smoking:** Exposing your baby to second-hand smoke isn't a good thing. It increases his risk of SIDS and respiratory problems. However, that doesn't mean you shouldn't breastfeed if you are a smoker. The baby of a mother who smokes will do better if he is breastfed than if he is formula-fed. Quit or cut back if you can, and avoid smoking indoors, but plan to stick with breastfeeding.

- **Herbal products:** It's also important to exercise caution where herbal products are concerned. They may be "natural," but many of these products contain pharmacologically active substances that could be harmful to your baby. Since there hasn't been a lot of research on the effects of many of these products on breastfed babies, your best bet is to exercise caution unless you know for certain that it's safe for a nursing mother to use a particular herbal product while she's breastfeeding.

I'm going to be taking a course one night a week and my partner is going to need to feed my baby while I'm gone. At what point should I think about introducing a bottle?

Lactation experts advise against introducing a bottle until breastfeeding is well established. (What does "well established" mean? It means that you are confident your baby is feeding well, that you are producing plenty of milk, and that your nipples are not sore.) Not only do you risk having your breastfed baby develop a preference for artificial nipples if you introduce a bottle too soon, but offering supplemental feedings of anything other than breast milk could also interfere with your milk supply.

You might want to bear in mind that there are alternatives to offering a bottle to a breastfed baby. These include offering expressed breast milk from a spoon, a dropper, a small cup, or via a lactation device taped to an adult's finger. (The baby latches on to the fleshy part of the adult's finger.) Unfortunately, none of these alternatives is quite as convenient as offering a bottle, which is why many parents choose to go the bottle-feeding route instead. (Of course, your baby may solve your bottle-feeding dilemma for you, refusing to have anything to do with a plastic nipple now that she's experienced "the real thing.")

If you do decide to offer a bottle, make sure you wait until your baby's an old pro at nursing (she's been nursing for at least a month and breastfeeding is well established) and be sure to heed the following bits of advice.

- Don't expect your baby to take a bottle if "the real thing" is nearby. Have your partner or another person offer the bottle of expressed breast milk rather than trying to feed your baby the bottle yourself. Otherwise, your baby may become confused and upset, wondering why you're shoving a plastic nipple in her mouth when she can tell by her acute sense of smell that your breasts are within latching distance.

- Offer the bottle at a time when your baby's more likely to be receptive. If you attempt to introduce the bottle when she's frantically hungry, she may become angry at the person offering the bottle, wondering why you're offering her a plastic "toy" to chew on when all she wants is food.

- Don't shove the nipple of the bottle in your baby's mouth—something that may cause her to gag and turn away. Instead, drip a bit of breast milk onto her lips and then wait for her to open her mouth and draw the nipple in herself. This is definitely one of those situations when slow and steady wins the race.

- Try a variety of different feeding positions. If your breastfed baby keeps looking for a breast whenever she is held in your usual breastfeeding position, have the person offering the bottle hold her in a different position instead. (Hint: Some parents find that breastfed babies are more likely to accept a bottle if the person offering the bottle stands and sways gently during the feeding. Strange but true . . .)

---

baby talk Don't heat breast milk in the microwave because the intense heat will quickly destroy many of its disease-fighting properties. And, just so you know, nothing for a baby should be heated in a microwave, due to the risk of hot spots. (Hot spots occur when food or liquid feels warm in one spot but is scalding hot in another.) Besides, babies do not need to have their liquids warmed up. You can take the chill off a bottle of breast milk by letting it sit in a cup of warm water, but that's the most that's required, and even that is not absolutely necessary.

mother wisdom Don't introduce a bottle just because your partner is eager to have a chance to feed the baby. Remind him that he'll have plenty of opportunities to play chef for the new arrival in a couple of months' time when the baby starts eating solid food. In the meantime, it's important for him to do whatever he can to support the breastfeeding relationship between mother and baby—even if that means missing out on some of the fun of feeding the new arrival for the time being. Once the whole concept of nipple confusion is explained to partners, they tend to back off a little on the bottle-feeding issue and find other ways to play an active role in their babies' lives.

- Listen to your baby if she gives the bottle the total thumbs-down. Either try reintroducing the bottle on another occasion or switch to another feeding method like cup feeding, finger feeding, or giving the baby milk from a dropper or spoon. And even if she does accept an alternative method of feeding when she's totally famished, don't be surprised if she tries to hold out for "the real thing" as long as possible. You may be astounded to arrive home one night and discover that your little darling has gone four or five hours without food because she's decided nothing but fresh breast milk will do.

baby talk The ongoing controversy about nipple confusion can be a source of, well, *confusion* to new parents, who may receive conflicting information about when (or if) they should introduce a bottle to a breastfed baby.

The Canadian Institute of Child Health offers these cautionary words in its *National Breastfeeding Guidelines for Health Care Providers*: "Sucking a bottle is fundamentally different from suckling at the breast, and lactation may be undermined by making the infant's suckling motions inappropriate for breastfeeding. For some babies this preference appears to be related to the instant flow of milk they obtain with minimal effort when bottle-feeding."

Most health-care practitioners prefer to err on the side of caution by making parents aware that the early introduction of the bottle could potentially result in such breastfeeding-related complications as breast refusal, a poor latch, or sore nipples. (A baby doesn't need to open her mouth as wide to bottle-feed as to breastfeed, so when the baby goes back to breastfeeding again, she may tend to latch on to the nipple rather than the areola.) Since it's impossible to predict which babies will be able to hop from breast to bottle with relative ease and which ones won't, if breastfeeding is important to you, it's probably best to delay introducing a bottle for as long as possible or even to avoid bottles altogether.

How long should I breastfeed my baby?

The Canadian Paediatric Society recommends that babies be exclusively breastfed for six months. After six months, a combination of breast milk and solid foods are required for proper nutrition. Breastfeeding can continue for up to two years and beyond as long as mother and baby are willing. While your baby is mastering the mechanics of eating solid food and getting used to all those new tastes and textures, breast milk will continue to be the mainstay of her diet.

Should I wean from breast to formula or straight to cow's milk?

It depends on your baby's age. Babies who stop breastfeeding before age 12 months should almost always switch to an iron-fortified infant formula rather than to cow's milk (unless your baby's doctor advises otherwise). A baby's system isn't mature enough to digest all the minerals and proteins in cow's milk, plus there's an increased risk that your baby will become sensitized (hypersensitive) to the milk protein in cow's milk if you switch to cow's milk too soon. After age 12 months, most babies can be weaned from the breast directly to homogenized (3.25 per cent) cow's milk.

By the way, you don't have to wean your baby simply because you're returning to work. A part-time breastfeeding schedule works well for many working moms, and many moms find that they cherish the time they spend breastfeeding and connecting with their baby during their non-working hours. (See related section on **breastfeeding and working**, which follows.)

How do you wean a baby?

The easiest way to wean a baby is to let her wean herself. Yes, they really do all wean, when they are ready. But if you decide that you'd like to wean your baby before she weans herself ("mother-led" rather than "baby-led" weaning), you'll want to make the weaning process as gentle as possible for both of you. Here are a few tips.

---

mother wisdom Don't let anyone pressure you into weaning your baby before you're ready just because your baby has reached a particular age or has passed the point at which you had originally planned to wean her. This decision should be entirely up to the two of you.

- Pay careful attention to your timing. Don't try to wean your baby at the same time that she's dealing with an ear infection, getting a new tooth, or trying to adjust to your return to work.
- Decide whether you want to wean your baby to a bottle or a cup.
- Eliminate one feeding at a time, starting with the feeding that your baby cares about least (or that is the least convenient for you). Most mothers find it works best to eliminate one feeding per week. Be sure to allow at least three days between dropped feedings, in order to give your milk production time to decrease comfortably and gradually and to reduce the risk of plugged ducts and mastitis. Don't feel obliged to stick to your pre-determined weaning schedule if you or your child find that you want to hang on to breastfeeding a little longer.
- Find other ways to show your love for your child to help ease the transition for her. Read stories together or have some quiet cuddling time at the end of the day. You don't want your baby to miss out on the special together time that you enjoyed while she was nursing just because you'll no longer be breastfeeding.
- Don't be surprised if you find yourself grieving the loss of your breastfeeding relationship, even if both you and your baby are ready to wean. There are few experiences in life as special as that of nursing a baby, so it's only natural to feel a little sad about saying goodbye to this chapter in your life.

While you might assume that your milk will dry up and disappear overnight once you've weaned your baby, it may take several months. Some women, in fact, are able to express a drop or two of milk from their breasts for up to several years after weaning. The only time you're likely to be troubled by a lot of leaking and pressure is if you wean your baby quickly—or, of course, if your baby weans you cold turkey, suddenly and permanently refusing the breast (which is more likely to be a nursing strike than real weaning). In this case, you'll want to wear a bra that provides plenty of support and express just enough milk to relieve your discomfort. (If you express too much milk, you'll continue producing milk.) You may also find that applying ice packs to your breasts several times a day helps to relieve any breast pain you're experiencing.

---

mom's the word "My daughter weaned herself by 13 months, and although my head was ready, my heart wasn't. Fortunately, she made the decision so I didn't have the guilt of cutting her off or the power struggle I've seen with friends' babies."
—JANE, 33, MOTHER OF TWO

It may also take several months for your breasts to return to their pre-pregnancy size, at which point you may be surprised to discover that they're a little less firm than when you set out on this adventure called motherhood. (Breastfeeding isn't to blame for these breast changes, by the way; they're an inevitable side effect of pregnancy, whether you breastfeed or not. Like the stretch marks that may now adorn your belly, they're souvenirs of your child-bearing years.)

BREASTFEEDING AND WORKING

If breastfeeding is well established and you and your baby are both enjoying this special part of your relationship, there's no need to stop nursing just because you're returning to work.

Finding a breastfeeding-friendly caregiver

One of the keys to successfully breastfeeding your baby after you return to work is choosing a breastfeeding-friendly caregiver. That means looking for someone who

- breastfed her own babies and/or has cared for a number of breastfed babies over the years;
- encourages you to breastfeed your baby when you drop your baby off, when you pick her up at the end of the day, and perhaps during your lunch hour as well;
- is aware of the challenges of caring for a baby who is breastfed (such as bottle refusal) and has creative ways of dealing with the situation (for example, feeding the baby with a cup or a medicine dropper instead); and
- has a repertoire of techniques for dealing with breastfed babies who are used to nursing when they're in need of soothing (easily the toughest part of caring for a breastfed baby).

What you are looking for is a caregiver who understands the benefits of breastfeeding to both mother and baby, and who will do whatever she can to support your decision to continue breastfeeding your baby after you return to work.

Most mothers who return to work before their baby's first birthday will need to pump or express milk at least once in order to maintain their milk supply and to continue to feel comfortable. If you don't have much time to pump or express milk, a double-horned breast pump will likely be your best bet. It will allow you to collect milk quickly from both breasts in minimal time.

Breastfed babies consume an average of 830 to 950 millilitres (28 to 32 ounces) of breast milk in a 24-hour period. If you're going to be away from your baby for eight hours, you should plan to leave at least 300 to 350 millilitres (10 to 12 ounces) with your baby's caregiver.

If you need to introduce a bottle to your baby, have someone other than you offer the bottle—perhaps your baby's caregiver. It generally works best to have the other person offer the bottle before the baby is too hungry and to help the baby understand right away that there is breast milk in the bottle. (Warm the bottle nipple in warm water and then dip it in breast milk to make it as appealing as possible.) Suggest that the caregiver offer the bottle when the baby is drowsy (as opposed to wide awake) and that she rock or walk with the baby to encourage the baby to take the bottle. If the baby becomes upset, try the bottle another time. A baby can be fed breast milk via medicine spoon, a small glass (shot-glass sized), or a sippy cup, if necessary.

Choosing a breast pump

In the market for a breast pump? Here are some points to keep in mind when you're trying to decide which model will work best for you.

- **Cost:** If you're going to be using your breast pump a couple of times a day, you'll want to spring for a high-end model. On the other hand, if you're only going to need a breast pump every now and again, it may be difficult to justify a pump purchase at all. You may be better off learning to hand-express. Don't overlook the fact that renting a breast pump may be an option, depending on where you live. (Contact your local La Leche League, your public health unit, or your local hospital to inquire about breast pump rental options in your community.)

- **Efficiency:** It's important to factor in how much time you will have for pumping at work. If you have a half-hour lunch break, a high-efficiency, double-horned electric model is probably your best bet since it will allow you to pump milk from both breasts at the same time.

- **Portability:** If you're going to be lugging the pump back and forth to work with you each day, you'll want to opt for a model that's relatively lightweight and easy to carry. You'll also want to think about where you'll be doing your pumping at work. Will you have easy access to an electrical outlet or would a battery-operated model be a better bet? Would hand-expressing be the best option of all?

- **Noise level:** How noisy is the breast pump you're considering? Unless you don't mind announcing to everyone in your office that it's pumping time again, you'll want to look for a relatively quiet model—or to stick with hand-expressing.

- **Easy maintenance:** Look for a model that's easy to clean (that features dishwasher-safe parts).

Pumping 101

It's one thing to own a breast pump; it's quite another thing to know how to use it. Here are some tips on putting your breast pump to work for you.

- Expect it to take a while to master the art of using a breast pump. Consider your first few sessions to be about mastering technique rather than collecting milk.

- Having a pump that fits is crucial. If the flange is too small, it can damage your nipple or breast and you won't get much milk; if it is too big,

TABLE 6.2

Hand-Expression versus a Breast Pump: Which Option Is Best for You?

Hand-expression	Breast pump
Advantages: Free. No equipment required. Milk ejection boost. The skin-to-skin contact triggers more effective milk ejections in some women (as compared to the sensation of plastic or glass on skin). Portable. No electricity or batteries required. Low-maintenance. Only your hands need to be washed afterward.	Advantages: Automatic pumps take care of the physical work of pumping. Double pumps are capable of expressing more milk in less time. Some mothers feel uncomfortable touching their own breasts. Hospital-grade breast pumps are more effective at establishing milk production when a baby is not yet breastfeeding.
Disadvantages: Practice is required. Physical effort is required. Can be time-consuming if you express milk from one breast at a time. Not as effective at establishing milk production as a hospital-grade breast pump if your baby is not yet breastfeeding. Not all women can express their milk very easily.	Disadvantages: High-end models are expensive and less-expensive models may not be as effective. Pump parts can break or be left behind. A power source (electricity, batteries) is required. Pumps can be noisy. Pump parts need to be washed.

you won't get a good seal or vacuum and won't get much milk. Some pumps come with several flanges; with other styles you may have to order another flange separately. One size does *not* fit all.

- There's no need to wash the pump after each use, especially if you are going to be using it again the same day. Just throw it in the fridge. Remember, human milk is antiseptic and kills bacteria. Washing it once every 24 hours is more than adequate.

- Store pumped milk in the refrigerator at work or in a cooler bag with ice packs if you can. Breast milk can be stored safely at room temperature for up to eight hours; but if you are able to chill it, it will keep longer. If you know that you'll be using the expressed milk within the next three to five days, keep it in the back of your refrigerator (away from

- the door, where there are greater temperature fluctuations), as opposed to freezing it. If you decide to freeze it, breast milk can be stored in the freezer compartment inside a refrigerator for two weeks, in a separate-door refrigerator freezer for three to four months, and in a deep-freeze for six to twelve months. Freezing does destroy some of the immune factors, so refrigerator storage is preferred.

- Freeze breast milk in small batches so you can defrost just a few ounces at a time. Use heavy plastic or glass containers or specially designed freezer bags. Disposable bottle liners aren't designed to tolerate the extreme change in temperature and they may spring leaks as a result. Note: If you're adding fresh breast milk to milk that has already been frozen, be sure to refrigerate the freshly pumped breast milk before adding it to the frozen breast milk, and make sure that the amount of milk that you're adding is less than the amount that's already frozen. This will prevent the warm milk from defrosting the frozen milk.

- Don't assume that your frozen breast milk has gone bad just because it's turned yellow. This is what breast milk looks like when it's frozen. Likewise, don't hit the panic button if you notice that the breast milk you collected has separated into layers. If this occurs, simply stir the breast milk thoroughly when it is defrosted.

---

mother wisdom Some mothers find that after their milk has been frozen (or even stored in the refrigerator for a few days) it has an unpleasant smell and a soapy taste. This is due to high levels of an enzyme that breaks down the milk during storage. It's not harmful, but many babies dislike the taste. You can't fix milk that has already become soapy-tasting, but you can prevent this from happening in the future by scalding your expressed milk (heating it to just below the boiling point) before putting it in the fridge or freezer.

- When you serve your baby breast milk, offer her just a couple of ounces at a time. You can always offer her more if she's still hungry.

- To thaw frozen breast milk, either allow it to thaw gradually in the refrigerator or place the container of breast milk in warm water.

- Once breast milk has been thawed, it should not be refrozen. It can, however, be safely stored in the refrigerator for up to 24 hours (unless it was defrosted in warm water, in which case it must be used immediately or discarded).

TROUBLESHOOTING COMMON PROBLEMS

Here's how to cope with some of the most common—and frustrating—breastfeeding problems.

Breast engorgement

If you go to sleep one night feeling like your usual self and wake up the next morning with a chest that could rival that of any porn star, chances are you're experiencing breast engorgement.

Breast engorgement is a temporary condition that is triggered by a rapid increase in blood circulation and milk production caused by postpartum hormones. It tends to be most severe in first-time mothers, decreasing in intensity following subsequent births. Your breasts feel hard, swollen, and extremely tender, and may be so full that your nipples are flattened against your breasts. Prolonged engorgement can lead to such unwelcome complications as cracked nipples and a decreased milk supply.

Most of the discomfort you experience from breast engorgement is the result of tissue swelling triggered by all the glandular activity during the first two or three days postpartum. The swelling will gradually go away on its own, but here's what you can do to stay comfortable in the meantime.

- Apply heat to your breasts right before feedings by applying washcloths soaked in warm water or by taking a warm shower. Then gently massage your breasts to encourage the milk to start flowing. (The combination of heat and massage promotes the dilation of your milk ducts, making it easier for the milk to start flowing.)
- Use cold compresses in between feedings to reduce the amount of swelling in your breasts.
- Put your baby to the breast. Note: If your breasts are so engorged that your areola is completely stretched out, your baby may have difficulty latching on. You can solve this problem by hand-expressing (see Table 6.3 for some tips on hand-expressing milk) to relieve the pressure. Note: If your breasts are painful to touch, be gentle when you're

expressing milk. Handling your breasts too vigorously may damage the underlying breast tissue—something that may make you more susceptible to mastitis. Note: Using a breast pump is not generally recommended while your breasts are engorged.

---

mother wisdom You can massage your entire breast using a standard hair comb that has been lubricated with a bit of soap or hand cream. Starting from the top of the breast, press the side of the comb firmly but gently against the skin and slowly "comb out" the breast, down toward the nipple. Bring the comb back up to the top of the breast, move it over to the next part and repeat until the whole breast has been combed. This method often works better then using your fingers to move milk through your breast.

- Encourage your baby to nurse as often and as long as possible at each feeding so that he will be able to extract the maximum amount of milk from your breasts.

- If your breasts are so engorged that you find it painful to put your baby to the breast at all, try taking a pain relief medication (acetominophen or ibuprofen) 20 minutes before your next nursing session. That should help to take the edge off the pain. Then express a bit of milk before your next feeding session to prevent any further breast trauma.

- Apply ice packs to your breasts for 10 minutes after each feeding to help reduce some of the swelling. You can either make your own ice packs by filling a zipper-style freezer bag with water or simply rely on a bag of frozen corn or peas. (For added comfort, wrap the ice pack or vegetables in a tea towel before applying them to your breasts.) Clean cabbage leaves tucked in your bra are another tried-and-true remedy.

- Avoid wearing a bra that is too tight. An overly tight bra will increase the pressure on your ducts and simply add to your engorgement woes. A bra that is too loose can also cause problems, especially if you have large breasts.

TABLE 6.3

Hand-Expressing Breast Milk

Here are the basic steps involved in hand-expressing breast milk.

- Find a sterile container (a wide-mouthed cup or jar or a mixing bowl tend to work best) that you can use to collect your breast milk as you express it.
- Sit in a comfortable chair, put on some relaxing music, or tune into your favourite show on television—anything to relieve the monotony of sitting there expressing milk. Some women find it helpful to have a photo of their baby close by to provide them with inspiration while they're pumping.
- Apply heat to your breasts (such as a warm washcloth) and then gently massage your breasts to encourage the milk to start flowing. You'll get the best results if you massage your breasts gently, one at a time, starting from the top. Gently move your fingers in a circular motion, making your way around the sides and bottom of the breast. Then stroke yourself lightly from the armpit, from above and below the breast, and from the middle of the chest toward the nipple. There's no need to massage the nipples themselves, by the way. They'll be stimulated by the rest of the breast massage.
- Hold the sterile container under your breast. (Note: To minimize the risk of contamination, the milk should run directly from the breast into the container without passing over your fingers.)
- Hold your breast with your thumb above and your first two fingers below the breast. Make sure your fingers and thumb are placed about an inch and a half back from the nipple. (In most cases, you'll be putting your fingers and thumb just outside the edge of the areola, but if you have an exceptionally wide areola, they may need to be on the areola itself. It's the distance to the nipple that counts.)
- Push your thumb and fingers together while simultaneously pushing back toward the chest wall.
- Gently roll the thumb and fingers forward to empty the milk pools. (Note: Do this gently but firmly to avoid bruising your breast tissue. And avoid squeezing or cupping the breast, sliding your fingers, or pulling out the skin on the breast, all of which may prove painful and counterproductive. If you're doing it right, it shouldn't hurt.)
- Repeat the sequence until you are no longer obtaining any milk from the breast, varying your position slightly to encourage the milk to continue to flow. (Don't be surprised if you find that some positions work better for you than others. This is perfectly normal.)
- Switch breasts at least once during each session—ideally twice to encourage maximum draining.
- To maximize the amount of milk expressed, aim for shorter, more frequent sessions.

mother wisdom — Some women find that leaning over a basin full of warm water helps to encourage their milk to let down. The heat from the water combined with the effects of gravity can bring tremendous relief if you're dealing with tender, swollen breasts.

Sore nipples

Sore nipples are another common breastfeeding problem. Most often these are caused by the baby not latching on well, either because he's not positioned well at the breast or because there are anatomical problems.

Sore nipples can also be caused by thrush (discussed later in this chapter), the use of soap or ointments on the nipples (which can dry and irritate your nipples and areola), a condition called Reynaud's syndrome, or other issues. Unfortunately, if the problem is not corrected quickly, sore nipples can sometimes progress into cracked nipples and/or a full-blown breast infection.

Here are some tips on coping with sore nipples.

- Breastfeed your baby frequently to prevent your breasts from becoming overly full, something that can lead to both engorgement and nipple soreness. If you're having problems with engorgement, you should be putting your baby to the breast at least 10 to 12 times each day.
- If you can hardly bear the thought of having anything touch your breasts, let alone a newborn baby with a vigorous suck, try taking some sort of pain relief medication approximately 20 minutes before your next feeding and/or numbing your nipples and areola with an ice pack right before you nurse your baby.
- Before you offer your baby the breast, use heat, breast massage, and/or manual expression to encourage the milk to start flowing. (If your milk has already let down by the time your baby latches on, she won't have to nurse as vigorously to get her feeding started.)
- Start nursing on the least sore side first.
- Feed your baby promptly when she first starts cueing you that she could be hungry rather than waiting for her to start crying. A hungry baby may be too impatient to latch on well.

- It may help to try a different position. The baby may latch on better in this new position, and it will put pressure on a different part of your nipple so the pain may decrease.

- Expose your nipples to two to three minutes of sunshine a day. Granted, this may be a bit difficult to pull off if it's February and there's a blizzard in progress, but, assuming that our harsh Canadian climate will cooperate, a little bit of sunshine can make a world of difference in terms of healing.

- Apply ultra-pure lanolin (a natural lubricant extracted from sheep's wool and then mixed with olive oil and water to produce an emulsion) or ask your lactation consultant about hydrogel dressings (soothing pads that are worn in your bra to help promote healing).

- Change your breast pads frequently. The constant wetness may interfere with healing. It's best to simply allow your nipples to air dry.

- If even the weight of your clothing has become excruciatingly painful, try wearing breast shells (not breast shields!) in an extra-large bra. The breast shells will hold the bra fabric away from your sore nipples, ensuring that nothing but air comes into contact with them. (Note: You should be able to purchase a set of breast shells from your lactation consultant, your local La Leche League leader, or the nearest medical supply store.)

- Avoid using nipple shields unless they are specifically recommended by your lactation consultant. Nipple shields tend to cause more problems than they solve. They can interfere with your baby's sucking pattern and reduce your milk supply significantly, due to decreased nipple stimulation. If you absolutely have to use one (for instance you have an extremely painful cracked nipple or a latching problem that can't be solved any other way), plan to stop using the nipple shield as soon as possible (ideally within a few feedings) and have your baby weighed frequently to ensure that she's gaining weight properly. It may also help to pump or hand-express after each feeding with the nipple shield. Then give the milk you get to the baby at the next feeding.

Flat or inverted nipples

Not every woman is born with the perky erect nipples that you see in all the breastfeeding books; about 10 per cent of women are born with nipples that are flat or inverted (nipples that retract into the breast tissue rather than protruding and becoming erect when they are stimulated).

While having flat or inverted nipples may pose a few breastfeeding challenges, in most cases these types of problems can be resolved once you've learned a few simple tricks, like rolling your nipples between your thumb and forefinger before a feeding (to help the nipples to stand out); expressing a few drops of breast milk at the start of each feeding (to encourage your baby to open her mouth wide); and supporting the breast and gently compressing the tissue behind the areola so that it's easier for your baby to latch on. Remember, babies breastfeed, they don't "nipple feed," so your baby doesn't really need protruding nipples to feed well. A lactation consultant may be able to suggest some other effective "tricks of the trade" for working with flat or inverted nipples.

---

mother wisdom If you have flat or inverted nipples, you'll want to make a point of nursing frequently in order to prevent your breasts from becoming engorged—something that could make it very difficult for your baby to latch on and that could ultimately result in other breastfeeding problems such as sore nipples.

Leaking

Don't be surprised if you find yourself leaking milk during or between feedings. This is a very common experience during the early weeks of motherhood. In fact, a study conducted by the Harvard School of Public Health found that fully 57 per cent of new mothers leak enough milk to soak through their clothes on a regular basis.

Fortunately, the problem tends to be relatively short-lived: the Harvard researchers discovered that most leaking stops by the 20th week postpartum. Here are tips on coping with the Great Milk Flood in the meantime.

- Get in the habit of wearing breast pads. That way, when you feel that tell-tale tingling sensation that indicates that your milk is about to let down (which can be triggered by something as simple as thinking about your baby), you won't have to worry about soaking your shirt in a matter of minutes. While breast pads with plastic or waterproof liners can help to minimize the amount of leakage, they also tend to contribute to sore nipples and breast infections, so you're better off sticking to the non-waterproof variety and changing them a little more frequently.

- Don't panic if you end up leaking breast milk on to your clothes. Unlike formula, breast milk doesn't stain clothes. And if you wear patterned rather than solid-coloured tops, or an unbuttoned shirt over a tank or T-shirt it'll be almost impossible for anyone to tell that you've experienced any leakage at all.

- If you find yourself caught without a breast pad and you want to minimize the amount of leakage, try this handy-dandy technique: fold your arms across your breasts and press firmly toward the chest wall or use your finger or thumb to provide pressure directly over the nipple. That will usually do the trick.

- Don't be surprised or embarrassed if you find yourself ejecting milk when you reach a sexual climax. This is a byproduct of the oxytocin that causes your uterus to contract during orgasm. (You might want to tip off your partner ahead of time about this unexpected extra during sex so that he or she isn't caught off guard!)

Plugged ducts

If you notice a lump in your breast that is tender to the touch, it's probably the result of a plugged duct. A duct can become plugged if the milk in your breasts is not being fully drained, something that can lead to both a buildup of milk and inflammation in the surrounding tissue.

A plugged duct typically develops gradually, only affecting one breast. While there's no increased warmth in the affected breast (a tell-tale sign of a full-blown breast infection), there is mild, localized pain, and in some cases there may be a white spot on the nipple at the location of the plugged milk duct.

It's important to treat a plugged duct promptly in order to prevent it from developing into mastitis (a breast infection). Here's what to do.

- Have a warm shower, apply warm washcloths, or snuggle up to a hot water bottle on the affected breast in an attempt to promote drainage.

- Massage the breast gently using both your fingertips and the palm of your hand to try to encourage milk circulation. You should focus particularly on massaging the area behind and over the lump.

- Breastfeed your baby more often, offering her the breast with the plugged duct first.

- Ensure that your baby is positioned to promote maximum drainage. This means pointing your baby's chin toward the plugged area.
- Massage your breast partway through the feeding as this will also help to encourage proper milk flow.
- Avoid tight or restrictive clothing, which may prevent the plugged duct from clearing. Go braless if at all possible.

Mastitis (breast infection)

If you wake up one morning with flu-like symptoms, including a fever, and your breasts feel firm, swollen, and painful and are red or red-streaked and hot to the touch, chances are you're dealing with mastitis (the inflammation of the breast tissue and/or the milk ducts in all or a portion of the breast).

According to a 2009 Cochrane Review, as many as one in three breastfeeding mothers may develop mastitis at some point. Mastitis can be caused by a sudden decrease in the frequency of feedings (for example, if your baby goes on a nursing strike), which can result in blocked ducts, cracked nipples, and/or inadequate milk drainage. Mastitis can also be caused by cracked or damaged nipples, because this allows bacteria to get into the breast. While mastitis can be miserable to deal with while it lasts, it usually clears up quickly if you continue to nurse your baby from the affected breast, get plenty of rest, drink plenty of fluids, and take an antibiotic if one is recommended by your doctor.

Here are some other important tips on coping with the misery that is mastitis.

- Increase the frequency of your baby's feedings, offering your baby the infected breast first in order to promote maximum drainage. Don't be concerned about passing the infection on to your baby; this is one thing you can scratch off your worry list right now.
- Apply heat to the infected breast (either by having a warm shower or by applying warm washcloths) and massage the affected area before and during each nursing session to encourage the milk to flow.
- Experiment with a variety of different nursing positions until you find the one that allows for maximum milk drainage.
- Take acetaminophen for the pain (it will also help to bring down your fever) and get in touch with your doctor if the infection hasn't eased up

within six to eight hours. Your doctor may want to prescribe some sort of antibiotic to help clear up the infection. Cabbage leaf compresses can bring considerable relief, too.

- Untreated or poorly treated breast infections occasionally develop into a breast abscess (a collection of pus in one area of the breast). You should suspect that you've developed a breast abscess if your mastitis symptoms continue even after you've been taking antibiotics for two or three days. If you're still feeling miserable at this point you will need to get in touch with your doctor right away. The abscess will need to be drained surgically. In the meantime, continue to breastfeed your baby as usual.

---

mom's the word "With my two boys, I developed mastitis. My body started aching, and there was a hard lump in my breast. I started running a fever and having chills and generally feeling the most ill I'd ever felt in my life. If you develop mastitis, it really helps to breastfeed often, especially on the infected side. You should also make sure you keep your breasts dry and that you change your breast pads often. Try massaging the hard lump in a warm bath and applying warm compresses and see if that helps, and call your doctor to see if an antibiotic is in order."

—CHRISTINA, 25, MOTHER OF TWO

Thrush (oral candidiasis)

Sometimes a breastfeeding mother and her baby will develop a breastfeeding-related yeast infection known as thrush (oral candidiasis). Symptoms in the mother include the sudden onset of persistently sore nipples (nipples that are red, itchy, sore, and/or burning) accompanied by shooting pains in the breast during or just after a feeding (these pains tend to be particularly acute during the milk-ejection reflex). Symptoms in the baby include white cottage cheese–like patches on the tongue and the sides of the mouth (oral thrush) and a red spotty diaper rash (a classic yeast-based diaper rash). Babies breastfed by diabetic mothers tend to be especially susceptible to thrush.

Both the mother and the baby should be treated for thrush. Treatment usually consists of the application of a topical anti-fungal ointment to the mother's nipples and areola; an anti-fungal liquid to the baby's tongue, gums, and mouth; and an anti-fungal ointment to the diaper area. Unfortunately, thrush can be rather difficult to get rid of, so you and your baby may have to try more than one type of treatment (Nystatin cream or ointment, Gentian violet, or anti-fungal cream) before you get any relief.

Here are some important pointers to keep in mind when you're dealing with thrush.

---

baby talk Both breastfed and formula-fed babies are susceptible to thrush. Babies are most likely to pick up thrush during the birth process (although symptoms usually aren't visible until seven to ten days after the delivery). It is possible, however, for breastfed babies to develop thrush at any age.

- Be sure to keep the ointments that have been prescribed for you and your baby separate to minimize the opportunities for cross-contamination. Note: Do not allow the dropper to come into direct contact with the baby's mouth or you will contaminate it.
- If you're also being treated for a vaginal yeast infection, your partner may need to be treated as well.
- If your doctor suggests that you and your baby use Gentian violet to clear up thrush, keep in mind that it's very messy stuff. Everything it comes into contact with will be stained bright purple. Rarely, it can also cause ulcers in the mouths of some babies, something to be on the lookout for if you happen to go the Gentian violet route.
- Pay extra attention to cleanliness. Hand-washing is critically important during this time, as is sterilizing anything that touches the breast or your baby's mouth (such as breast pump parts or a pacifier).
- Prolonged sucking of a bottle or pacifier can prolong thrush by causing minor abrasions in the lining of the mouth—an important point to keep in mind if your baby uses a bottle or a pacifier on a regular basis. Note: Once you clear up the thrush, you'll want to get rid of any bottle nipples or pacifiers that were in use while your baby was infected. The last thing you want to do is trigger a recurrence.

- Thrush and other yeast infections tend to be more common after a course of antibiotics. You can reduce your risk of developing such an infection by eating yogurt with acidophilus (live yogurt cultures, known as probiotics) while you're taking antibiotics, or by taking acidophilus in capsule form. (You'll find acidophilus tablets in the health food store.)

Be prepared for thrush to recur, even with the best management. Multiple courses of treatment may be required. However, eventually, the thrush will go away for good, usually by the time your baby reaches 6 months of age.

BREASTFEEDING UNDER SPECIAL CIRCUMSTANCES

Some mothers and babies face some special challenges getting breastfeeding off to a good start. Here's what you need to know about:

- breastfeeding a premature baby;
- breastfeeding a baby with a congenital problem that affects her ability to breastfeed;
- breastfeeding after adoption;
- breastfeeding after breast enhancement or breast reduction surgery; and
- breastfeeding multiples.

Breastfeeding a premature baby

There are tremendous health benefits to breastfeeding a premature baby. Not only is a premature baby less capable of fighting off infection than a full-term baby, many premature babies end up living in an environment (the special-care nursery) where antibiotic-resistant infectious diseases may be easily transmitted. Breast milk can make a world of difference to a premature baby with an already compromised immune system. It can literally be lifesaving.

Here's another benefit to breastfeeding a premature baby: your breasts instinctively know how to produce the type of milk your baby needs at this stage of his development—milk that contains higher-than-average amounts of protein, nitrogen, sodium, chloride, iron, and fatty acids. And, as your baby matures, the composition of your breast milk changes to meet your baby's changing nutritional requirements. By the time your original due date rolls around, your breast milk will contain the unique blend of nutrients needed by full-term babies.

You'll also want to learn about the benefits of kangaroo care (skin-to-skin contact) and connect with other parents of premature babies.

If your baby is very small, she will probably be fed by a nasogastric tube (a tube that extends through the baby's nose or mouth and into the baby's stomach) until she's able to remain stable outside the isolette for short periods of time and learns how to coordinate her sucking and swallowing reflexes (something that typically happens around 32 weeks' gestation).

Note: You don't have to wait until the sucking and swallowing reflexes kick in before you start preparing your baby to breastfeed—your baby can lick or nuzzle against your breast prior to this time. And, of course, you can express breast milk for your baby right from Day 1. If your baby is a large premature baby, she may be fed by a cup, spoon, or syringe rather than a nasogastric tube. Even if your baby is not yet able to latch on and breastfeed, you should plan to offer the breast regularly and practise kangaroo care as often as possible in preparation for future breastfeeding. If you are going to be pumping breast milk for your premature baby, you should plan to pump at least as often as your baby would normally be nursing—at least eight times per day or more. You don't have to feel pressured to provide your baby's entire food supply (although that, of course, is the ideal): any amount of breast milk that you can provide will be beneficial to your baby. It's also something that only you can do for your baby—something that you may find tremendously rewarding and reassuring during this stressful time in your life. As Tamara Eberlein notes in *When You're Expecting Twins, Triplets, or Quads*, "My breast milk was a lifeline that I—and only I—could throw to my babies, via nasogastric tubes, as they faced their sink-or-swim struggles in the NICU. Considering how much of their care I was forced to entrust to others, providing this unique form of nourishment helped me feel more like a real mother."

---

baby talk According to the Canadian Institute of Child Health, breastfeeding has been shown to be the single most effective means of preventing necrotizing enterocolitis (NEC) in a premature baby—a disease that is six times more common in bottle-fed babies than in breastfed babies.

Breastfeeding a baby with a congenital problem

Some babies are born with congenital anomalies that make breastfeeding difficult or even impossible. In most cases, these babies will still derive tremendous benefits from breast milk, even if they aren't actually able to nurse at the breast. Consider these words of wisdom from Dr. Jack Newman and Teresa Pitman, co-authors of *Dr. Jack Newman's Guide to Breastfeeding*: "Some medical professionals feel that if the baby is not perfect, the baby needs formula, while in truth the opposite approach should prevail."

Here's what you need to know about some of the most common types of congenital problems that can interfere with breastfeeding.

- **Baby who is tongue-tied:** If your baby makes clicking sounds while he is nursing, has trouble staying on the breast, or has poor weight gain, or you experience a great deal of nipple pain even though your baby's latch appears to be good, it's possible that your baby is tongue-tied. This means that your baby's frenulum (the stringy piece of membrane under his tongue) is unusually short. Your baby's pediatrician or another doctor can clip your baby's frenulum to treat this problem. Because there aren't many nerves and blood vessels in the frenulum, it's a fairly simple, painless, and almost blood-free procedure.

- **Cleft lip and cleft palate:** Most babies with cleft lip are able to breastfeed if you use your thumb to plug the opening in the lip, or if your breast is large enough to block the opening. However, if the alveolar ridge (the ridge where the teeth will eventually be) is also affected by the cleft, breastfeeding may be much more difficult. It's also very challenging—and sometimes impossible—to breastfeed a baby with a cleft palate. But even if breastfeeding itself isn't possible, breast milk can be expressed and fed to the baby using other feeding methods.

- **Down syndrome:** Babies with Down syndrome may have difficulty breastfeeding because they have lower muscle tone than other babies and because they have smaller-than-average sized mouths with typical-sized tongues, which causes protruding—two factors that can interfere with a proper latch. They may also have related health problems (such as cardiac problems and intestinal blockages) that may prevent them from taking anything by mouth until they've had corrective surgery.

Alternative feeding methods can be used until the baby is able to nurse, and breast milk that is expressed during this waiting period can be frozen for future use.

- **Cystic fibrosis:** Babies with cystic fibrosis have difficulty digesting food because they have unusually low levels of the enzymes responsible for breaking down fats and proteins. They also have breathing problems due to a buildup of thick secretions in the lungs. To breastfeed a baby with cystic fibrosis, the mother expresses some breast milk and mixes it with digestive enzymes. This special "mixed drink" is then fed via a lactation aid at the breast while the baby nurses as usual.

- **Phenylketonuria (PKU):** Babies with PKU lack the ability to metabolize phenylalanine (an amino acid), which can lead to a buildup of this substance in the blood, eventually causing mental retardation, seizures, and other problems. Doctors at the Hospital for Sick Children in Toronto have pioneered some techniques that now allow babies with PKU to receive both low-phenylalanine formula (the standard food for babies with PKU) and breast milk (rather than only low-phenylalanine formula). The treatment, however, requires careful monitoring and supervision by health-care workers experienced in dealing with babies with PKU.

Breastfeeding after adoption

If you are planning to breastfeed an adopted baby, you should start preparing your breasts for lactation as soon as possible. You can find detailed instructions on techniques that have proven successful for stimulating milk production in adoptive mothers in *Dr. Jack Newman's Guide to Breastfeeding* by Dr. Jack Newman and Teresa Pitman. While it is not always possible for an adoptive mother to fully breastfeed her baby, the baby will derive significant health benefits from any amount of breast milk she is able to provide, and both mother and baby will enjoy significant emotional benefits as well.

Breastfeeding after breast enhancement or reduction surgery

Your odds of being able to breastfeed a baby if you've had breast enhancement surgery at some point in your life are quite high, unless, of course, you required the surgery for treatment of hypoplastic immature breasts, which may not fully lactate. The surgical techniques used to increase the size of a woman's breasts generally do not interfere with the glandular development of the breasts or lactation, so breastfeeding is still quite possible.

Your odds of being able to breastfeed a baby after breast reduction surgery aren't quite so good, although they increase significantly if your nipple was transposed (moved without completely detaching it from the breast) rather than transplanted (completely removed). Transposing a nipple reduces the likelihood that ducts and nerve endings essential for breastfeeding will be severed. While it is rare for a woman who has been through breast reduction surgery to be able to totally breastfeed her baby, partial breastfeeding may be possible. Note: Even if you were unable to breastfeed your first baby, you might want to try breastfeeding your second and subsequent babies. The hormonal changes of pregnancy and menstruation may cause enough glandular tissue to regenerate to allow your attempts to be successful the next time around.

Breastfeeding multiples

Breastfeeding multiples is largely a matter of getting organized, ensuring an adequate milk supply, and lining up plenty of support.

If you're breastfeeding twins, the simplest way to share the milk around is to offer each baby one breast during a particular feeding. Then, when the next feeding rolls around, switch sides. (According to Barbara Luke and Tamara Eberlein, co-authors of *When You're Expecting Twins, Triplets, or Quads*, it's important to remember to switch sides. Otherwise you limit the amount of visual stimulation that each baby is receiving and, what's more, you may end up with lopsided breasts and a diminished milk supply on one side if one of your babies has a smaller appetite.) In the beginning, while the babies are learning, it's usually better to feed each baby separately, but once breastfeeding is established, some mothers prefer to put both babies to the breast at the same time—a tremendous timesaver given that it can take between 10 and 15 hours daily to feed twins if you feed them one at a time! You can either put both babies in the cradle hold, both babies in the football hold, or use the combination position (one baby in the cradle position and one baby in the football position)—whatever works best for you. You'll either need a mountain of pillows to support two babies or a special nursing pillow designed for moms of twins.

mother wisdom Keep track of which baby nursed on which breast during which feeding by moving a safety pin on your shirt from side to side or by keeping written records—whatever works best for you and requires the least amount of effort.

chapter 7

THE OWNER'S MANUAL: NEW BABY CARE

> "I think if you really want to be a parent, then your curiosity and thirst for knowledge go a long way toward preparing you. I think if you accept that you won't always know what to do or how to do it, you are 'prepared.'"
>
> —JEANNINE, 35, MOTHER OF TWO

It's one of those jokes that comedy writers tend to recycle again and again: the fact that toasters and flashlights come with more detailed instructions than new babies. But it's hardly a laughing matter if you're a first-time parent who's wondering how on earth you're going to figure out how to take care of your brand-new baby for the next 18 *days*, let alone the next 18 *years*.

While it's completely understandable why Mother Nature chose not to package a baby instruction manual along with Baby (real estate is, after all, fairly tight inside the uterus), it certainly would be helpful to be able to get your hands on an instruction manual that would carefully explain how your baby works and how to troubleshoot the more common operating problems.

That brings us to the subject of this chapter—caring for your new baby. We're going to cover a variety of different topics: everything from diapering to bathing to dressing your baby. (If you didn't have a younger sibling and you never took a babysitting course, this is brand new turf for you—and you'd probably like someone to cover off the basics for you at some point.)

I'm also hoping that this particular set of instructions will prove to be at least a little more interesting than the instructions that came with your new barbecue—and a lot more helpful than the so-called help feature on your computer.

THE CARE AND HANDLING OF BABIES

You've no doubt had at least one well-meaning advice-giver warn you about the dangers of touching your baby's fontanelle or failing to support his neck properly—a lecture that probably left you afraid to do anything but hold on to your baby for dear life. Fortunately, babies aren't nearly as fragile as some people make them out to be—which goes a long way toward explaining how the human species has managed to survive this long, fontanelles and all!

Still, it's always best to err on the side of caution when you're handling a baby. Not only does exercising that extra bit of care reduce the risk of injury, but gentle handling will make your baby feel more secure. As you may recall from our discussion in Chapter 1, newborn babies come programmed with a number of reflexes, including the aptly named startle reflex. To avoid startling your baby each time you change his position, you need to move slowly and deliberately and ensure that his entire body is supported. If his head or limbs are allowed to dangle, he may feel as if you're about to drop him—something that will cause him to fling out his arms and legs in a classic "startle" response and start to wail. If you get in the habit of supporting his head and neck with one hand and his bottom and thighs with the other, and holding him close to your body when you're carrying him around, he'll feel much more secure about the world around him.

You might be wondering why babies are born with this particular reflex. It makes perfect sense if you consider it from a survival perspective. The startle reflex prompts a baby human (or other baby animal) who feels like he is about to be dropped to grasp on to his mother and cling to her before he tumbles to the ground.

---

mother wisdom — Just as you always suspected, there is a trick involved in putting down a sleeping baby without waking him up or causing him to startle.

- √ Move slowly and gently, carefully putting your baby's head down first and then gradually laying the rest of his body down until he is lying flat on his back.
- √ Carefully remove one hand and then the other so that your baby has a chance to adjust to his new surroundings before you let go of him entirely. If you're lucky, he'll stay asleep rather than startling himself

into wakefulness (a major drawback to this whole startle reflex business). Some babies tend to flail their arms and wake themselves the moment you lay them down.

√ Don't exit stage left the moment your arms are finally free (as difficult as it may be for your sleep-deprived body to resist the almost magnetic pull of the closest horizontal surface). Instead, stand beside your baby for a minute or two so that you can give him a reassuring pat or speak to him in a soft and soothing voice if he begins to stir. Then, as soon as you're convinced he's really and truly settled, get some sleep yourself.

THE DIRT ON DIAPERS

Don't have a clue how to put a diaper on a baby? Don't sweat it: according to a figure cited in a 2008 National Geographic Channel documentary, you'll have at least 3,796 times to perfect your technique before your baby's toilet-trained.

The first thing you need to do, of course, is to ensure that you have all the necessary diapering paraphernalia on hand. Once you start changing your baby's diaper, you've reached the point of no return. If you discover that the items you need to clean your baby's bum are across the house, you'll have to drag him with you, poopy bottom and all. Here's what you'll want to have within grabbing distance before you take the fateful step of removing your baby's dirty diaper: a change pad and/or a soft towel to lay the baby down on, diapers, diaper liners, diaper cream (if you decide to use any—some parents do, others don't), a bowl full of lukewarm water, and a baby washcloth or two. (You can replace the last three items with a box of disposable baby wipes, if you prefer, but bear in mind that baby wipes tend to be expensive, they take a hefty environmental toll over time, and they may be irritating to your baby's tender skin.)

mother wisdom If you are using cloth diapers and diaper cream, you may want to get in the habit of using diaper liners. Whether paper or cloth, inserts catch stool and make diapers easier to clean. Diaper cream can be a pain to remove from cloth diapers.

TABLE 7.1

Baby Care Essentials

You'll want to round up these baby care essentials during your next trip to the baby department or drug store:

- diaper cream (if you decide to use it)
- moisturizing lotion (natural, unscented)
- soap (natural, mild, unscented)
- shampoo (optional)
- soft washcloths
- thermometer (digital)
- nasal aspirator (for removing mucus from baby's nose)
- calibrated medicine dropper or a syringe or spoon for measuring and administering medication
- baby nail scissors or clippers
- antibacterial ointment
- acetaminophen (infant drops)
- vitamin D drops

---

mom's the word "One thing we learned that nobody ever told us was that you really have to move up to the next size of diaper way before the weight limit on the package. Claire started to have blowouts up the back of the diaper almost every diaper she had."

—TAMMY, 32, MOTHER OF ONE

Once you've assembled all the necessary gear, take a moment to read the instructions on the package of cloth or disposable diapers. (Hey, why make life more difficult for yourself than it has to be? The instructions are your friend.) Here's what to do next.

- Place a clean diaper or receiving blanket under your baby's bottom to help contain any leaks that may occur as you remove the diaper. (Expect the unexpected when you're changing a baby.)
- Remove the dirty diaper and set it out of Baby's reach (otherwise, your baby will somehow find a way to dip his legs in the poop while you're busy putting the new diaper on). If your baby is a boy, drape a baby washcloth across his penis immediately or you're likely to get squirted

at some point during the diaper change. (Here's another tip: if you open your son's diaper and his penis is erect, hold the diaper over the penis and wait for a warm sensation—a sign that he has urinated. Then proceed with the diaper change.)

---

mother wisdom Trying to figure out how many cloth diapers to have on hand for your newborn? You should plan to have at least two dozen diapers on hand. (You should figure on 10 to 12 diaper changes each day during the early weeks, and you'll want to have at least a two-day diaper supply on hand at all times.) In addition to diapers, you'll need diaper liners, diaper inserts (which increase the absorbency—a must-have for overnight diapering), diaper covers, and cloth wipes.

It can be more than a little daunting to try to figure out how to put a diaper on a newborn baby the first time around, even if you've dutifully practised on a doll or stuffed animal as your prenatal instructor suggested. It's one thing to wrap a diaper around an inanimate object. It's quite another to accomplish the same feat when you're dealing with a wiggly baby who's likely to fill his new diaper the moment you finish putting it on.

- If your baby's diaper is wet rather than soiled, you can skip the next step entirely.
- Use some toilet paper (moistened in warm water) or a wet washcloth to wash away as much stool as possible from your baby's bottom. Then take a clean washcloth, dip it in warm water, and wash your baby's bottom and genital area with a bit of soap. Rinse thoroughly, using another washcloth.
- If the diaper is just wet, dip a baby washcloth in water and use it to wipe your baby's bottom and genital area. Again, you might want to use soap, but keep an eye on how your baby's skin reacts. <u>Plain water works just fine.</u> Remember to use gentle motions when you're washing your baby's bottom. Avoid any vigorous scrubbing or your baby's skin may become irritated. Rinse thoroughly.

- When you're finished washing your baby, pat his bottom dry with a clean and dry baby washcloth or let it air-dry for a couple of minutes. Then apply diaper cream (such as zinc oxide ointment, for example) if you choose to. The experts continue to disagree about whether it's really necessary to routinely apply diaper cream after each diaper change as a means of preventing diaper rash or whether it should only be used if a baby shows some early signs of developing a rash. Bottom line? You'll probably have to experiment a little to find out whether your baby's skin does better with or without any added gunk.

- If your baby is a girl, be sure to wipe from front to back when you're cleaning the diaper area. This will help to prevent germs from getting inside her vagina and causing an infection.

- If your baby is a boy, remember not to attempt to retract his foreskin or clean underneath it. You could damage the delicate tissues underneath. (The foreskin will gradually detach from the glans—generally during the first few years of life.) Simply wash your baby boy's penis as you would any other part of his body.

- Put on the new diaper, doing up the fasteners so that it is tight enough to contain leaks but not so tight as to pinch the baby's legs or be uncomfortably snug around the middle. If your baby is a boy, you'll want to ensure that his penis is pointed downward as you close the diaper. Otherwise, when he urinates, he may end up drenching the front of his undershirt.

- Dress your baby and put him in a safe spot while you clean up the change area. Note: If the change pad happened to get splattered while you were changing your baby, you'll want to give it a quick wipe-down with a mild disinfecting spray (if it's a waterproof change pad) or throw it in the washing machine (if it's a cloth change pad).

- Remember that it's important to change your baby often—whenever your baby's diaper is wet or soiled. That means you could be changing your baby's diaper 10 to 12 times a day (or even more often) during the newborn stage. Frequent diaper changes decrease your baby's chances of developing a diaper rash. Diaper rash can be triggered through contact with digestive agents in the stool or with chemicals that are formed as the urine decomposes in the diaper—both of which can be tremendously irritating to a baby's skin.

mother wisdom During the seventeenth and eighteenth centuries, urine was believed to possess disinfecting qualities. Rather than wash urine-soaked diapers, a mother simply lay her baby's diapers to dry in front of the fire. And instead of washing the urine off a baby's bottom, his bottom was powdered with the dust of worm-eaten wood—the baby powder of centuries gone by.

mother wisdom You can eliminate some of the lingering odour on your baby's cloth diapers by pre-rinsing the diapers with vinegar before running them through the regular wash cycle.

Rash decisions

The term diaper rash is used to describe any sort of skin inflammation in the diaper area—whether it's slight redness that is accompanied by heat or severe inflammation involving sores or pustules.

Certain babies are more prone to diaper rashes than others.

- **Babies who are 8 to 10 months of age.** Babies this age are more prone to diaper rashes because they spend so much time sitting—something that allows for extended contact with wet or dirty diapers—and because they tend to be consuming a wider variety of solid foods than younger babies, which can alter the acidity level in their stools, causing irritation.

- **Babies who are just starting to eat solid foods.** Babies who are new to the world of solid foods are more prone to diaper rashes because of digestive process changes triggered by the introduction of new foods.

- **Babies who have frequent stools.** Babies who have frequent stools are more susceptible to diaper rashes because their bottoms are likely to spend more time in contact with stool—particularly if they pass their stools at night when they are sleeping and it's a couple of hours before their next feed and diaper change.

- **Babies who aren't changed frequently.** Babies who are changed infrequently spend more time with their skin in contact with urine and feces—something that can be highly irritating to a baby's skin.
- **Babies who are formula-fed.** Formula-fed babies are more susceptible to diaper rashes than their breast-fed counterparts.
- **Babies who are being treated with antibiotics.** Antibiotic use can encourage the growth of yeast organisms that can infect the skin. (Note: Breastfed babies whose mothers are taking antibiotics are also susceptible to yeast-based diaper rashes.)

The key to treating a diaper rash is to start dealing with the problem as soon as you detect any initial signs of redness or soreness. Once your baby's skin has become irritated, it's susceptible to becoming even more irritated or infected as a result of contact with urine and feces. Here are some tips on managing diaper rash.

- Change your baby's diaper as soon as possible after a bowel movement, and check your baby's diaper frequently to see if he is wet and in need of a diaper change.
- Stop using baby wipes. Once a rash has started to develop, baby wipes can be extremely irritating to your baby's skin. Instead, use a squirt bottle (the same type they gave you in the hospital to rinse your perineum after the delivery) to squirt warm water on your baby's bottom and then gently pat your baby's bottom dry.
- Expose your baby's bottom to air on a regular basis by scheduling some "bare bum time" every day (or, at the very least, time with just a cloth diaper and no plastic cover or barrier). You can minimize messes by placing your baby on a waterproof change pad or by taking him outside (weather permitting, of course). Not only will messes be less of a concern, your baby will benefit from being exposed to fresh air. Just be sure to avoid direct sun exposure so that your baby doesn't end up with a sunburn.
- Avoid using rash creams that contain boric acid, camphor, phenol, menthyl salicylate, or compound of benzoin tincture—all of which may be harmful to a baby's tender skin.

baby talk According to the College of Family Physicians of Canada, you should have your baby's diaper rash checked by a doctor if

- √ the rash occurs when your baby is less than 6 weeks of age;
- √ the rash shows signs of becoming infected (for example, some pimples, small ulcers, large bumps, or nodules have developed);
- √ your baby has a fever, is losing weight, or isn't eating well;
- √ the rash starts spreading to other areas of your baby's body; or
- √ the rash hasn't improved despite your best efforts to treat it on your own for a week. (Note: Some other experts suggest that you make that call a little sooner—within two to three days.)

- Don't apply baby powder to your baby's bottom in the hope that it will ease your baby's rash. Not only does baby powder tend to be ineffective, it could be hazardous to your baby's health if he happens to breathe some in. (There are health risks associated with inhaling talc, a key ingredient in most types of baby powder.) If you really feel the need to put some sort of powder on your baby's bottom, stick to plain, old-fashioned corn starch. (Just one quick word of warning where this is concerned: be sure to wash away any corn starch powder that accumulates in baby's skin folds as this can create a breeding ground for bacteria that can lead to infections.)

- If you're using cloth diapers, make sure that you're using a baby-friendly laundry detergent and that the diapers are cleaned and rinsed properly. (For best results, use half the recommended amount of detergent, add vinegar to the first rinse cycle, and then rinse the diapers a second time in plain water. Avoid fabric softener and dryer sheets.)

- If your baby is having recurrent problems with diaper rash, try boiling the diapers for 15 minutes after washing to get rid of soap residue and germs, and then hang the diapers to dry in the sun. Alternatively, add 1/2 cup (125 millilitres) of bleach or Borax to your next load of diapers and allow the diapers to soak for at least six hours before running the diapers through the wash and spin cycles twice.

- Learn how to spot the signs of a yeast infection so that you can seek medical treatment for your baby sooner rather than later. Unlike garden-variety diaper rashes, yeast infections won't go away on their own. Here's how to tell the difference: rashes caused by yeast infections tend to be limited to the thighs, genitals, and lower abdomen rather than the actual buttocks. And yeast infections typically have small red dots around the edge of the rash.

---

baby talk According to the College of Family Physicians of Canada, cloth diapers washed by a diaper service are less likely to cause diaper rashes than diapers that are washed at home. This is because diaper services tend to use hotter water than what is available in a typical residence—which helps to kill germs and remove chemicals that might otherwise be irritating to a baby's skin.

Elimination communication (diaper-free)

Some parents take a different approach to their babies' elimination needs, choosing to bypass diapers entirely (or as much as possible). These families practise "elimination communication," which is based on a few core beliefs: that babies are aware of their elimination needs from birth and communicate those needs through sounds and body language; that babies should be respected rather than coerced when it comes to a biological function as basic as elimination; and that when parents tune into their babies' elimination signals, they strengthen the communication with their child and enhance their bond with the baby.

If you visit www.diaperfreebaby.org, you can learn more about the reasons many families are choosing elimination communication as an alternative to infant diapering and traditional toilet training methods.

CARING FOR A CIRCUMCISED BABY

If you had your newborn son circumcised shortly after birth, you'll need to apply some protective lubricant to his circumcision site each time you change his diaper for the first few days. Don't be surprised if his penis looks swollen and then develops a yellowish scab on it: this is a normal part of the healing process. If, however, your baby's entire penis is red, warm, and swollen, and/or the surgical site is draining pus, you'll need to get in touch with your baby's doctor to arrange for treatment as it's likely that your baby's penis has become infected.

UMBILICAL CORD CARE

In most cases, the plastic clamp that was used to seal your baby's umbilical cord is removed within 24 hours of the birth. At that point, your baby's cord stump may look swollen and jellylike but, over the next few days, it will start to dry and shrivel up. It should fall off entirely within a week or two—an event that most parents welcome both because the umbilical cord stump is anything but a thing of beauty and because it can also get a little stinky over time!

While parents used to be told to swab their baby's umbilical cord stump with rubbing alcohol at each diaper change in order to prevent infection and encourage the stump to fall off, a study of 1,800 newborns conducted by researchers at McMaster University in Hamilton, Ontario, found that umbilical cord stumps fall off sooner if they are simply left alone. It took an average of ten days for the alcohol-swabbed umbilical cord stumps to dry up and fall off, compared with eight days for the cord stumps that were unswabbed. None of the infants involved in the study—swabbed or not—developed an infection. The researchers concluded that the alcohol may kill off "good" bacteria that help the cord to dry up and fall off.

To avoid irritating your baby's umbilical cord stump while it is healing, leave the cord stump exposed to the air. (Don't cover it with a diaper, in other words.) You may have to roll your baby's diaper down a little to prevent it from covering up or rubbing against the cord stump (something that isn't harmful to your baby, but that can cause a bit of bleeding that is nonetheless worrisome).

Here's something else to keep in mind until your baby's umbilical cord stump dries up and falls off: most experts agree that it's best to avoid immersing your baby in water until the stump has fallen off and the umbilical cord site is fully healed, due to the risk of infection. So for the first week or two of your baby's life, you'll want to sponge-bathe your baby rather than pop him into his bathtub. You'll find more tips on bathing your newborn later in this chapter.

baby talk It's not unusual for a baby's umbilical cord stump to get a little "ripe" over time and start giving off a mildly unpleasant odour. If, however, your baby's cord develops a particularly offensive odour or a pus-like discharge, get in touch with your baby's doctor. The doctor may want to apply silver nitrate to the umbilical cord site to encourage drying and healing.

A BABY FOR ALL SEASONS

You need to make a concerted effort to protect your baby's tender skin against the harsh elements in the environment around him. And when it comes to harsh elements, there are few countries that can rival the good old Canadian climate. We have both blistering hot summers and bone-numbingly cold winters—and about three weeks of good weather in between each spring and fall. (Okay, it's not quite that bad, but we are famous for our weather extremes.) Here's what you need to know to protect your baby's skin from season to season.

During the spring and summer:

- Keep babies under one year of age out of the direct sunlight. Not only are babies this age at risk of developing a sunburn, they're also highly susceptible to both dehydration and sunstroke. If you're going to take your baby outside for any length of time, make sure he's dressed appropriately (he's wearing a wide-brimmed hat and long-sleeved clothing made from tightly woven lightweight fabrics that block out a lot of ultraviolet rays) and he's kept out of the direct sun (something that's particularly important during the hours of peak ultraviolet light intensity, from 10 a.m. to 4 p.m.).

- Use sunscreen where appropriate. According to the Canadian Dermatology Association, it's safe to use sunscreen on babies over the age of 6 months. When you're shopping around for a sunscreen, be sure to look for one with an SPF rating of at least 15 and to avoid ones that contain alcohol, which may burn and sting your baby's skin and eyes. (Consult the Environmental Working Group's Skin Deep Cosmetics Database (www.ewg.org/skindeep/) to find out the hazard score given to known and suspected hazards associated with the ingredients found in various products.) Be sure to test your baby's skin for a possible allergic reaction before you start to use the product. (To test for a possible reaction, simply apply a small amount of sunscreen to your baby's inner forearm and allow the sunscreen to remain on the skin for several hours while watching for signs of any possible reaction.) Note: It's best to minimize the amount of sunscreen you use on a baby. Reserve it for the areas of her body that you can't protect from the sun via clothing and shade. Apply sunscreen 30 minutes before you take your baby outdoors. Suncreen doesn't work right away; it needs time to be absorbed by the skin. Remember to reapply sunscreen every two hours. (You won't want to keep your baby out in the sun for hours at a time, but it's an important point to keep in mind if you bring your baby outside again later in the day.)

---

baby talk Babies have super-sensitive skin and can react to substances that don't prove bothersome to most adults: things like the chemicals in brand-new clothing or the detergent residue that can build up on clothes that have been washed. That's why it's a good idea to wash baby clothes thoroughly before your baby wears them and to wash and double-rinse any item that is going to come into contact with your baby's tender skin: clothing, blankets, change pads, stroller liners, car seat covers, and so on.

- Don't overlook the hazards of reflected light. According to the Canadian Dermatology Association, up to 85 per cent of the sun's harmful ultraviolet B rays can be reflected by sand, snow, water, and concrete. This means that your baby can still get a great deal of sun exposure even if she's sitting in the shade.
- Keep in mind that cloudy days can pose a problem, too. Up to 80 per cent of the sun's rays manage to penetrate the cloud cover—something that can result in a nasty burn on an anything-but-sunny day. For this reason, you should make a point of using sunscreen on exposed skin every day, whether it is sunny or not.
- If your baby does end up getting a sunburn, you'll need to seek medical attention. Sunburns in infants this age can be quite serious.

During the fall and winter:

- Bundle your baby well when you're going outdoors, both to prevent frostbite and to protect your baby's skin. A baby's skin is thinner, is more sensitive, and contains less protective keratin than the skin of an adult, so it tends to be particularly susceptible to the drying effects of the cold and the wind.

- If you're going to have your baby outside for an extended period of time, you might want to dab a bit of sunscreen on his face to prevent him from getting a burn. Sunburns can even happen in minus 30 degree weather.

- Pay careful attention to the temperature of your baby's bath. The warmer the bath water, the greater the amount of moisture that will be removed from baby's skin. You should also make a point of using the mildest soap you can find (or skipping the soap altogether) and then applying a baby-friendly (non-allergenic) moisturizing cream to your baby's skin after he's been toweled off, but while his skin is still damp. (Don't add baby oil to your baby's bath: it doesn't absorb or lubricate as well as lotion, and it can make your baby even slipperier to handle in the tub.)

- Use a cool-mist humidifier in your baby's room to add moisture to the air. (Just be sure to clean it after use to prevent harmful moulds and bacteria from building up inside the humidifier and being transmitted into the air. To clean a humidifier, wipe it down with a solution of 10 per cent bleach—that is, one part bleach to nine parts water.)

---

mother wisdom

You don't need a shelf full of toiletries to care for Baby's tender skin. All Baby really needs is a bar of mild soap (for getting clean at bath time), some shampoo (assuming your baby has enough hair to need shampoo and you choose to use shampoo as opposed to soap), some diaper cream (see the previous discussion), and a small amount of non-allergenic moisturing lotion (to retain the skin's moisture in dry weather and to apply to any patches of dry skin that develop). Choose products that are free of perfumes and other additives and that are made from the most natural ingredients you can find. Your baby's skin will thank you for it.

mother wisdom — Breast milk contains docosahexaenoic acid—an essential fatty acid that acts as a natural skin moisturizer. Feel free to squirt some on to any dry skin areas your baby might have.

- Watch for signs that your baby could be developing eczema (reddened skin that becomes dry and itchy) and then talk to your doctor about ways of treating this common skin condition in babies. (See Chapter 8 for more information.)

NAIL CARE

As you've no doubt discovered by now, babies have unbelievably small fingernails and toenails—so small, in fact, that you may have to squint to see them. But even though your baby's nails are very soft, they can still scratch his face quite badly if he tends to rake at his face a lot. That's why you'll want to keep his fingernails well trimmed. You can either file your baby's nails with an emery board, use nail clippers or scissors that are especially designed for use on babies, or gently bite his fingernails off. The best time to give your baby a manicure is when he's sleeping. Gently push the pad of his finger away from each nail as you trim his nails in order to reduce the risk that you will accidentally nip his finger. If you do happen to draw blood—which will leave you feeling like the worst parent ever—simply apply light pressure to the cut. The bleeding will stop. Note: Don't put a bandage on the cut. Your baby could stick his fingers (and the bandage) into his mouth. That could pose a choking risk.

Babies' nails grow quickly. Chances are you will need to trim your baby's toenails once or twice a month and your baby's fingernails once or twice a week.

DENTAL CARE

It may seem strange to be thinking about dental care before your baby even has any teeth, but according to the Canadian Dental Association, it's never too soon to start practising good oral hygiene. (You may not be able to see your baby's teeth right now, but your baby already has 20 primary teeth.) Here's what you need to know in order to take good care of those precious soon-to-be pearly whites during his first year of life.

Before your baby's teeth come in

You can expect your baby to remain toothless for the first six months of his life—and perhaps a little longer than that. As Table 7.2 indicates, there's considerable variation from baby to baby when it comes to the timing of the eruption of that first tooth. While some babies are actually born with a tooth or two, others manage to celebrate their first birthdays still sporting a toothless grin! But once those teeth start coming in, you should expect your baby's teeth to appear in roughly the following order: central incisors (the teeth at the front of the mouth: bottom first, then top); lateral incisors (the teeth that are directly beside the central incisors on either side); first molars (the second last teeth at the back of the mouth); canines or cuspids (the teeth in between the lateral incisors and the molars); and finally second molars (the teeth at the very back of the mouth).

---

baby talk Early childhood tooth decay can be caused by going to bed with a bottle or cup of formula, cow's milk, or juice. Early childhood tooth decay can result in toothaches, feeding difficulties, and the premature loss of the baby teeth (which can, in turn, result in speech problems, jaw development problems, and the need for orthodontic work). The most severe tooth damage tends to occur in the areas where liquid can build up in the baby's mouth: around the fronts and backs of the upper front teeth. The earliest warning sign that there could be a problem is the presence of tiny white spots or lines on the teeth. (These spots are sometimes so small that they can only be detected by a dentist.) Dark teeth are also an indication that your child's teeth are suffering from tooth decay. If you notice any signs of tooth decay, make an appointment for your child to see a dentist right away.

You don't have to worry about tooth decay in a baby who is exclusively breastfed. However, once your baby starts eating solid food, you need to be more concerned about your baby's oral hygiene. Breast milk can interact with any food particles or plaque left behind on your baby's teeth, causing cavities. For this reason, it is a good idea to brush and clean your baby's teeth thoroughly at bedtime once he starts eating solid food.

While you're waiting for your baby's first tooth to make its way through the gum, get in the habit of wiping your baby's gums down at least once a day. Simply cradle your baby in your arms, wrap a piece of gauze around your finger, dip your finger in some warm water, and wipe down your baby's gums.

TABLE 7.2

When Your Baby's Teeth Will Come In

Wondering when you'll be able to spot your baby's first tooth and which tooth will come in first? The following chart outlines approximately when your baby's teeth will start to appear and in what order they'll make their grand entrance.

Teeth	Location	When they come in
Central incisors (lower)	Front of mouth on lower jaw	6 to 10 months
Lateral incisors (lower)	Teeth directly beside central incisors on lower jaw	7 to 16 months
Central incisors (upper)	Front of mouth on upper jaw	7 to 12 months
Lateral incisors (upper)	Teeth directly beside central incisors on upper jaw	7 to 13 months
First molars (lower)	Second last tooth at the back of the mouth on either side of the lower jaw	12 to 18 months
First molars (upper)	Second last tooth at the back of the mouth on either side of the upper jaw	13 to 19 months
Canines (cuspids, upper)	The teeth in between the lateral incisors and the molars on the upper jaw	16 to 22 months
Canines (cuspids, lower)	The teeth in between the lateral incisors and the molars on the lower jaw	16 to 23 months
Second molars (lower)	The teeth at the very back of the mouth on the lower jaw	20 to 31 months
Second molars (upper)	The teeth at the very back of the mouth on the upper jaw	25 to 33 months

Source: Canadian Dental Association website (www.cda-adc.ca)

Once your baby's teeth come in

Once your baby's teeth have started to appear, you should start using a soft-bristled baby toothbrush with a pea-sized amount of fluoride toothpaste to clean your baby's teeth. Teach your baby to spit out the toothpaste rather than swallowing it. Excessive consumption of fluoride, including the fluoride in toothpaste, can lead to a condition called dental fluorosis, which can affect the enamel on your baby's teeth. If you're using a special "baby toothpaste," make sure that it contains fluoride. Not all baby toothpastes do. You should clean your baby's teeth at least once or twice daily—ideally after the first and last meals of the day. Clean your baby's teeth by making gentle circles with the toothbrush, cleaning every surface of every tooth as you go along. Don't scrub too hard or you could injure your baby's gums. Be sure to replace your baby's toothbrush on a regular basis—every three to four months (sooner if your baby has been ill).

Something else you need to think about as soon as your baby has teeth is whether or not he needs a fluoride supplement. If your community has fluoridated water, your baby's fluoride needs are already being fully met, but if your water supply doesn't contain fluoride, your doctor may recommend that your child receive some sort of fluoride supplement.

---

baby talk Discourage your baby from using a bottle as a pacifier (for example, taking small sips for comfort throughout the day rather than having a drink and then putting the bottle away). Provide him with a cup instead, and encourage him to sit down to have a drink (something that eliminates the risk of an injury caused by falling with a bottle or a cup in his mouth).

Plan to make the switch from a bottle to a cup as soon as possible after your baby's first birthday, if not sooner. Drinking from a cup doesn't cause liquid to collect around the teeth in quite the same way as drinking from a bottle, and consequently it is less likely to contribute to tooth decay.

DRESSING THE PART

If you opt for easy-to-wear baby garments (see recommended clothing picks listed in Table 7.3), dressing your baby is going to be a breeze. You

TABLE 7.3

The Canadian Baby Layette

2 to 3 sleep sacks (wearable sleeping bags that are used instead of a blanket; see Chapter 8 for more on safe sleep)
6 sleepers
6 other one-piece outfits (short-sleeved or long-sleeved daytime wear or more sleepers: your choice)
6 diaper shirts ("onesies"—undershirts that include a diaper cover-up portion)
3 pairs of socks: To keep baby's feet warm on days when he wears outfits without built-in feet. Skip the fancy shoes for now (unless you live for shoes). They're more trouble to get on and off than they're worth and your baby won't be walking for a while.
4 large bibs (only necessary if you're intending to formula-feed or if your baby spits up a lot)
Hats: At least one wide-brimmed hat, regardless of the season (to protect baby's tender skin). You'll also want at least one hat to keep baby's head warm (again, regardless of the season).
Seasonal outerwear: a snowsuit, a sweater with leggings, or whatever the season dictates
12 extra-large receiving blankets (you'll use these for everything *except* as blankets in your baby's bed: see Chapter 8 for more on safe sleep)
1 dozen or more baby washcloths
2-3 hooded baby towels
3 or more fitted crib sheets

won't have to struggle with sleepers that have such ridiculous features as buttons down the front or zippers up the back—or turtlenecks, which are likely to give your baby flashbacks to the trip down the birth canal. Yep, the key to dressing a baby with minimum fuss is to have the right clothing on hand. (Remember how tough it was to get your Barbie doll's arm to fit down her pencil-thin sleeve? That's nothing compared with the art of wrestling a newborn into one of those super-cute baby outfits featuring skin-tight sleeves and a million and one buttons or—worse—hook-and-eye fasteners. Who invents these clothes anyway? It certainly isn't anyone who's been anywhere near a real baby.)

Here are some tips on choosing the right types and quantities of clothing and linens (sheets, towels, receiving blankets) for your baby.

- **Don't spend a fortune on brand-name baby wear.** Your baby will be growing at a phenomenal rate during the upcoming weeks, so it doesn't make sense to spend a lot of money on items that she may only be able to wear once, if at all. If you've got your heart set on buying your baby some sort of designer togs, buy them in size 24 months or larger. By the time she fits into that size, her rate of growth will have slowed considerably, so she'll be able to get more wear out of the garment. (Besides, you're likely to receive all kinds of cute outfits in the newborn and 6-month size once friends and family members get a peek at the new arrival.)

- **Gratefully accept any offers of second-hand baby clothing.** Then sit down and figure out which items you actually need. Spend your dollars filling in the blanks on your baby layette shopping list.

- **Don't overbuy.** Your baby needs something to wear, but she doesn't need dozens of outfits in each size. If you're willing to do laundry daily or every other day, you may be able to get away with even fewer items of clothing than what I've listed in Table 7.2. (It will all depend on how much laundry your baby generates in a day.)

---

mom's the word "You don't need a fraction of the stuff that you are told you need. Only buy the bare essentials until you see how big your baby is. There is no point in having a pile of clothes to fit a newborn, only to give birth to a 10-pound baby who won't be able to fit into any of them."

—LISA, 35, MOTHER OF THREE

- **Don't assume that you need doubles of everything if you have twins.** You can probably get away with having one-and-a-half times as much clothing on hand. And, if you connect with your local chapter of Multiple Births Canada (www.multiplebirthscanada.org), you should be able to outfit your babies for just a fraction of the cost of buying everything new. (This non-profit group for parents of multiples is famous for its parent-to-parent clothing sales.)

- **Don't load up on too many items in the newborn size, but do make sure you have at least one newborn-sized outfit on hand.** (If your baby ends up being smaller than anticipated, she'll get lost in a size 6-months sleeper.)

- **Don't take the size labels on children's clothing too literally.** Make a point of judging the size of each garment for yourself. Sizes vary tremendously from manufacturer to manufacturer, so it's better to let your eye be your guide rather than relying on some arbitrary number on a clothing label.

- **Look for items that will fit your baby for the longest possible period of time.** Certain brands of sleepers are designed to grow with your baby, such as those that feature adjustable foot cuffs. And certain styles of clothing can be worn longer than others due to their cut and fit.

- **Be careful when you're shopping for end-of-season clothing.** While you might assume that your chubby-cheeked 6-month-old will be a perfect candidate for that size-2 snowsuit next winter, it's hard to predict what size he'll be at that time—and that snowsuit won't be the bargain it initially appeared to be if the only time it fits him is in the midst of an August heat wave.

- **Get in the habit of shopping for children's clothing at stores that offer wear guarantees.** That way, if your child wears out an item of clothing before he outgrows it, the store will replace it free of charge.

- **Keep your baby's safety and comfort in mind.** Avoid baby clothes with buttons (a potential choking hazard) and garments with drawstrings any longer than 20 centimetres (7 inches). Watch for loose threads and fringes that could trap your baby's fingers. And make sure that any sleepwear you purchase for your baby conforms to federal regulations. According to Health Canada, loose-fitting sleepwear should be manufactured from polyester, nylon, or polyester/nylon blends, but tight-fitting styles such as sleepers may be made from cotton or cotton blends. Note: Be sure to follow the care instructions on your children's sleepwear in order to maintain the products' flame-resistant properties.

- **Buy garments that are suited to your baby's developmental stage.** "Shoes and socks for a newborn are a waste of time," insists Marguerite, a 37-year-old mother of two. "Use sleepers with feet instead." The same deal applies when you're shopping for clothing for older babies, adds Lisa, a 35-year-old mother of three. "Avoid dresses for crawling babies!"

- **Look for items that appear to have been designed with the needs of mothers and babies in mind—as opposed to those that appear to have been thought up by some fashion designer who's never even set eyes on a baby.** "My pet peeve is undershirts that go over the head," exclaims Holly, a 34-year-old mother of two. "If the baby poops all over the undershirt, you have to haul it over their back and their head. Needless to say, it doesn't exactly make for ease in cleanup!"

---

mother wisdom The "layered look" is still very much in vogue for babies: adding or subtracting a layer or two of clothing and/or blankets is the easiest way to keep your baby at a comfortable temperature.

Now that you've acquired some baby fashion sense, you'll want to master these insider tips on dressing a baby.

- Don't be surprised if your baby kicks up a bit of a fuss when you attempt to change his clothes. He's not objecting to your taste in clothing (although, frankly, that could be a factor if you insist on dressing him in those horrible little sailor suits), but rather the fact that he hates being naked and alone. (If he is going to be naked, he wants skin-to-skin contact.) You can solve that problem by keeping a towel or a receiving blanket on top of him once you've stripped him down to the buff.

- Choose your changing position wisely. It's easier to change a baby's clothes when he's lying down than when he's sitting on your lap. Otherwise, you'll end up using both hands to support him and you won't have any hands left for changing his clothes.

- Keep in mind that you have to do everything for a baby. He won't be able to put his arm through his sleeve just because you hold the armhole toward him. You have to guide his arm into the sleeve and make sure his arm comes out the other end without catching any of his fingers along the way. (Hint: Sometimes it's easiest to stick your fingers through the bottom of the sleeve and then gently pull your baby's arm through the arm hole rather than try to feed his arm through the entire length of the sleeve.)

- If Aunt Mildred gave you an outfit that has to go over your baby's head, pull it over the back of his head and then use one hand to block your baby's face so that the fabric doesn't end up scratching him as it passes across his face. (If you're lucky, the outfit in question will have a snap or two in the shoulder area to make the neck hole a little bit larger.)

- Pass on the shoes for now. According to the Canadian Paediatric Society, babies do not need shoes until they start to walk. In fact, there is growing evidence to suggest that wearing shoes in early childhood may interfere with the development of a normal longitudinal arch.

- Keep the weather in mind when you're deciding how to dress your baby. Babies require one more layer than adults. (This rule doesn't necessarily apply during the dog days of summer, when you might not want to put anything more on your baby than a diaper. And it also doesn't apply to premature babies, who typically need two additional layers until they reach the weight of a typical full-term newborn—7.5 pounds or so.)

BATH TIME BASICS

If there's one baby-care task that tends to strike terror into the hearts of first-time parents, it's the thought of bathing a baby for the very first time. Fortunately, new parents get off easily in that department for at least the first week or two. Until the baby's umbilical cord site has healed up, the only type of bath a baby should be having is a bath on dry land—a sponge bath.

How to sponge-bathe a baby

Here's what's involved in sponge-bathing a baby.

- Spread a change pad on your bathroom counter, your baby's change table, or whatever other surface you'll be using for your baby's sponge bath, and make sure that the room is sufficiently warm—about 24 degrees Celsius (75 degrees Fahrenheit). (If you're going to be sponge-bathing your baby in the bathroom, you can warm it up by turning on the shower for a couple of minutes to create some warm steam or by turning on a small space heater for a couple of minutes to take the chill out of the room.)

- Cover the change pad with a hooded baby towel, laying the hood part at the point on the change table where you'll be placing your baby's head.
- Keep a second baby towel or a receiving blanket handy so that you can use it to cover up the parts of your baby that aren't being washed at that time. (Babies hate the feel of cold air on their bodies at the best of times, let alone when they're dripping wet.)
- Line up all the other paraphernalia you'll need to do your baby's bath: a basin of water, a couple of baby washcloths, and some mild baby soap (optional).
- Remove any jewellery that could accidentally scratch your baby. (Watches and rings tend to be perennial offenders.)
- Start by cleaning your baby's face—you won't need any soap for this part of his body, by the way—and then, if you're using soap, proceed to wash the rest of his body with soap, finishing up with his diaper area. Make sure that you do a good job of cleaning all your baby's creases: the ones under his arms, behind his ears, and in his genital area. Also take care to rinse your baby thoroughly so that you don't leave an irritating soapy residue all over his body. If your baby has highly sensitive skin, you may have to use the soap sparingly (every few days only or on the diaper region only). Pay careful attention to how your baby's skin is tolerating the soap (and use the gentlest soap you can find), and proceed accordingly.
- Limit your cleaning activity to your baby's external body parts. Your baby's nose and ears are self-cleaning devices—the mucus in your baby's nose and the wax in his ears are designed to carry any dirt away. And as for your baby's eyes? You don't have to worry about doing anything to keep them clean (other than giving a gentle wipe to your baby's eyelids when his eyes are closed). His tears will take care of the rest of the housecleaning.

baby talk When you're washing your baby's eyes, be sure to use a fresh section of washcloth on each eye. That way, you won't accidentally spread any minor infections from eye to eye.

baby talk About 5 per cent of healthy infants are born with a blocked tear duct (where the tear duct is either fully or partially obstructed). The key symptom is excessive tearing or yellow crusty discharge, especially after a nap. In 90 per cent of cases, the problem resolves itself by the time a child is 18 months of age and no treatment is required. Note: Some doctors recommend a technique called tear duct milking (to help ease tear drops out of the blocked duct). Others recommend a minor surgical procedure in which the duct is unblocked with a wire probe if the duct remains plugged by the time a baby reaches one year of age.

Some babies and toddlers develop eye infections as a result of having a blocked tear duct (the eye white turns red and the discharge turns green), in which case eye ointments may need to be prescribed.

- Go easy with the baby shampoo. Your baby's hair only needs to be shampooed once or twice a week (if you're using baby shampoo at all; if your baby has very little hair, a mild bar soap may be a better bet). The best way to wash your baby's hair, by the way, is to hold her football-style under your arm, with her head held over a sink. Use your hand or a small cup to pour water over her head and then lather her head. Rinse her head thoroughly and towel-dry her hair immediately to prevent any water from dripping down her face. Then comb her hair with a soft-bristled brush or a rounded-edge comb.

- Don't overdo it with the baths. If you're washing your baby's diaper area regularly, there's no need to give him a full sponge bath more often than two or three times a week. Overbathing may cause your baby's skin to become dry and flaky.

- When you're finished bathing your baby, wrap him in a hooded towel and gently pat him until he's dry.

Your baby's first real bath

Once your baby's umbilical cord site has healed and/or your baby's health-care provider has given you the go-ahead, you can start bathing your baby in a baby bathtub. There are a variety of different baby bathtub styles to choose from: tubs with a sloped back similar to what you would find in a car seat; tubs with mesh slings designed to support a newborn; convertible tubs; sink or sling inserts. Just don't make the mistake of trying to bathe your newborn in the big bathtub all by himself just yet. He isn't quite ready for that....

Here's what's involved in giving your baby his first real bath (in other words, actually putting him in water).

- Make sure the bathroom (or whatever room you choose for the bath) is sufficiently warm. You may want to rely on some of the room-warming tricks we discussed above.
- Remove any jewellery that could inadvertently scratch your baby.
- Fill the baby bathtub or sink with two to three inches of warm—not hot—water. (Hint: Use the inside of your wrist to test the temperature. If it feels too warm to you, it will definitely feel too warm to your baby's sensitive skin.)
- Using one hand to support your baby's head and neck and the other to support his bottom and thighs, gently lower your baby into the tub.
- Use a baby washcloth to wash your baby's face (no soap) and then soap and rinse the rest of his body. Pour warm water over your baby's body to help keep him warm.
- Wash your baby's hair, massaging his entire scalp, including the area over the fontanelles (soft spots). (If your baby's almost bald, you can get away with using plain bar soap; if he has a full head of hair, you'll find baby shampoo a lot easier to work with.) If your baby is willing to wear a shampoo visor (a strange-looking contraption that's designed to keep the shampoo from running down the baby's face), then use one; otherwise, use a cup to pour water down the back of his head until all the shampoo has been rinsed away. If you accidentally get some soap or shampoo in your baby's eyes, take a wet washcloth and wipe his eyes with lukewarm water to get rid of the soap or shampoo.
- If your baby seems to enjoy his bath, allow him to relax in the tub for a few minutes after you've finished washing him. Just be careful not to let the water cool down to the point that he starts to get cold.
- If, on the other hand, your baby hates his bath, you might consider going back to sponge baths for a couple of weeks and then reintroducing

the bathtub again. At this stage of his life, your baby really isn't getting all that dirty: after all, he hasn't mastered the art of grinding squash and peas into his hair just yet. (All in good time!)

---

mother wisdom Worried that you won't be able to keep a good enough grip on your baby while you're giving him his bath? Trying slipping on a pair of cotton gloves first. Not only do you end up with a better grip, you'll have a built-in washcloth on each hand.

- When you're finished bathing your baby, wrap him in a hooded towel and gently pat him until he's just a little damp. At that point, you might want to rub a little baby lotion (all-natural, non-allergenic) on his skin to replenish some of the moisture he lost during the bath.

Moving up to the "big tub"

Most babies aren't ready for baths in a full-sized bathtub until they are somewhere between three and six months of age—the age by which most babies have begun to develop good head and neck control.

It's very important to pay attention to safety when you're bathing a baby in a full-sized tub. That means

- ensuring that you use a rubber bath mat to minimize the risk of slipping;
- filling the tub *before* you put your baby in the water and keeping your water heater turned down to 50 degrees Celsius (120 degrees Fahrenheit) to reduce the risk of scalding; and

---

mother wisdom You can help your baby adjust to being bathed in a full-sized bathtub by placing her baby bathtub inside the tub for a while before she "graduates" to the big tub. You might also try taking a bath or two with her yourself. (Just make a point of keeping the water a little cooler than you normally like it since what feels nice and toasty to you will probably feel too hot to her.)

- never leaving your baby unattended in the bathtub for even a minute. (If the phone or the doorbell rings, either ignore it or quickly wrap the baby in a towel and take her with you while you dash off to answer it.)

Warning: According to Health Canada, babies in bath rings (plastic rings with suction cups that help to support the baby in a seated position) have drowned when the suction cups became loose and the seat tipped over, when the baby slipped through a leg opening of the seat, or when the baby tried to climb out of the seat. *If parents choose to use a bath ring, a baby must be kept in sight and within arm's reach at all times.* A bath ring should never be used with a baby who is unable to sit on his or her own or with a baby or toddler who is capable of standing up on his or her own.

A final bit of advice on the business of bathing babies: be prepared to get soaked. Even if you throw a towel over your shoulder when you're taking your baby out of the tub, you're bound to get wet—assuming, of course, that you aren't already. (Some babies love to kick up a storm in the tub, drenching everything, and everyone, in sight.) Of course, if you've opted for bathing with your baby (as many parents do), this is a non-issue. You planned to get wet right from the get-go.

With any luck, your baby's bath time will become an enjoyable time for both you and your baby—a fun and relaxing time to play together and enjoy one another's company.

INFANT MASSAGE

You've no doubt heard how beneficial infant massage is to babies, but what you might not realize is that infant massage is highly beneficial to parents, too. Studies have shown that parents who massage their babies tend to be more sensitive to their baby's needs, more confident in their own parenting abilities, and more responsive and more attached to their babies than parents who do not practise infant massage.

Of course, the health benefits of massage for babies are reason enough to start practising infant massage. Studies have shown that infant massage encourages the release of growth hormones from the pituitary gland; improves food absorption and digestion; improves blood circulation; lowers levels of stress hormones, resulting in improved immune function; improves sleep; and improves weight gain and motor development in premature babies.

Here are some tips on getting started with infant massage.

- Wait for the right opportunity to introduce your baby to infant massage. Choose a time when she's calm and contented—in a quiet, alert state.
- Eliminate any outside distractions before you get started. Turn off the phone and put on some soothing music to block out any jarring background noises that might disturb you or your baby.
- Make sure that the room where you will be conducting the massage is warm enough (at least 24 degrees Celsius or 75 degrees Fahrenheit). Your baby won't be able to enjoy her massage if she's shivering the entire time.
- Remove any jewellery and ensure that your nails are well trimmed so that you won't accidentally scratch your baby during her massage.
- Wash your hands thoroughly before you get started. If you use warm water, you'll be able to warm up your hands at the same time.
- Remove your baby's clothing and lay her on her back on a soft blanket or towel, talking to her in a calm, soothing voice. Ask her permission to start the massage. If she expresses distress at some point during the massage, take that as a sign that she wants to stop.
- To minimize potentially irritating friction from the massage, put a small amount of cold-pressed edible oil (grapeseed, olive, sunflower) on your hands before you begin to massage your baby. (Note: You don't need to use any oil on your baby's face. In fact, some parents find that oil isn't needed at all. If you do use oil, remember that a little goes a long way.)
- Use your fingertips and the palms of your hands to massage your baby. Use a light touch at first, gradually increasing the amount of pressure you use as your baby becomes accustomed to being massaged. (See Table 7.4 for tips on some basic infant massage techniques.)
- Keep your massage sessions short and sweet: about 15 minutes or so. You can, of course, increase the length of each massage session if your baby seems to be eager for more, or cut it short if your baby's telling you that she's had enough. Respecting her likes and dislikes is another way of showing your love for your baby.

How to Massage Your Baby

Legs: Gently roll his legs between your hands, moving from the knee to the ankle. Then gently squeeze and knead each leg.

Arms: Lift each arm and gently stroke his armpits. Then gently squeeze and run your hand along his arm from the shoulder to the hand, much like what you'd do if you were sliding your hand up and down a baseball bat.

Chest: Lay both hands on his chest with your two thumbs side-by-side in the middle of the chest. Gently push out to either side. Then, without lifting your hands off his chest, gently bring them back together using a heart-shaped motion.

Abdomen: Place the side of each hand on his tummy, working in a water-wheel-like motion with one hand moving behind the other. Then walk your fingers across his tummy in a right-to-left motion. Variation: Hold your baby's legs with your left hand and grasp his ankles. Your baby's knees should be bent and his legs should be a few inches off the ground. Use the same water-wheel-like motion, but this time use your right hand only.

Face: Use your thumbs to make a smile with the upper lip and then the lower lip. Then massage your baby's temples and walk your fingers across his forehead.

Ears: Rub your forefinger and your thumb from the bottom of the ear lobe to the top of each ear.

Back: Place your two hands together at the top of his back at right angles to his spine. Move your hands in opposite directions: one hand should travel down his back toward his bottom while the other should travel up his back toward his shoulders. Reverse and repeat.

chapter 8

THE HEALTH AND SAFETY DEPARTMENT

> "Knowing what to fear, and what not to—the 'capacity to fear accurately,' as psychoanalyst Erik Erikson described it in his landmark work *Childhood and Society*—is key to good parenting (and also to staying sane as a parent)."
>
> —JOEL BAKAN, *CHILDHOOD UNDER SIEGE*

If there's a Murphy's Law that applies to parenting, it has to be this one: "The seriousness of your baby's illness will always be inversely proportional to the ease with which you can get in touch with your baby's doctor." In other words, you can expect your baby to come down with a raging fever exactly 10 minutes after the doctor's office shuts down for a holiday weekend. While you always have the option of finding an after-hours clinic or dragging your sick baby down to the hospital emergency department, that usually means sentencing yourself to an interminably long wait in a stuffy room that is overflowing with sick and crying children and their totally stressed-out parents—definitely a less than ideal state of affairs.

In this chapter, we're going to talk about the important role you play in keeping your baby healthy. We'll start out by talking about the importance of "well-baby checkups" (your child's non-emergency visits to the doctor's office) and immunizations for ensuring your child's continued good health. Then we'll look at ways of treating some of the most common types of childhood illnesses and swap strategies for staying sane if your baby ends up being hospitalized. At that point, we'll move on to a detailed discussion about infant and child safety, including "environmental childproofing," keeping baby safe when you're travelling by car, and reducing the risk of sudden infant death syndrome (SIDS).

mother wisdom — One of the key challenges you'll face as a parent is in finding a way to balance the need to keep your child safe and healthy against the need to allow him to explore his world and develop new strengths and capabilities.

mom's the word — "Before you can drive a car, you get a lot of practical experience with a driving instructor. It's not like there's a baby school where you can go for a week or two and practise with other people's babies. But maybe there should be!"
—JOYCE, 41, MOTHER OF TWO

HOW OFTEN SHOULD YOUR BABY SEE THE DOCTOR?

Your nine months of prenatal checkups were mere training for what lies ahead: years and years of kid-related doctor's appointments. While there may be times when you feel less than enthusiastic about hanging out in the doctor's office, it's important to keep the big picture in mind: well-baby checkups allow your doctor to keep tabs on your baby's overall health and troubleshoot any problems that arise sooner rather than later.

What happens at a well-baby checkup

At each appointment during your baby's first year of life, you can expect your doctor to check your baby's height, weight, and head circumference (a measurement around your baby's head); to give him a head-to-toe examination to ensure that he is healthy; to ask you questions about his eating habits, his sleeping habits, and any developmental milestones he may have achieved since the last visit (rolling over, sitting up by himself, starting to say words); and to provide immunizations at the appropriate intervals (see immunization section that follows). These visits provide you with the ideal opportunity to ask any baby-related questions of your own. (Trust me, there are bound to be plenty—so many, in fact, that you might want to get in the habit of keeping a running list of questions to bring to your baby's next checkup. Of course, if it's a pressing question, you'll want to call your health unit or your doctor's office right away rather than wait for the next checkup to roll around.)

As a general guideline, you can expect your baby to visit the doctor's office during the first week after the birth, and at age 2 months, 4 months, 6 months, 9 months, and 12 months, although, of course, you'll be trekking to the doctor's office more often than this if your baby ends up being susceptible to ear infections or other such illnesses.

THE FACTS ON IMMUNIZATIONS

Immunizations continue to play a vital role in helping to protect children against disease—so vital, in fact, that both the Canadian Paediatric Society and the National Advisory Committee on Immunization have spoken out strongly in favour of the current practice of routinely immunizing Canadian infants against a number of potentially life-threatening diseases.

That said, there are three situations in which an individual *definitely should not* receive a vaccine, two of which may be applicable to infants:

1. Anyone who has had a severe allergic reaction to a vaccine or a component of a vaccine should not receive the same vaccine again. The invidividual should be referred to an allergist so that the specific cause of the allergic reaction can be determined, along with which vaccines should be avoided and for how long.

2. Individuals with severely compromised immune systems should avoid live viral or bacterial vaccines.

3. Pregnant women should avoid live viral or bacteria vaccines unless their risk from an illness is greater than the potential risk from the vaccine.

---

mother wisdom How *you* react during your baby's immunization affects your baby's ability to cope. (If you fall apart, odds are your baby will, too.) "A matter-of-fact, supportive, nonapologetic approach" is recommended. Researchers with the Pain Relief Program at the Connecticut Children's Medical Center in Hartford, Connecticut, and the Centre for Research in Pediatric Pain at the IWK Health Centre in Halifax, Nova Scotia, have discovered that humour and distraction tend to decrease distress, while excessive parental reassurances, empathy, and apologies tend to increase distress. So bring along a few of your baby's favourite toys, as a means of distracting baby, and you'll make that immunization easier on your little one.

How immunizations work

Immunizations help the body produce antibodies against a particular disease. Depending on the type of immunization, the immunization may be injected or given orally. Still, as much as they have revolutionized pediatric health, they aren't always 100 per cent effective. (Of people who have been immunized against measles, 99.7 per cent will be immune to measles, while 99 per cent of people who have been immunized against polio will be immune to polio.)

Here's what you need to know about the most common early childhood vaccinations and the 13 diseases that they prevent. (See Table 8.1 for a schedule outlining when these immunizations typically occur and in which combinations.)

The 5-in-1 vaccine: Diphtheria, pertussis, tetanus, polio, haemophilus influenzae type b

The 5-in-1 vaccine (DTAP-IPV) immunization provides protection against five different diseases:

- diphtheria (a disease that attacks the throat and heart and that can lead to heart failure or death);
- pertussis or whooping cough (a disease characterized by a severe cough that makes it difficult to breathe, eat, or drink and that can lead to pneumonia, convulsions, brain damage, and death);
- tetanus (a disease that can lead to muscle spasms and death);
- polio (a disease that can result in muscle pain and paralysis and death); and
- haemophilus influenzae type b (Hib) (a disease that can lead to meningitis, pneumonia, and a severe throat infection (epiglottis) that can cause choking).

Immunization side effects are generally mild. The vast majority of children who experience some sort of reaction to the needle don't experience anything more serious than some pain and redness at the injection site or a low-grade fever.

TABLE 8.1 Recommended Immunization Schedule for Canadian Children

	2 months	4 months	6 months	12 months	18 months	4–6 years	14–16 years
Diphtheria, tetanus, acellular pertussis, and inactivated polio virus vaccine (DTAP-IPV)	X	X	X		X	X	
Haemophilus influenzae type b conjugate vaccine (Hib)	X	X	X		X		
Measles, mumps, and rubella vaccine (MMR)				X	X or	X	
Varicella vaccine (Var)				X			
Rotavirus vaccine	X (oral) at 6 weeks; X (oral) at 15 weeks						

(continued)

	2 months	4 months	6 months	12 months	18 months	4–6 years	14–16 years
Hepatitis B vaccine (HB)	3 doses during infancy or 2–3 doses during preteen/teen years						
Pneumococcal conjugate 7-valent vaccine (Pneu-C-7)	X	X	X	X (12–15 mo)			
Meningococcal C conjugate vaccine (Men-C)	X	OPTIONAL DOSE	X	or X (if not yet given)			X (if not yet given)
Influenza vaccine (Inf)			X 1–2 doses: 6–23 months				

Note: Exact immunization schedule varies by province or territory. You can obtain a copy of the most up-to-date immunization schedule for your province or territory by visiting www.phac-aspc.gc.ca/im/is-pi-eng.php. Or you can use the immunization tool at www.phac-aspc.gc.ca/im/iyc-vve/is-cv-eng.php to generate an immunization schedule that is customized to reflect your child's age and your province or territory. Some provinces and territories also immunize for baccillus Calmette-Guerin (a vaccine that protects against tuberculosis).
Note: Some Canadian children are now receiving the MMRV vaccine, which combines the varicella vaccine with the measles, mumps, rubella vaccine.

baby talk — Worried about something you've read about immunizations causing autism? A British physician raised this possibility in a much-talked-about 1998 study published in the medical journal the *Lancet* that ended up being thoroughly discredited. Other concerns regarding a possible link between the perservative thimerosal (used in certain types of vaccines) and autism were also investigated, but no such link was found. According to the Centers for Disease Control and Prevention, the misconception that there is a link between vaccination and autism likely persists because of "the coincidence of timing between early childhood vaccinations and the first appearance of symptoms of autism."

Measles, mumps, rubella (MMR) vaccine

This vaccine provides protection against three diseases:

- measles (a disease that involves fever, rash, cough, runny nose, and watery eyes and that can cause ear infections, pneumonia, brain swelling, and even death);
- mumps (a disease that can result in facial swelling, meningitis—the swelling of the coverings of the brain and spinal cord—and, in rare cases, testicular damage that may result in sterility); and
- rubella (a disease that can result in severe injury to or even the death of the fetus if it is contracted by a pregnant woman).

baby talk — You should talk to your doctor about MMR vaccination if your baby:

√ is taking a medication or has a disease like HIV that affects the immune system;

√ has received blood products or immune globulin within the past year;

√ is allergic to eggs (particularly if he experiences hives, wheezing, difficulty breathing, or a swelling of the face or the mouth after eating eggs); or

√ is allergic to an antibiotic called neomycin.

While most children who have the MMR vaccine experience few, if any, side effects (a slight fever, fussiness, redness or soreness at the injection site), in rare cases, children may develop a fever and/or rash seven to twelve days after the immunization. In one out of 3,000 cases, this fever may lead to convulsions. This type of reaction is more common in children who have reacted to a previous immunization or whose parents or siblings have experienced convulsions following an immunization. In rare cases, a child may develop meningitis (an infection of the fluid lining covering the brain and the spinal cord) or swelling of the testicles in response to the mumps portion of the vaccine.

Note: While the measles, mumps, and rubella vaccines are typically packaged together in a single injection, they can also be given separately—something to bear in mind if, for whatever reason, your child is not a good candidate for one of the individual vaccines.

Varicella vaccine

Chicken pox is a generally mild and non-life-threatening disease that can, in some cases, lead to a number of potentially serious complications, including pneumonia (an infection of the lungs) and encephalitis (an infection of the brain). An unborn baby who is exposed to chicken pox prior to birth faces a risk of birth defects, pneumonia, brain damage, or even death. Newborn babies, adults, and people with compromised immune systems are at risk of experiencing serious complications if they contract chicken pox.

The varicella (chicken pox) vaccine can be given to your child shortly after his first birthday (at the same time that the MMR vaccine is administered, but using a separate syringe and a separate injection side), or as part of a combined vaccine (MMRV).

It is not recommended for babies under one year of age. It's also not recommended for babies who are allergic to any of the vaccine compounds (including gelatin and neomycin); who have a blood disorder or any type of cancer that affects the immune system; who are taking medications to suppress the immune system; who have active, untreated tuberculosis; or who have a fever.

The chicken pox vaccine has only minor side effects: redness, stiffness, soreness, and/or swelling at the immunization site. Occasionally, babies may develop a mild chicken pox–like rash (typically 50 spots or fewer, as compared with the up to 500 spots that can accompany a full-blown case of chicken pox) one to two weeks after having the vaccine.

Note: In September 2010, Canada's National Advisory Committee on Immunization (NACI) began recommending that healthy children between the ages of one and twelve should receive two doses of varicella-containing vaccine.

Rotavirus

Rotavirus is a virus in the stool that is spread through person-to-person contact. It is the most common cause of diarrhea outbreaks in childcare centres.

The National Advisory Committee on Immunization is now recommending that healthy infants receive an oral vaccine to protect them against rotavirus in two doses: one dose at 6 weeks and the other dose at 15 weeks. All doses of the vaccine should be completed by the time the baby is 8 months old.

If you are pregnant, you don't have to worry about having your baby receive the rotavirus oral vaccine. According to NACI, "Because most women of childbearing age have pre-existing immunity to rotavirus through natural exposure, the risk of infection and disease from vaccine virus is low. Additionally, rotavirus infection during pregnancy is not known to pose a risk to the fetus."

If your baby has a history of anaphylactic reaction to any ingredient in the rotavirus vaccine or its oral applicator (which contains latex), your baby should not be vaccinated. Talk to your health-care provider.

---

baby talk Severe allergic reactions (breathing problems such as wheezing; swelling and blotchy skin on the body or around the mouth) following any vaccination are extremely rare. Typically these reactions occur within minutes of getting the vaccine, which is why your health-care provider will ask you to stay for at least 15 minutes after your baby receives a vaccination. If it is confirmed that your child has experienced an allergic reaction, seek advice from a pediatrician or allergist about which vaccines your child should receive and which vaccines your child should avoid in future.

Hepatitis B

Hepatitis B is a contagious disease that is spread from person to person via body fluids, including blood and breast milk. Hepatitis B attacks the liver, resulting in liver cancer or other serious liver problems.

Side effects of the vaccine are usually very mild. Your child may have a slight fever and there may be redness and soreness at the injection site. These side effects—which typically occur within 12 to 24 hours of the immunization—usually disappear within a few days.

Pneumoccocal vaccine

Pneumoccocal disease is a bacterial disease that can lead to meningitis (brain infection), bacteremia (bloodstream infection), pneumonia (lung infection), and otitis media (middle ear infection). Complications from pneumoccocal disease can result in lifelong damage to the brain, the ears, and major organs.

Side effects of the vaccine are usually very mild and include a slight fever and/or redness and soreness at the injection site. These side effects—which typically occur within 12 to 24 hours of the immunization—usually disappear within a few days.

Meningococcal meningitis vaccine

Meningococcal meningitis is a disease that can cause meningitis (an inflammation of the lining around your child's spinal cord and brain). It can also cause septicemia (infection of the bloodstream). It is spread by the meningococcal germ, a germ carried by one in five healthy teenagers and adults.

Side effects of the vaccine are usually very mild. Your child may have a slight fever and/or redness and soreness at the injection site. These side effects—which typically occur within 12 to 24 hours of the immunization—usually disappear within a few days. About one in ten older children and adults may experience a headache.

Flu shot (seasonal influenza)

Seasonal influenza (flu) is a common, contagious respiratory infection. It is spread via droplets that are coughed or sneezed by someone who has the flu. It typically starts with a headache, sore throat, and cough. Other symptoms include fever, loss of appetite, muscle aches and fatigue, runny nose, sneezing, watery eyes, and throat irritation. Children with the flu often experience nausea, vomiting, and diarrhea as well. They are also at risk of developing complications from the flu, including pneumonia.

The National Advisory Committee on Immunization recommends that all healthy children over the age of 6 months receive an annual flu shot to prevent illness and reduce spread of the flu to those who are more vulnerable. If there are children under the age of 2 in your home, everyone living in your home should receive a flu shot. Note: If your child is less than 9 years old and receiving a flu shot for the very first time, two doses are required, spaced about a month apart. From this point onward, a single flu shot is all that is required. Visit www.fightflu.ca for more information about seasonal flu. (Note: Children between the ages of 6 months and 23 months previously received a lower dose per injection, but will now receive the same dose as everyone else.)

Your child may have a slight fever and/or redness and soreness at the injection site. These side effects—which typically occur within 12 to 24 hours of the immunization—usually disappear within a few days. Once your child reaches age 2, your doctor may suggest a nasal spray form of the flu shot (FluMist) as an alternative to the flu shot itself, in order to reduce the number of injections your child receives (assuming, of course, that this option is available in your part of Canada).

Note: The best time to get a flu shot is in the fall (between October and December), before the number of flu cases in Canada peaks. The shot is still effective, though, even if you get it later in the season. It takes about two weeks after immunization for the flu shot to provide full protection.

HOW WILL I KNOW IF MY CHILD IS SICK?

Most first-time parents live in fear that they will mistakenly assume that their baby's runny nose is caused by nothing more sinister than the common cold when, in fact, it's actually a symptom of some life-threatening disease. Just in case this is one of those fears that have you tossing and turning in the middle of the night, allow me to reassure you.

Believe it or not, your parent radar is more highly developed than you realize. Mother Nature has programmed your baby with a series of symptoms that are designed to tell you that he's developed some sort of illness. (They're not unlike the error messages that show up on your computer screen from time to time, alerting you to the fact that your computer is anything but happy.) But unlike the nice, neat little text box that shows up on your computer screen, baby-related error messages tend to be a whole lot messier. You can expect your baby to experience one or more of the following symptoms if he's doing battle with some sort of illness:

Respiratory symptoms

- **Runny nose:** Your baby's nose starts secreting clear, colourless mucus that may become thick and yellowish or greenish within a day or two. A runny nose is usually caused by a viral infection such as the common cold, but it can also be caused by a reaction to a food or something else in the baby's environment. Note: Your baby should be checked by a doctor if the runny nose continues for longer than 10 days in order to rule out these causes and to check for the presence of a sinus infection.

- **Coughing:** Your baby starts coughing because there is some sort of infection in the respiratory tract—anywhere from the nose to the lungs. Common causes of coughing include the common cold, allergies, and chemical irritations (such as exposure to cigarette smoke). Rare but more serious causes of coughing can include cystic fibrosis and other chronic lung diseases, or because he has inhaled and aspirated an object that's causing him to cough.

- **Wheezing:** Your baby makes wheezing sounds that are particularly noticeable when he's breathing out (exhaling). Wheezing is caused by both the narrowing of the air passages in the lungs and the presence of excess mucus in those major airways (bronchi) or the lungs, most often triggered by a viral infection. (The more rapid and laboured your child's breathing, the more serious the infection.)

- **Croup:** Your baby's breathing becomes very noisy (some babies become very hoarse and develop a cough that sounds like a seal's bark) and, in severe cases, his windpipe may actually become obstructed. Typically, the more laboured and noisy your baby's breathing, the more serious the infection. Croup is caused by an inflammation of the windpipe below the vocal cords. See the section on treating croup later in this chapter.

---

mom's the word "One thing that really scared me was my babies' breathing. All of my kids seemed to be so congested when they were newborns—it was almost like they had a cold for the first couple of weeks. They found it difficult to breathe and had a lot of mucus in their noses, which I had to remove using a baby nasal aspirator."

—LORI, 30, MOTHER OF FIVE

Gastrointestinal symptoms

- **Diarrhea:** Your baby's bowel movements become more frequent and/or their texture changes dramatically (for example, they become watery or unformed). Just bear in mind that the colour and texture of a breastfed baby's bowel movements can vary considerably—and that breastfed babies can have a lot of bowel movements: eight to ten in a single day is not usual. What you're looking for, when you're monitoring your baby's bowel movements, is a pattern that is unusual for your baby—possibly accompanied by other signs that your baby could be ill.

    Diarrhea is often accompanied by abdominal cramps or a stomach ache and is triggered when the bowel is stimulated or irritated (often by the presence of an infection). It can lead to dehydration if it is severe or continues for an extended period of time, so you'll want to monitor your baby for any possible signs of dehydration. Note: See the section on treating diarrhea elsewhere in this chapter.

- **Dehydration:** Your baby has a dry mouth, is urinating less often than usual, and doesn't shed any tears when he cries. He may also be experiencing vomiting and/or diarrhea and probably isn't drinking as much as usual. Dehydration is commonly triggered by the presence of an infection and results in reduced blood circulation. Dehydration can occur quite rapidly in infants with diarrhea, so you'll want to watch your baby carefully if he's suffering from this problem—especially if he's also experiencing some vomiting. Signs that your baby's dehydration may be severe include lethargic or irritable behaviour; sunken eyes; a sunken soft spot (fontanelle); a dry mouth; an absence of tears; pale, wrinkled skin; highly concentrated urine (urine that is dark yellow rather than pale in colour); and infrequent urination. Note: See the section on dealing with dehydration elsewhere in this chapter.

- **Vomiting:** Vomiting is more common in children than in adults and tends to be less bothersome to children than adults. It can be caused by specific irritation to the stomach or, more commonly, is simply a side effect of another illness. It is generally only worrisome if your child vomits often enough to become dehydrated or if your child chokes and inhales vomit. The combination of high fever and vomiting in a young child should prompt a medical visit, particularly if the child is not drinking well. This combination of symptoms may indicate pneumonia or a kidney infection. Note: See the section on managing vomiting elsewhere in this chapter.

But before you panic, it's important to understand that vomiting is not the same thing as "spitting up." It's normal for a baby to regurgitate (spit up) some milk during or after a feeding. This regurgitated milk smells like sour milk and looks like thick milk with a few lumps of cottage cheese. Babies tend to spit up if they eat quickly, consume a lot of milk, or swallow a lot of air, and/or if the valve (the lower esophageal sphincter) that is supposed to keep the contents of their stomachs from being regurgitated hasn't fully matured (as is the case for about one-quarter of babies). In this situation, as long as your baby is gaining weight normally, there is generally no cause for concern.

Skin changes

- **Change in skin colour:** Your baby suddenly becomes pale or flushed, or the whites of his eyes take on a yellowish or pinkish hue. Your child may have developed some sort of an infection, whether it be a systemic infection (such as stomach flu or jaundice) or a more localized infection (such as pink eye).
- **Rashes:** Your baby develops some sort of skin rash. It could be the result of a viral or bacterial infection, or an allergic reaction to a food, medication, or other substance. Note: See the section on skin rashes later in this chapter.

Other symptoms

- **Behavioural changes:** Your baby becomes uncharacteristically fussy and irritable or sleepy and lethargic. It's possible that some sort of illness or infection is responsible for these changes in your baby's usual behaviour. You know your baby best, so you may tune into these behavioural changes sooner than someone who doesn't know your baby quite so well. If you feel that your baby is sick, trust your instincts and get your baby checked out. You were given those instincts for a reason.
- **Fever:** Your baby's temperature is higher than normal—something that often indicates the presence of an infection, but that can also be caused by a reaction to an immunization or the fact that baby is wearing too many layers of clothing.

baby talk

Fever can also be a sign of heat stroke—an important point to keep in mind on a hot day.

MORE ABOUT FEVER

Before we move on to our discussion of the most common types of childhood illnesses, let's take a moment to talk about babies and fevers—a perennial cause of concern to parents.

Fever is not the bad guy: The illness is

The first thing you need to know about fevers is that the fever in and of itself is not dangerous. Contrary to popular belief, fever does not cause brain damage. In order for brain damage to possibly occur, your baby's temperature would have to shoot to above 42 degrees Celsius (107.6 degrees Fahrenheit) for an extended period of time. Fevers that are caused by an infection rarely manage to climb above 40.5 degrees Celsius (105 degrees Fahrenheit) unless a child is overdressed or in an extremely hot environment. So that's one fever-related worry you can strike off your list relatively easily.

Fever can, in fact, be a *good* thing, even though it can make your baby (and consequently you) feel downright miserable for a while. The presence of a fever is usually a sign that the body is hard at work fighting off an infection (typically a common illness such as a cold, a sore throat, or an ear infection). Most of the bacteria and viruses that cause infections in humans thrive at our normal body temperature, so one of the body's key strategies for defending itself is to elevate its temperature by a couple of degrees. Add to that the fact that fever helps to activate the immune system—boosting the production of white blood cells, antibodies, and many other infection-fighting agents— and you'll see that there's no need to sweat it when your child gets a fever.

---

baby talk — A rapid increase in temperature can cause seizures in some babies.

---

mother wisdom — Mother knows best—well, at least 75 per cent of the time. Studies have shown that mothers who put a hand on their child's forehead can determine whether or not their child has a fever approximately three out of four times.

---

baby talk Don't make the mistake of assuming that your baby's high fever is the result of teething. While teething can produce a mild fever as a result of inflammation caused by the pressure of the teeth against the soft gums, it rarely causes a fever of more than 38 degrees Celsius (101 degrees Fahrenheit). If your baby is teething and develops a fever, don't ignore the fever, figuring it's part of teething. And remember: a fever in a young baby (under three months) *definitely* needs to be checked out by a doctor.

This does not compute

Something else you need to know is that the height of the fever is not necessarily directly related to the severity of your child's illness. In other words, even though your child may have a relatively high fever, it's possible that she's only mildly ill. On the other hand, a child with a relatively low fever can, in fact, be quite ill, which is why it's important to pay attention to your child's other symptoms. Instead of getting hung up on the number on the thermometer—an easy trap to fall into, by the way—concentrate on how sick your child is acting and look for symptoms of any underlying infection. (See Table 8.2.)

TABLE 8.2

Common Illnesses That Can Cause a Fever

Symptoms	What could be causing these symptoms
Fever, cough, runny nose, trouble breathing, sore throat, sore muscles	Common cold, influenza, other respiratory infections
Fever, earache, discharge from ears, dizziness from pain	Ear infection
Fever, swollen glands, sore throat	Tonsillitis, streptococcal or viral infection, mononucleosis
Fever, nausea, vomiting, diarrhea, and/or cramps	Infectious gastroenteritis (stomach flu)

What type of thermometer to use

If you've checked at your local drugstore lately, you already know that there are all kinds of different makes and models of thermometers on the market today—everything from basic digital thermometers to high-tech tympanic (ear) thermometers.

You have two basic choices when it comes to taking the temperature of a young baby: taking your baby's temperature rectally or taking an axillary temperature (under the armpit). Temperatures of children under 4 years of age should not be taken orally.

- **Rectal temperatures** tend to be the most accurate, but they aren't exactly the temperature-taking method of choice for parents (who can feel a bit squeamish about inserting anything into their babies' bottoms). Here's what's involved in taking your baby's temperature rectally:
  - Place your child on his back and position him so that his knees are bent over his abdomen.
  - Coat the tip of the thermometer with water-soluble lubricant and insert it approximately 2.5 centimetres (1 inch) into your baby's rectum.
  - Hold the thermometer in place until the digital thermometer beeps to indicate that the final temperature reading has been obtained—something that typically takes about two minutes.
  - Keep in mind that rectal temperature readings tend to be about 0.5 degrees Celsius higher than temperatures taken orally: a "normal" range for a rectal temperature is 36.6 to 38 degrees Celsius (97.9 to 101 degrees Fahrenheit).
  - Clean the thermometer thoroughly using soap and warm water.

mother wisdom Today's digital thermometers are every bit as accurate as the glass thermometers of yesteryear. What's more, they offer a few additional advantages: they are faster to use; they beep when the maximum temperature has been reached; they are easier to read; and the same thermometer can be used for both oral and rectal temperatures. (You'll want to hold off on taking your child's temperature orally until she's at least 4 years old.)

mother wisdom Avoid using fever strips (strips that are placed on a child's forehead to take the child's temperature). According to the College of Family Physicians of Canada, they aren't sufficiently accurate. You'll also want to take a pass on that flashy tympanic (ear) thermometer, since these types of thermometers are only recommended for use in children over the age of 2 due to concerns about the quality of the readings they produce when they are used on infants.

- **Axillary temperatures** (temperatures that are taken under the armpit) tend to be slightly less accurate, but they're much easier to take. Here's what's involved in using this method of taking your baby's temperature:
  - Place the bulb of the thermometer under your baby's arm so that it's nestled in his armpit, and then hold your baby's arm against his body so that the bulb is thoroughly covered.
  - Hold the thermometer in place until the digital thermometer beeps to indicate that the final temperature reading has been obtained—something that typically takes about two minutes.
  - Clean the thermometer thoroughly using soap and warm water.
  - Keep in mind that axillary temperature readings tend to be about 0.3 degrees Celsius lower than temperatures taken orally: a "normal" range for an axillary temperature is 34.7 to 37.3 degrees Celsius (94.5 to 99.1 degrees Fahrenheit).

What you need to know about febrile convulsions

Febrile convulsions (seizures) tend to occur when a baby's temperature shoots up very suddenly. They occur in children ages 6 months to 6 years, and they're more likely to occur in families with a history of febrile convulsions. They occur in approximately 4 per cent of children.

While febrile convulsions are relatively common and generally quite harmless, they can be extremely frightening to watch. If your baby has a febrile convulsion, he may breathe heavily, drool, turn blue, roll his eyes back in his head, and/or shake his arms and legs uncontrollably.

If your baby has a febrile convulsion you should lay him on his back or side, ensuring that he's far away from anything he could hurt himself on, and then gently turn his head to one side so that any vomit or saliva can drain easily. If possible, you should time how long the febrile convulsion lasts—anywhere from 10 seconds to 10 minutes. (See the tips on managing your child's fever later in this chapter.) You should call 9–1–1 if your baby's seizure lasts for more than five minutes, your baby is having difficulty breathing, you suspect that your baby's seizure is being triggered by an underlying illness (perhaps pneumonia or meningitis), or another seizure starts shortly after the first one ended. Any baby who is experiencing febrile convulsions should be seen by a doctor as soon as possible to rule out the possibility of more serious illness.

When to call the doctor

While most fevers are harmless, you should plan to get in touch with your baby's doctor right away and/or seek emergency assistance if

- your baby's fever is too high for a child his age, regardless of whether or not he actually appears to be very ill (see Table 8.3);

TABLE 8.3

How High Is Too High?

According to the College of Family Physicians of Canada, you should call your baby's doctor if his temperature becomes higher than the maximums recommended for a child his age.

Age	Temperature
Under one month of age	It's always best to err on the side of caution when you're dealing with a fever in a child of this age. You may want to call your doctor's office even if your child has a very low-grade fever (see guidelines on the previous page for information on what constitutes a normal range for a rectal temperature), since the doctor may want to check your baby for signs of streptococcal meningitis.
One to three months of age	A rectal temperature of 38.6°C (101.4°F) or higher
Three months to two years of age	A rectal temperature of 39°C (103°F) or higher

- your baby has had a fever for a couple of days and his temperature is not coming down;
- he is crying inconsolably or seems cranky or irritable, or he's whimpering and seems weak;
- he's having difficulty waking up or seems listless and confused;
- he's limp;
- he's having convulsions;
- the soft spot (fontanelle) on his head is beginning to swell;
- he appears to have a stiff neck or a headache;
- he is acting as if he is experiencing stomach pain;
- he has purple (not red) spots on the skin or large purple blotches (possible signs of meningitis, an infection of the brain);
- he has developed a skin rash;
- he is noticeably pale or flushed;
- he's having difficulty breathing (a possible sign of asthma or pneumonia);
- he is refusing to drink or nurse (this is probably the most important);
- he has constant vomiting or diarrhea;
- he is unable to swallow and is drooling excessively (a possible sign of epiglottitis, a life-threatening infection that causes swelling in the back of the throat); or
- you know that he has a weakened immune system, due to a pre-existing condition.

baby talk Don't expect your doctor to prescribe an antibiotic to ward off your child's fever unless there's a specific underlying infection that requires treatment. According to the Canadian Paediatric Society, the vast majority of children with fevers have non-bacterial (viral) upper respiratory infections that don't require antibiotics. That means your first line of defence against fever is likely to be none other than acetaminophen.

Treating a fever

Of course, it's not necessary to rush off to the emergency ward every time your baby's temperature shoots up by a degree or two.

The majority of fevers can be managed at home. Here's what you need to know.

- The best way to treat a fever is by administering acetaminophen—an analgesic that helps to bring down your child's fever while relieving some of his discomfort. (Note: See Table 8.4 for a complete list of items that should be in the family medicine chest while you have a young baby at home.) If your baby is under the age of 3 months, you'll want to have your baby checked by a physician first before you automatically reach for the acetaminophen bottle. It's important to have the cause of the fever determined in a baby this age before you start treating the symptoms.

- It's dangerous to exceed the recommended dose of acetaminophen, so make sure that you use a medication syringe or dropper to measure your child's dose and that you stick to the recommended schedule for administering the medication.

TABLE 8.4

Medicine Chest Essentials

Keep the following items on hand at all times so that you'll have them in the event of illness or injury:	
acetaminophen	nail clippers (baby-safe type)
adhesive tape	nasal aspirator
antibiotic ointment	nose drops (saline)
bandages	oral electrolyte solution (to treat dehydration)
cotton balls	
flashlight	Q-tips
gauze	scissors (blunt ended)
hydrogen peroxide	syringe
ice packs (the instant type don't require refrigeration)	thermometer (digital)
	tongue depressors
infant dropper or medicine	tweezers

baby talk — In December 2008, Health Canada issued an advisory recommending that over-the-counter cough and cold medications no longer be given to children under age 6. The advisory was the result of a review of the use of cough and cold medications in young children. The researchers concluded that there was "limited evidence supporting their effectiveness" and that "reports of misuse, overdose, and very rare serious side effects" raised concerns about the use of these products in children under age 6.

baby talk — Studies have shown that giving a child twice the recommended dose of acetaminophen over a period of days can be toxic. If your child becomes nauseated, starts vomiting, and experiences some abdominal pain, you should try to determine whether or not he might have been given too much acetaminophen and seek medical attention.

- If your baby spits up within a matter of minutes of taking his acetaminophen, ask your doctor if you should repeat the dose. It generally takes between 30 and 45 minutes for a medication to be absorbed by the intestine. If the medication has been in your child's stomach for more than a few minutes, don't risk giving him any extra without obtaining medical advice first. It's simply too difficult to determine how much of the original dose he managed to keep down. You can find some other helpful tips on administering medication to a baby in Table 8.5.
- Give your baby plenty of fluids in order to help bring his body temperature down and to help protect against dehydration.
- Avoid overdressing your child. Instead, dress him in loose, lightweight cotton clothing with only a sheet or light blanket for covering.
- Keep your baby's room cool, but not cold. If your child gets too cold, his body will start shivering—something that will cause his body temperature to rise.

- You can also try to lower your child's temperature by sponging him down with lukewarm water (a sponge bath) or giving him a lukewarm bath. (Don't use cold water or he'll start shivering.) Instead of drying him off, let the water evaporate from his skin. This will help to cool him down. Whatever you do, don't add alcohol to the water in some mistaken belief that this will somehow help to bring down your baby's temperature. Doing so could lead to serious—even life-threatening—complications.

---

mother wisdom Don't rely on your memory when it comes to administering your baby's medications. It's easy to make mistakes. Instead, get in the habit of writing down the time that the medication was given and the dose that was administered. (This is particularly important if more than one person will be responsible for administering the medication.) And if you're likely to forget to give your child his medication, set the alarm on your phone to go off the next time he's due for a dose.

TABLE 8.5

Administering Medication to a Baby

Forget about the spoonful of sugar: what it really takes to get the medicine to go down is a proper technique. Here are some tips on administering some of the types of medication that your doctor might prescribe for your baby.

Oral Medications

Use a syringe or an oral dropper to administer medication to an infant. A spoon is too awkward to use: you and your baby will both end up wearing the medication.

Slowly squirt the medication into the area between the baby's tongue and the side of his mouth, pausing between squirts so that he has a chance to swallow. Otherwise, he'll start to gag and spit the medication out, and you'll be back at square one.

Avoid squirting the medication into the back of your baby's throat or you'll trigger his gag reflex. And try to avoid hitting the taste buds at the front and centre of your baby's tongue. (Should the medication not meet with his exacting standards for taste, he will use his tongue to push the medication right back out!)

(continued)

Oral Medications (*continued*)

Avoid adding any sort of medication to a full bottle of milk or bowl of cereal. If your child only wants part of his milk or his cereal, he'll miss out on some of the medication. If you absolutely have to mix your child's medication with some sort of food because he refuses to take it any other way, make sure that you use a very small amount of food or liquid—a quantity that you know your child will have no trouble eating or drinking. (Obviously, this tip only applies to babies who have already started eating solid food.)

Let your doctor know if your child vomits repeatedly after taking a particular medication or if he has a stomach flu that makes it impossible for him to keep anything down. Your doctor might decide to prescribe an injection or suppository instead.

If you miss a dose, administer the next dose as soon as you remember. Don't double up on doses unless your doctor specifically tells you to do so. Be sure to get in touch with your doctor if your child ends up missing an entire day's worth of medication.

Ear Drops

Lay your child down.

Remove any medication that may have built up on the outer ear from past treatments before you administer the next dose.

Turn your baby's head to one side and gently pull the middle of the outer ear back slightly. This will allow fluid to enter the ear canal more readily. You may find it works best to give your baby his ear drops while he is breastfeeding.

Eye Drops/Ointments

Lay your baby on his back with his eyes closed. Drop the eye drop into the corner of his eye. When your child opens his eyes, the drop will roll into his eye.

Skin Ointments or Creams

Apply some of the ointment or cream to a tissue or gauze pad.

Using the tissue, apply the ointment or cream to your child's skin. To reduce the chances of contaminating the ointment or cream, discard the used tissue and use a fresh tissue if more ointment or cream is required.

COPING WITH COMMON CHILDHOOD ILLNESSES AND INFECTIONS

Since there are literally hundreds of illnesses and conditions that can occur during early childhood, we aren't going to be able to touch on each and every one in this chapter. Due to space constraints, I had to limit myself to the more common ones—pediatric medicine's greatest hits, so to speak. If you want to find out about an illness that isn't covered here, you might want to visit one of the many excellent pediatric health websites listed in Appendix B.

baby talk According to the Canadian Institute of Child Health, approximately one-third of babies who are hospitalized during the first year of life are hospitalized as a result of respiratory problems.

Respiratory and related conditions

Condition: Allergies

Cause: Allergies can be caused by pollens, animal dander, moulds, dust, and other substances.

Signs and symptoms: A clear runny nose and watery eyes, sneezing fits, constant sniffling, nosebleeds, dark circles under the eyes, frequent colds or ear infections, a cough that is bothersome at night, a stuffy nose in the morning, and/or noisy breathing at night.

What you can do:

- Eliminate or limit exposure to the substances that seem to trigger your baby's allergies.

- If the allergy is to dust, animal dander, et cetera, you can "allergy-proof" your baby's room by using allergy-proof zippered covers, purchasing non-allergenic bedding, removing stuffed animals from your baby's room (they should already be out of your baby's bed, due to the risk of sudden infant death syndrome: see section at the end of this chapter), removing all room deodorizers and baby powders, vacuuming the mattress and washing all of your baby's bedding at least once every two weeks, avoiding plush carpet (if possible), keeping your baby's windows closed during allergy season, investing in a high-efficiency particulate remover (HEPA filter), and only vacuuming your baby's room when he's out of the room since vacuuming tends to stir up dust. One final tip: If you haven't done so already, make your home smoke-free. Not only does smoke aggravate allergies, it increases the risk of SIDS.

- Keep your child comfortable by treating his symptoms (for example, using a nasal aspirator to clear his nose) and/or running a cold-air humidifier in his room. (Clean the humidifier once or twice a week.)

mother wisdom — Here are some important questions to ask your doctor or pharmacist when he prescribes a medication for your child for the very first time:

- ✓ How will this medication help my child?
- ✓ What is the correct dosage?
- ✓ Do I need to shake the bottle before administering the medication to my child?
- ✓ How often do I give my child the medication? Does it have to be administered at a particular time of day?
- ✓ How long does my child have to take the medication? Will the prescription be repeated or is this a "one-shot" deal?
- ✓ Should the medication be taken on a full or empty stomach?
- ✓ Are there any foods or drinks my child needs to avoid while taking this medication?
- ✓ Should the medication be stored in the refrigerator or at room temperature?
- ✓ Is it necessary to wake my child in the night to administer this medication?
- ✓ Are there any side effects to this medication that I need to know about?
- ✓ Is there any chance that my child could have an allergic reaction to this medication? If so, what warning signs should I watch out for?

Condition: Asthma (a lung condition that affects the bronchial tubes)

Cause: Most commonly triggered after a viral respiratory infection inflames the lining of the bronchial tubes in the lungs. Asthma can also be caused by irritants such as cigarette smoke, paint fumes, and chemicals found in common household cleansers; allergens such as pollens, mould spores, animal dander, house dust mites, and cockroaches; and inhaling cold air. In some older children, exercise may also be a trigger for asthma.

Signs and symptoms: Coughing and/or high-pitched wheezing or whistling as your baby breathes. The cough typically gets worse at night or if your baby comes into contact with an irritant such as cigarette smoke. In cases of severe asthma, your baby's breathing may become very rapid and laboured, his heart rate may increase, or he may become very tired and slow-moving and cough all the time (in which case he requires immediate medical attention).

What you can do:
- Try to eliminate anything that could be triggering your baby's asthma problems, including any irritants or allergens.
- Work with your doctor to come up with a game plan for preventing and treating future asthma attacks through medication and/or lifestyle modifications.

Condition: Bronchiolitis (an infection of the small breathing tubes of the lungs, not to be confused with bronchitis, which is an infection of the larger, more central airways)

Cause: Caused by a virus (frequently the respiratory syncytial (RSV) virus) that results in swelling of the small bronchial tubes. It is typically picked up as a result of being exposed to someone with an upper respiratory tract illness. Bronchiolitis is most common in children under the age of 2 and is most likely to occur during the winter months. Note: According to the American Academy of Pediatrics, almost half of babies who develop bronchiolitis will go on to develop asthma later in life.

Signs and symptoms: Triggered by a virus that results in swelling of the bronchioles, which, in turn, leads to reduced air flow through the lungs. It starts out like a normal cold with a runny nose and sneezing, but after a couple of days a baby with bronchiolitis starts coughing, wheezing, and having trouble breathing. Your baby may also be irritable and may experience difficulty eating due to the coughing and breathing problems.

What you can do:
- Keep your baby comfortable by using a nasal aspirator or a vaporizer. (Just make sure that you clean the vaporizer on a regular basis—ideally once or twice a week—to prevent it from becoming a breeding ground for bacteria.)
- Watch for signs of dehydration, as babies with bronchiolitis can become dehydrated.

- Get in touch with your doctor to find out whether any additional treatment may be required. Some babies who have a lot of difficulty breathing may require medication to open the bronchial tubes. A few will also need to be hospitalized so that oxygen and fluids may be administered until the baby's breathing improves.

Condition: Common cold
Cause: Spread from person to person via airborne droplets containing the cold virus or via contaminated hands and/or objects (such as toys). It is most contagious from one day before to seven days after the onset of symptoms, which helps to explain why your baby managed to pick up a cold at play group even though every child in the room appeared to be the absolute picture of health.

---

baby talk According to the Canadian Paediatric Society, there are more than 200 viruses that cause colds. Unfortunately, being infected by a particular virus once doesn't provide you with any protection against getting that virus again—something that goes a long way toward explaining why the common cold is so, well, *common*!

Signs and symptoms: Runny nose, sore throat, cough, decreased appetite. May also be accompanied by a fever, in which case your child may also experience muscle aches and/or a headache. While a cold typically lasts for five to seven days in an adult, children's colds tend to drag on a little longer—bad news, I know, if your baby is waking up every hour on the hour, totally enraged because his nose is clogged up.

What you can do:
- Keep your baby comfortable. You might want to clear out your child's runny nose by using a nasal aspirator or—if his nose is really stuffed up—by placing a vaporizer in his room. (Note: Be sure to clean the vaporizer frequently, at least once or twice a week.)
- Nasal drops and sprays (saline only) can also be used to soften up the mucus in your baby's nose so that he can breathe more easily.
- Keep your baby's face clean. Infections of the face can occur as a result of prolonged exposure to nasal secretions, and your baby

- could end up with yellow pustules or wide, honey-coloured scabs (impetigo).
- Expect feedings to take a little longer when your baby has a cold, and don't be surprised if your baby ends up drinking less than he normally would. Your baby may have difficulty nursing if his nose is really stuffed up—something that can quickly result in a hungry, gassy, unhappy baby.
- Watch for signs that your child's cold could be developing into something more serious. You'll want to get in touch with your doctor if your child develops an earache or a fever over 39 degrees Celsius (102.2 degrees Fahrenheit); if she becomes exceptionally sleepy, cranky, or fussy; if she develops a skin rash; if her breathing becomes rapid or laboured; or if her cough becomes persistent or severe.

Condition: Croup, or laryngotracheitis (an inflammation of the voice box or larynx and windpipe or trachea)

Cause: Usually caused by a viral infection in or around the voice box. Children are most susceptible to croup between 6 months and 3 years of age. As children get older, their windpipe gets larger, so swelling of the larynx and trachea is less likely to result in breathing difficulties. There are two types of croup: spasmodic croup (which comes on suddenly and is caused by a mild upper respiratory infection or allergy) and viral croup (which results from a viral infection in the voice box and windpipe and which may be accompanied by noisy or laboured breathing—a condition known as "stridor").

Signs and symptoms: A cough that sounds like a seal-like bark and/or a fever.

What you can do:
- Keep your baby comfortable by using a cool-mist vaporizer in his room; by filling your bathroom with hot steam from the shower and letting your baby breathe in the moist vapours; or by taking your child for a walk in the cool night air.
- Get in touch with your doctor if the croup seems to be particularly severe or if your baby shows the following types of symptoms: fever higher than 39 degrees Celsius (102 degrees Fahrenheit); rapid or difficult breathing; severe sore throat; increased drooling; refusal to swallow; and/or discomfort when lying down.

Condition: Ear infections (otitis media)

Cause: Caused by a virus and/or bacteria, and typically occurs in the aftermath of a cold. Because a child's eustachian tube (the tube that connects the middle ear to the back of the nose) is very short and narrow, children are highly susceptible to ear infections. A study of all children born in southwestern British Columbia between 1999 and 2000 found that just under half (48.6 per cent) paid at least one visit to the doctor because of an ear infection by the time they reached age 3.

Signs and symptoms: Fussiness and irritability, difficulty sleeping (because lying down tends to increase ear pain), difficulty nursing or drinking a bottle (because sucking and swallowing can result in painful pressure changes in the middle ear), difficulty hearing (for example, your baby stops responding to certain types of sounds), fluid draining from your baby's ear, and fever and cold symptoms. Note: If there is pus coming from your baby's ear, this means that your baby's eardrum has burst—something that may require treatment with antibiotics or antibiotic drops.

---

baby talk Certain babies are more susceptible to ear infections than others. According to the College of Family Physicians of Canada, a baby is more likely to develop an ear infection if he's exposed to cigarette smoke, he has had one or more ear infections in the past (particularly if those infections occurred before his first birthday), he is formula-fed rather than breastfed, he attends daycare, or he was born prematurely or was a low-birthweight baby, and if he is male. What's more, other research indicates that babies who use pacifiers face an increased risk of ear infections. Not only can pacifiers be breeding grounds for germs, some experts believe that the constant sucking motion associated with using a pacifier may cause fluid to be pulled from the nose and throat into the middle ear.

What you can do:

- Keep your baby comfortable by treating his fever and cold symptoms (see earlier sections of this chapter) and by offering him acetaminophen to treat his earache. Note: Heating pads are *not* recommended for babies due to the risk of overheating. Overheating is a risk factor for SIDS.

- Get in touch with your doctor to arrange for your baby's ears to be checked. Your doctor may want to prescribe an antibiotic to clear up the infection. (Note: In most cases, there's no need to rush off to the emergency ward in the middle of the night to seek treatment for an ear infection. Simply treat your baby's pain with acetaminophen during the night and then call your doctor's office in the morning to set up an appointment.)

- Even if your baby's ear infection has already been diagnosed by a doctor, you should call your doctor's office again if your baby develops one or more of the following symptoms: an earache that worsens even after your baby is on antibiotics; a fever that's greater than 39 degrees Celsius (102 degrees Fahrenheit) after treatment begins, or a fever that lasts more than three days; excessive sleepiness; excessive crankiness or fussiness; a skin rash; rapid or difficult breathing; or hearing loss.

  See that your child's ears are checked again in two to four weeks (after he's finished the antibiotic) to ensure that there's no fluid remaining in his ear. (Fluid in the ear can lead to further infections and/or hearing problems down the road.) Note: If your child has recurrent problems with ear infections, your doctor may recommend that your baby stay on antibiotics for a long period of time to prevent ear infections from developing, or that myringotomy tubes be inserted in your child's ears to help balance the pressure between the middle ear and the ear canal, thereby allowing the fluid that accumulates in the middle ear to drain. The tubes are inserted while your child is under general anaesthetic and generally stay in place for 6 to 9 months, at which point they typically fall out on their own. Some children need a second set of tubes.

---

baby talk Not everyone agrees that antibiotics should be prescribed for children with uncomplicated ear infections. A recent study sponsored by the Agency for Healthcare Research and Quality (AHRQ) revealed that almost two-thirds of children with garden-variety ear infections recover from pain and fever within 24 hours of diagnosis without any treatment and that over 80 per cent recover spontaneously within one to seven days. (When children are treated with antibiotics, 93 per cent recover within the first week.)

Condition: Influenza

Cause: Caused by a respiratory virus that is spread from person to person via droplets or contaminated objects.

Signs and symptoms: Fever; chills and shakes; extreme tiredness or fatigue; muscle aches and pains; and a dry, hacking cough. (It's different from the common cold in that a baby with the common cold only has a fever, a runny nose, and a small amount of coughing.)

What you can do:

- Keep your baby comfortable by treating his fever and cold symptoms (see relevant sections above). Young children, or children with underlying health conditions, may need anti-viral therapy (Tamiflu).

Condition: Pink eye (conjunctivitis)

Cause: A bacterial or viral infection spread from person to person as a result of direct contact with secretions from the eye. Pink eye is contagious for the duration of the illness or until 24 hours after antibiotic treatment has been started.

Signs and symptoms: Redness, itching, pain, and discharge from the eye.

What you can do:

- Get in touch with your doctor to see if antibiotic eye drops should be prescribed (if your child's eye discharge is yellowish and thick, indicating a bacterial infection that will respond to antibiotics).

- Keep your child away from other people until the antibiotic eye drops have been used for at least one full day.

Condition: Pneumonia (infection of the lung)

Cause: Spread from person to person via droplets or by touching contaminated objects. The infectious period varies according to the cause. Pneumonia can be caused by both viruses and bacterial infections.

Signs and symptoms: Rapid or noisy breathing possibly accompanied by a cough and/or flaring of the nostrils; pale or bluish skin colour; shaking or chills; high fever; vomiting; decreased appetite and energy.

What you can do:

- Get in touch with your doctor so that the cause of the pneumonia can be determined and an appropriate course of treatment can be mapped out. Viral pneumonias are typically treated with acetaminophen (for fever) and bronchodilators (to minimize wheezing). Bacterial pneumonias, on the other hand, respond to treatment that includes antibiotics, fluids, and humid air. Note: Children under the age of 6 months are often hospitalized when they develop pneumonia.

- Monitor your child's symptoms carefully if he's being cared for at home and report any changes in his condition to his doctor. Your child may require emergency assistance if he is having difficulty breathing.

Condition: Respiratory syncytial virus (RSV)
Cause: A virus with an incubation period of five to eight days.
Signs and symptoms: A raspy cough, rapid breathing, and wheezing.

What you can do:
- Keep your baby comfortable by using a nasal aspirator or a vaporizer.
- Watch for any signs of dehydration.
- Get in touch with your doctor to talk about treatment options. Some babies who have a lot of difficulty breathing may require medication to open the bronchial tubes. A few will also need to be hospitalized so that oxygen and fluids can be administered until the baby's breathing improves.

Condition: Strep throat
Cause: Strep throat is a bacterial infection. It is transmitted via droplets or by touching contaminated objects. It is contagious until 24 to 36 hours after the start of antibiotic treatment. Fortunately, strep throat is more common in children over the age of 3, so hopefully this is one infection your baby won't have to deal with during his first year of life.

---

baby talk Antibiotics are powerful medications that can be used to treat life-threatening illnesses like meningitis as well as less serious infections such as impetigo. Because they are so effective, they tend to be used widely—something that has unfortunately led to the emergence of antibiotic-resistant strains of bacteria. You can do your bit to prevent antibiotic-resistant strains of bacteria from becoming more of a problem by ensuring that you follow your doctor's instructions for antibiotic use carefully and seeing that your child finishes taking any antibiotic he starts.

---

baby talk — Don't be surprised if your child's temperature remains high for the first day or two after he starts antibiotic treatment. It takes time for the antibiotics to start working their magic.

Signs and symptoms: Sore throat, fever, swollen glands in the neck. (Note: If a skin rash is also present, the condition is known as scarlet fever.)

What you can do:
- Get in touch with your baby's doctor to arrange to have a throat swab taken to determine whether or not your baby has strep throat. If your baby does have strep throat, an antibiotic will be prescribed to help kill off the strep germ. If left untreated, strep throat can result in kidney disease or rheumatic fever (a serious condition that can cause heart damage and joint swelling). It can also lead to skin infections, bloodstream infections, ear infections, and pneumonia.
- Offer liquids and bland foods (if your baby is old enough for solid foods) and watch for signs of dehydration.

Condition: Tonsillitis
Cause: Can be bacterial or viral in origin.
Signs and symptoms: Fever, swollen glands under the jaw, a very sore throat, cold symptoms, and abdominal pain.
What you can do:
- Treat your baby's fever and cold symptoms. (See earlier sections of this chapter.)
- Have your baby examined by your doctor to see if an antibiotic should be prescribed.

Condition: Sinusitis (sinus infection)
Cause: The mucus in your child's sinuses becomes infected with bacteria, usually as the result of a lingering cold.
Signs and symptoms: Persistent green or yellow nasal discharge lasting more than a week, fever, a cough that gets worse at night, tenderness in the face, dark circles under the eyes, puffy lower eyelids, bad breath, fatigue.

What you can do:
- Get in touch with your baby's doctor to talk about whether your baby should be on some sort of antibiotic. If he prescribes one, don't be surprised if he prescribes a four- to six-week supply! Sinus infections can take time to clear up.
- Keep your child comfortable. (See tips in section above on treating the common cold.)

Condition: Whooping cough

Cause: Caused by a bacterial infection. The incubation period is seven to ten days.

Signs and symptoms: Cold-like symptoms that linger. About two weeks into the illness, the cough suddenly worsens. When the baby coughs, thick mucus is dislodged, causing the baby to gasp for his next breath (the "whoop" in whooping cough). The baby turns red in the face during the cough and then vomits afterwards. Whooping cough typically lasts for three to twelve weeks (it is often called "the cough that lasts 100 days") and is considered to be a serious illness in a baby under age one.

What you can do:
- Offer your baby plenty of fluids.
- See if a cool-mist vaporizer will help with your baby's cough.
- Seek immediate medical attention if your child becomes exhausted or is having difficulty breathing. Most babies under one year of age end up being hospitalized so that they can be treated with oxygen (and antibiotics in the hope of preventing the illness from spreading).

Skin and scalp conditions

Condition: Boils

Cause: Usually caused by staphylococcus bacteria from an infected pimple.

Signs and symptoms: Swellings on the skin that are raised, red, tender, and warm. Most commonly found on the buttocks.

What you can do:
- Apply hot compresses to the boils 10 times daily in order to bring them to a head, and then continue applying them for a few days after the

boils pop and drain. Avoid picking at or squeezing your baby's boils as this may result in scarring and spreading.

- Get in touch with your baby's doctor. If the boils don't drain on their own, they may need to be incised and drained by your doctor. A topical antibiotic or systemic antibiotics may also be required.

Condition: Cellulitis

Cause: Usually caused by a bacterial infection such as staphylococcus or streptococcus.

Signs and symptoms: Swollen, red, tender, warm areas of skin that are usually found on the extremities or the buttocks. They often start out as a boil or a puncture wound but then become infected. They are typically accompanied by a fever and swollen and tender lymph glands.

What you can do:

- Give your baby acetaminophen to help control the fever and pain.
- Contact your baby's doctor. This condition will need to be treated with antibiotics (oral, injected, or intravenous).

Condition: Chicken pox

Cause: Caused by a viral infection that is spread from person to person. The incubation period is two to three weeks. It is very difficult to control the spread of chicken pox because it can be spread through direct contact with an infected person (usually via fluid from broken blisters), through the air when an infected person coughs or sneezes, and through direct contact with lesions (sores) from a person with shingles (a possible complication of chicken pox). Outbreaks are most common in winter and in early spring.

Signs and symptoms: A rash with small blisters that develops on the scalp and body and then spreads to the face, arms, and legs over a period of three to four days. A child can end up with anywhere from less than a dozen to more than 500 itchy blisters that dry up and turn into scabs two to four days later. Other symptoms of chicken pox include coughing, fussiness, loss of appetite, and headaches. Chicken pox is contagious from two days before to five days after the rash appears.

What you can do:

- Keep your baby's nails trimmed so that he'll be less able to scratch at his chicken pox. If that doesn't seem to do the trick, then you might want to consider putting cotton mitts on his hands. (If you want to entertain him at the same time, look for a set of sock-style foot rattles and put those on his hands instead.)

- Try to minimize the amount of itching your baby experiences by giving him oatmeal or baking soda baths or by dabbing calamine lotion on his spots. (Note: Don't apply calamine lotion to the spots in his mouth. Calamine lotion is for external use only.)

- Give your baby acetaminophen to help bring down his fever and eliminate some of his discomfort. Note: Do not give children Aspirin or any drug containing salicylate at any time as Aspirin use during certain illnesses—including chicken pox— has been linked to Reye's syndrome, a potentially fatal disease that affects the liver and the brain.

---

baby talk If your child has an immune system problem, you'll want to get in touch with your doctor as soon as possible if you suspect that your child may have been exposed to chicken pox. He may recommend that your child receive a dose of a special immune globulin (VZIG) that can help to prevent chicken pox.

- Be sure to get in touch with your doctor if your baby's fever lasts longer than four days or remains high after the third day after the spots appear; if your baby shows signs of becoming dehydrated; or if your baby's rash becomes warm, red, or tender.

Condition: Cradle cap (seborrheic dermatitis)
Cause: A relatively common skin condition in the newborn.
Signs and symptoms: A yellowish, scaly buildup on the baby's head that may also be accompanied by red areas in the creases (neck, armpits, groin, behind the ears). It typically disappears by the time a baby is one year old, but it can be difficult to control in the meantime.

What you can do:
- Gently massage olive oil into the affected areas and then gently comb your baby's scalp to remove some of the crusty scales that have built up. (Non-food-grade oils such as baby oil may contain fragrances and/or other ingredients which may be irritating to baby's skin.)
- If the scaly patches become infected or begin to seep clear or cloudy fluid, get in touch with your baby's doctor to find out if she recommends that you apply a cortisone cream to the most severely affected areas.
- Pay attention to what soaps and shampoos you're using to keep your baby clean—and how often you're bathing him. Overdoing it in the cleanliness department can make your baby's skin problems worse. Soaps and creams designed for use on a baby should contain food-grade ingredients, and fragrances should be avoided. Fragrance is a proprietary ingredient which is not subject to the same rigorous standards as food-grade products.

Condition: Eczema

Cause: Unknown, but it tends to be worse in winter when your baby's skin is driest. It is no longer believed to be triggered by allergies. Eczema is not contagious.

Signs and symptoms: Extreme itchiness that results in a rash in areas that are scratched, especially the cheeks, wrists, elbows, knees, and belly.

What you can do:
- Keep your baby's skin well moisturized by applying a non-allergenic moisturizing lotion a couple of times each day.
- Dress your child in cotton and other breathable fabrics.
- Keep your baby's nails trimmed so that he'll be less likely to infect his skin through scratching.
- Give your baby an oatmeal bath. (Don't open the cereal cupboard; you need colloidal oatmeal, a product that can be purchased in the drugstore.)
- Your doctor may prescribe a steroid cream (such as cortisone) if your baby's eczema is particularly severe, but she will recommend that you use it sparingly.

Condition: Fifth disease (erythema infectiosum)

Cause: Caused by a virus known as parvovirus B19. Outbreaks are most common in the spring. Once the rash appears, the disease is no longer likely to spread.

Signs and symptoms: A "slapped cheek" rash on the face accompanied by a red rash on the trunk and extremities. The child may also have a fever and sore joints. Fortunately, this illness is more common in school-aged children than in younger children.

What you can do:

- Get in touch with your baby's doctor as soon as possible if your child has sickle-cell anemia or some other form of chronic anemia. Fifth disease may heighten anemia in children who are already anemic.
- There is no treatment for fifth disease, nor is there any vaccine available. This is one of those diseases that you simply have to "wait out," but the prognosis for the condition is excellent.

Condition: Hand, foot, and mouth syndrome

Cause: Caused by the coxsackie virus—a contagious virus with an incubation period of three to six days.

Signs and symptoms: Tiny blister-like sores in the mouth, on the palms of the hands, and on the soles of the feet that are accompanied by a mild fever, a sore throat, and painful swallowing. Lasts approximately seven to ten days and is contagious from one day before until one day after the blisters appear.

What you can do:

- Give your baby plenty of liquids and, if he's old enough, soft foods as well. Note: Popsicles can ease some of the discomfort of the sores in the mouth while ensuring that your child remains well hydrated.
- Keep your baby comfortable by treating him with acetaminophen until his symptoms start to subside.

Condition: Herpangina (inflammation of the inside of the mouth)

Cause: Caused by the coxsackie virus (the same virus responsible for hand, foot, and mouth syndrome), a contagious virus that has an incubation period of three to six days.

Signs and symptoms: Numerous painful greyish-white ulcers on the baby's tongue and on the roof of the baby's mouth toward the back; painful swallowing; a fever of 38.9 to 40 degrees Celsius (102 to 104 degrees Fahrenheit); diarrhea; and a pink rash on the trunk. The symptoms last about seven days and the illness is highly contagious until the ulcers are gone.

What you can do:

- Take your baby to the doctor to have the diagnosis confirmed.
- Give your baby plenty of fluids, but avoid acidic juices that may make his mouth ulcers sting. If your baby refuses to eat, offer soft food and liquids to prevent dehydration.
- Give your child acetaminophen to help bring down his fever and reduce the pain associated with the mouth ulcers.

Condition: Impetigo (an infection of the skin)

Cause: Caused by a bacterial infection.

Signs and symptoms: A rash featuring oozing, blister-like honey-coloured crusts that may be as small as pimples or as large as coins. Outbreaks of impetigo typically occur below the nose or on the buttocks or at the site of an insect bite or scrape.

What you can do:

- Have your baby seen by a doctor so that the rash can be diagnosed and an antibacterial ointment and/or an oral antibiotic can be prescribed.
- Trim your baby's nails to prevent her from scratching the rash, and keep the sores covered to minimize the chance that they will spread to other parts of the body and other people.

Condition: Measles (rubeola)

Cause: Spread by a virus that has an incubation period of eight to twelve days.

Signs and symptoms: Cold, cough, high fever (40 degrees Celsius, or 104 degrees Fahrenheit), and bloodshot eyes that are sensitive to light. Around the fourth day of illness, a bright red rash erupts on the face and spreads all over the body. (Even the inner cheeks will have spots, which will be white in colour.) At around the time that the spots break out, the baby starts feeling quite ill. The infectious period lasts from three to five days before the rash appears until after the rash disappears (typically four days after the rash appears).

What you can do:
- Have your baby seen by your doctor so that the illness can be properly diagnosed and any complications (pneumonia, encephalitis, ear infections, et cetera) can be treated.
- Give your child acetaminophen to manage his fever and plenty of fluids to keep him well hydrated.

Condition: Ringworm

Cause: Caused by a fungus that is spread from person to person through touch.

Signs and symptoms: An itchy and flaky rash that may be ring-shaped and have a raised edge. When the scalp is affected, a bald area may develop. Ringworm is highly contagious until treatment has commenced.

What you can do:
- Take your baby to see the doctor so that oral medications and/or topical ointments or creams may be prescribed to treat the outbreak.

Condition: Roseola

Cause: Caused by a virus with an incubation period of five to ten days. Roseola is very common in babies from 6 to 24 months.

Signs and symptoms: High fever that shows up suddenly in a previously well baby, and which may result in febrile convulsions. The fever breaks on the third day and is then followed by a faint pink rash that appears on the trunk and the extremities and lasts for one day.

What you can do:
- Treat your baby's fever (see previous Fever section) and give her plenty of fluids to prevent dehydration.

Condition: Rubella (German measles)

Cause: Caused by the rubella virus—a virus that has an incubation period of 14 to 21 days and that is contagious from a few days before until seven days after the rash appears.

Signs and symptoms: A low-grade fever, flu-like symptoms, a slight cold, and a pinkish-red spotted rash that starts on the face, spreads rapidly to the trunk, and disappears by the third day. Also accompanied by swollen glands behind the ears and in the nape of the neck.

What you can do:
- Have your child examined by a doctor to confirm that he has developed rubella. Sometimes only a blood test can confirm that the rash and other symptoms have been caused by rubella as opposed to some other illness.
- Keep your child away from women who are or could be pregnant. Rubella can be very dangerous to the developing fetus.

Condition: Scarlet fever

Cause: Caused by streptococcus bacteria. Has an incubation period of two to five days.

Signs and symptoms: Sunburn-like rash over face, trunk, and extremities, including a moustache-like gap of unaffected skin around the mouth; sandpaper-like skin; fever; tonsillitis; vomiting. The rash usually disappears in five days. Despite its scary name, it is usually no more serious than strep throat, but it is contagious until one to two days after antibiotic treatment has begun. It is more common in school-aged children than in infants.

What you can do:
- Have your baby seen by your doctor so that antibiotic treatment can be started. (Note: Other members of your family may also be treated at the same time, even if they haven't actually developed the illness.)
- Offer liquids and bland foods (if your baby is old enough for solid foods) and watch for signs of dehydration.

Condition: Shingles

Cause: Caused by the zoster virus—the same virus that is responsible for chicken pox. Very rare in children.

Signs and symptoms: A rash with small blisters that begin to crust over; intense itching. Shingles is very contagious while the rash is present: it's possible to spread the disease to anyone who has not had chicken pox.

What you can do:
- Follow the guidelines for treating chicken pox. (See earlier section of this chapter.)

Gastrointestinal conditions

Condition: Campylobacteriosis

Cause: Source of infection may be poultry, beef, unpasteurized milk, or other food. The germ that causes this condition is excreted in the stool, so your child is infectious while he has symptoms.

Signs and symptoms: Fever, diarrhea, blood in stool, and cramps.

What you can do:
- Get in touch with your baby's doctor to see if a stool sample is required in order to confirm that your baby has been infected with campylobacteriosis.
- Keep your baby away from other children while you treat the illness.
- Give your child acetaminophen to reduce his discomfort and treat his fever. Also, see tips under Diarrhea (next page) for advice on managing your child's diarrhea.

Condition: Constipation

Cause: Too little water in the intestines and/or poor muscle tone in the lower intestines and rectum. The problem can be triggered by a change in diet (for example, switching from breast milk to formula or formula to cow's milk; starting infant cereals).

Signs and symptoms: Abdominal discomfort and large, hard, dry stools that may be painful for your baby to pass (for example, your baby draws up his legs to his abdomen, grunts, and gets red-faced) and that may be streaked with blood when they finally emerge.

What you can do:
- Up your baby's intake of water, prune juice, prunes, pears, plums, and peaches—nature's stool softeners. Warmed fruit compote (for example, three to four pieces of dried apricot that is warmed or stewed with a small amount of water) will really help to get your baby's bowels moving. If these methods aren't effective, ask your doctor about the pros and cons of using non-prescription stool softeners or laxative suppositories.
- Limit the number and quantities of constipating foods that your baby eats (such as white rice, rice cereal, bananas, milk, and cheese) while adding fibre to your baby's diet. (Good sources of fibre for older babies include bran cereals, wholegrain breads and crackers, and fibre-rich vegetables such as peas and beans.)

baby talk Many babies over the age of 6 weeks experience infrequent bowel movements. A bowel movement once a week is not uncommon for babies this age. This is not the same thing as constipation. (You can tell the difference because the bowel movements are soft, not hard.)

Condition: Diarrhea

Cause: Caused by gastrointestinal infections (especially gastroenteritis), colds, food intolerances, and/or antibiotic treatments.

Signs and symptoms: Frequent watery, often green, mucous, foul-smelling, explosive, and occasionally blood-tinged stools. Diarrhea is frequently accompanied by a bright red rash around the anus. A baby with diarrhea can also be expected to show other signs of a viral infection. Note: Because each child's pattern of bowel movements is different, what you're looking for is a change in the consistency of your baby's bowel movements. (See Table 8.6 for further information on bowel movements in babies.)

What you can do:

- Start tracking the frequency and quality of your baby's stools and note whether he's vomiting or not, how much food and liquid he's been taking in, and how ill he seems. This information will help your doctor to assess whether your baby is at risk of becoming dehydrated.

- Try to figure out what has triggered the diarrhea: illness, a change in diet, antibiotic treatment (for an ear infection, for example), or if it is simply due to an oversupply of milk (see Chapter 6 for tips on troubleshooting common breastfeeding problems).

- If you're breastfeeding, continue to breastfeed on demand. If your baby is becoming dehydrated, consult your doctor about the advisability of offering an oral electrolyte solution such as Pedialyte.

- If you're not breastfeeding, continue to feed your baby his normal diet. If your baby is becoming dehydrated, consult your doctor about the advisability of offering an oral electrolyte solution such as Pedialyte.

TABLE 8.6

The Poop on Baby Poop

Type of Stool	What It Looks Like	When It Occurs	What You Need to Know
Meconium	Greenish-black sticky mucus that is present in the baby's bowels before birth.	Most babies pass their meconium within 24 hours of the birth, although some babies pass meconium prior to or during the birth. (Note: Passing meconium prior to birth may be an indication of fetal distress and may result in the baby inhaling some of the meconium into her lungs—something that could result in respiratory difficulties in the newborn. So don't be surprised if your doctor or midwife gives your baby an extra-thorough checkup if your baby happened to pass meconium prior to birth.)	If your baby hasn't passed any meconium by the second day of life, be sure to let your baby's doctor know as this could be a symptom of a bowel obstruction.
Transitional stool	Greenish brown to bright green; either semi-fluid or full of curds and mucus.	During the first few days.	Your newborn may have three to nine transitional stools per day. There may be a small amount of blood in the first few stools—likely the result of blood from the mother that may have been swallowed during the delivery, but you should check with your doctor just to be sure.

(continued)

Type of Stool	What It Looks Like	When It Occurs	What You Need to Know
Regular stool (breastfed baby)	Mustard yellow; creamy in texture; may contain seed-like particles; may have a mild yeasty smell.	By day five.	Initially, breastfed babies have bowel movements more often than formula-fed babies, but by age 2 months, the number of bowel movements may drop to two a week (or even fewer). This is because your body has switched from producing colostrum, which is thought to have a laxative effect, to producing mature breast milk. Since there is very little waste material in mature breast milk—it's not in Mother Nature's best interest to throw in a lot of filler, after all—your baby simply doesn't need to eliminate waste as often as a formula-fed baby does.
Regular stool (formula-fed baby)	Yellowish, tan-coloured, or brown stools that are relatively solid (e.g., peanut butter–like consistency); foul smell.	Once the transitional stools end (within the first month of life).	A typical formula-fed baby will have a bowel movement up to five times per day. Formula-fed babies sometimes have problems with constipation (the infrequent and painful passage of a hard stool). If you are certain that you're preparing the formula correctly (using the correct proportions of formula and water), you might want to talk to your baby's doctor about the pros and cons of switching to another type or brand of formula. (See section elsewhere in this chapter on dealing with constipation.)

Note: You should get in touch with your baby's doctor immediately if your baby's stools become black after the passage of the initial meconium (a possible indication of upper gastrointestinal bleeding), putty coloured or chalky white (a possible indication of liver trouble), very mucous (a possible indication of inflammation or infection), or bloody (a possible indication of infection or internal bleeding, although it's likely to just be the result of maternal blood swallowed during the delivery if the bloody stools show up during the first few days of life).

Your baby's stools will change dramatically during the first few weeks of her life. What you might initially take for diarrhea could, in fact, be a perfectly normal bowel movement for a young baby. Here's what you need to know about infant bowel movements.

From six to 24 hours:
- Keep giving your child the oral electrolyte solution.
- Once the vomiting stops, reintroduce your baby's usual formula or whole milk and offer small quantities of favourite, simple foods throughout the day. (Avoid fruit juices and other sugary foods until the diarrhea has stopped or it may worsen again.)
- Don't be alarmed if your baby has more frequent bowel movements once you reintroduce these foods. It may take seven to ten days or even longer for her stools to go back to normal again. The bowel is relatively slow to heal.
- Don't give your baby any diarrhea medication unless you are specifically advised to do so by your doctor. These medications—which slow down the action of the intestines—can actually worsen diarrhea by allowing the germs and infected fluid to stagnate in the gut.

---

baby talk While mothers a generation ago were told to treat diarrhea by giving their children ginger ale, juice, and sugar water, doctors no longer recommend that these beverages be given because their salt content is too low and their sugar content is too high—something that can actually aggravate the child's diarrhea. Add to this the fact that certain types of fruit juices can have a laxative effect—the last thing your baby needs when she's battling diarrhea—and that many types of soda pop contain caffeine (a diuretic that can cause your baby to become dehydrated) and you can see why oral electrolyte solutions (also known as oral rehydration solutions) are becoming the first-line defence against diarrhea. Breast milk is, of course, even more effective. Believe it or not, even plain water isn't recommended for a baby who is becoming dehydrated because it can result in a lowering of the amount of salt or sugar in the blood.

> **baby talk**
>
> According to the College of Family Physicians of Canada, you should call your doctor if your baby.
>
> √ has diarrhea and is less than 6 months of age;
>
> √ has diarrhea and a fever of over 38.5 degrees Celsius (101.3 degrees Fahrenheit) and is over 6 months of age;
>
> √ is exhibiting some of the signs of dehydration (irritability, decreased appetite, less frequent urination, more concentrated urine, weight loss, dry mouth, thirst, sunken eyes, lack of tears when crying, sunken fontanelle, skin that isn't as "springy" as usual);
>
> √ has stools that are bloody and slimy or has blood in his vomit;
>
> √ is bloated, listless, and/or unusually sleepy;
>
> √ has had abdominal pain for more than two hours; or
>
> √ hasn't passed urine in eight hours.

- Assess the severity of the diarrhea and watch for any signs of dehydration, particularly if your baby is also experiencing a lot of vomiting. Diarrhea can throw your baby's balance of salts (called electrolytes) and water out of whack—something that can affect the functioning of his organs.

- Make sure that you apply a barrier cream at each diaper change to prevent your baby's bottom from developing a diarrhea-related rash. (These can be incredibly painful for a baby.)

- Once the diarrhea subsides, start reintroducing other foods, starting with formula, diluted if necessary if your baby is formula-fed. Keeping your baby on a clear fluid diet for too long may itself produce diarrhea (aptly named "starvation stools"). In rare situations, your doctor may recommend that you use a non-lactose, soy-based formula since your baby's intestines may have difficulty tolerating lactose for up to six weeks. Ditto for any potentially irritating foods. Your best bet is to stick to simple foods like the so-called BRAT diet at first: bananas, rice, applesauce, and toast—assuming, of course, that your baby's already eating solid foods.

- If you notice the diarrhea starting up again, you might want to back off and stick to foods that you know he can tolerate well. If the diarrhea continues to be a problem, get in touch with your doctor: he may want to order stool cultures to see if there's a parasite such as giardia responsible for your baby's misery.

- Call your baby's doctor or go to the hospital immediately if your baby is less than 6 months of age and is having bloody or black stools; has been vomiting for more than four to six hours; has a fever of 38.5 degrees Celsius (101.3 degrees Fahrenheit) or greater; or is showing some signs of dehydration. (See section on dehydration elsewhere in this chapter.)

Condition: Escherichia coli (E. coli)

Cause: Can be picked up from poultry, beef, unpasteurized milk, or other food sources.

Signs and symptoms: Fever, diarrhea, blood in stool, and cramps. The germ that causes this condition is excreted in the stool, so your child is infectious while he has symptoms.

What you can do:

- Get in touch with your baby's doctor to see if a stool sample is required to attempt to confirm that your baby has been infected with E. coli.

- Keep your baby away from other children while you treat the illness. (See previous tips on managing diarrhea.)

- Give your child acetaminophen to reduce his discomfort and treat his fever.

Condition: Food poisoning

Cause: Caused by eating contaminated food.

Signs and symptoms: Nausea, vomiting, cramps, and diarrhea. Not infectious, but symptoms may be shared by all members of the family who ate the same food.

What you can do:

- Contact your baby's doctor if your child's symptoms are severe. Otherwise, offer plenty of fluids and follow the tips on treating vomiting and diarrhea that you'll find elsewhere in this section.

Condition: Giardia (a parasite in the stool that causes bowel infections)

Cause: Spread from person to person.

Signs and symptoms: Most children have no symptoms, but some may experience loss of appetite, vomiting, cramps, diarrhea, very soft stools, and excessive gas. This condition is infectious until cured.

What you can do:

- Get in touch with your baby's doctor to see if a stool sample is required to attempt to confirm that your baby has been infected with giardia.
- Keep your baby away from other children while you treat the illness.
- Give your child acetaminophen to reduce his discomfort and treat his fever. Also, see tips under Diarrhea for advice on how to manage your child's diarrhea.

Condition: Hepatitis A (a liver infection)

Cause: A virus in the stool that can be spread from person to person or via food or water.

Signs and symptoms: Most children exhibit few symptoms. Where symptoms are present, they include fever, reduced appetite, nausea, vomiting, and jaundice (a yellowish tinge to skin and eyes). Hepatitis A is infectious from two weeks before to one week after the onset of jaundice.

What you can do:

- Get in touch with your baby's doctor. He may want to order an immune globulin vaccine for all members of your family, including your baby.

Condition: Norwalk virus

Cause: Spread from person to person via the air.

Signs and symptoms: Vomiting for one to two days. Contagious for duration of illness.

What you can do:

- Get in touch with your baby's doctor to see if a stool sample is required to attempt to confirm that your baby has been infected with Norwalk virus.
- Keep your baby away from other children while you treat the illness.
- Give your child acetaminophen to reduce his discomfort and treat his fever. Also, see tips under Diarrhea for advice on how to manage your child's diarrhea.

Condition: Rotavirus

Cause: Caused by a virus in the stool that is spread through person-to-person contact. The most common cause of diarrhea outbreaks in childcare centres.

Signs and symptoms: Fever and vomiting followed by watery diarrhea. Can lead to rapid dehydration in infants. Contagious for duration of illness.

What you can do:

- Get in touch with your baby's doctor to see if a stool sample is required to attempt to confirm that your baby has been infected with rotavirus.
- Keep your baby away from other children while you treat the illness.
- Give your child acetaminophen to reduce his discomfort and treat his fever. Also, see the section earlier in this chapter on managing your child's diarrhea.

Note: The rotavirus vaccine is now routinely recommended to prevent this illness.

Condition: Salmonella

Cause: Acquired mainly by eating food that has been contaminated with salmonella. Such foods typically include eggs, egg products, beef, poultry, and unpasteurized milk.

Signs and symptoms: Diarrhea, fever, and blood in stool. Infectious while symptoms persist.

What you can do:

- Contact your baby's doctor if your child's symptoms are severe. Otherwise, offer plenty of fluids and follow the tips on treating vomiting and diarrhea that you'll find elsewhere in this section.

Condition: Shigella

Cause: Caused by a virus in the stool that can be spread from person to person.

Signs and symptoms: Diarrhea, fever, blood and/or mucus in stool, and cramps. Highly contagious for duration of illness.

What you can do:

- Get in touch with your baby's doctor to see if a stool sample is required to attempt to confirm that your baby has been infected with shigella.

- Keep your baby away from other children while you treat the illness.
- Give your child acetaminophen to reduce his discomfort and treat his fever. Also, see tips under Diarrhea for advice on how to manage your child's diarrhea.

---

baby talk Persistent green-stained projectile vomiting can be a symptom of an intestinal obstruction—a serious condition that requires emergency surgery. You should suspect this possibility if your baby is experiencing intermittent abdominal pain, has pale and sweaty skin, isn't having any bowel movements, and shows signs of getting sicker rather than better.

---

baby talk If your baby is diagnosed with gastroesophageal reflux (GER), you may find that your baby's symptoms lessen if you burp your baby at regular intervals during feedings; prop your baby at a 30-degree angle on his stomach for 30 minutes after a feeding (but do not leave your baby unsupervised, due to the risk of SIDS); offer the breast more often (with the goal being smaller, more frequent feedings); elevate the head of your baby's crib so that his head is elevated while he is sleeping on his back; try to minimize the amount of time your baby spends crying (babies reflux more when they're crying); and talk to your baby's doctor about whether a medication designed to neutralize stomach acids or to speed up their removal from the esophagus would help to ease your baby's discomfort. Sometimes eliminating dairy products from the breastfeeding mother's diet can make a difference. Switching infant formulas (in the case of a formula-fed baby) may also be helpful, but it's a good idea to discuss formula changes with your baby's doctor first. In most cases, GER becomes less of a problem by the time a baby is 6 months of age and disappears entirely by the baby's first birthday.

Condition: Vomiting

Cause: Vomiting can be caused by a viral infection, food poisoning, or a medical condition such as pyloric stenosis (projectile vomiting caused by a partial or complete intestinal blockage that requires surgical correction) or gastroesophageal reflux (GER, a condition in which stomach acids are regurgitated into the esophagus, frequently resulting in forceful regurgitation through the nose).

Signs and symptoms: Vomiting can be accompanied by diarrhea or other symptoms depending on the underlying cause.

What you can do:

- If the vomiting is caused by infection: offer small, frequent servings of fluid to prevent dehydration. If your baby is old enough to eat a Popsicle, you might want to try making your own from an oral electrolyte solution such as Pedialyte to see if this makes it easier for her to keep the fluid down.

- If the vomiting is caused by GER or pyloric stenosis: see other sections in this chapter and consult your baby's doctor.

Other conditions

Condition: Meningitis

Cause: Can be bacterial or viral in origin. Bacterial meningitis can be fatal. The incubation period is usually 10 to 14 days. Fortunately, bacterial meningitis is very rare in preschool children over the age of six weeks who have been fully immunized.

Signs and symptoms: Bacterial meningitis (spinal meningitis) may begin like a cold, flu, or ear infection, but the child becomes increasingly ill and very lethargic; develops a fever of 38.9 to 40 degrees Celsius (102 to 104 degrees Fahrenheit); and has a stiff neck and a bulging fontanelle. With viral meningitis, the baby exhibits similar symptoms but isn't quite as ill.

What you can do:

- Contact your doctor immediately. Your doctor will want to do a spinal tap to determine whether the meningitis is bacterial or viral in origin. The sooner the illness is diagnosed and treated, the better the outcome.

- If the meningitis turns out to be bacterial in origin, your doctor will want to treat the illness with intravenous antibiotics for at least seven days. Your baby will need to be hospitalized during this time.
- If the meningitis turns out to be viral in origin, the illness will be treated like the flu.

Condition: Mumps

Cause: Spread by a virus that has an incubation period of seven to ten days.

Signs and symptoms: Flu-like symptoms and an upset stomach initially; then tender swollen glands beneath the ear lobes two or three days later. Your child may look as if he has chipmunk cheeks and may find it painful to open his jaw. He may also have a low-grade fever. Mumps typically last for seven to ten days and the illness is contagious until the swelling is gone.

What you can do:
- Feed your child liquids and soft foods.
- Apply cool compresses to the neck.
- Administer acetaminophen to relieve discomfort and pain.
- Call your doctor's office immediately if your child becomes drowsy, starts vomiting repeatedly, becomes dehydrated, or develops a stiff neck.

Condition: Pinworms

Cause: Caused by a parasite (intestinal worms).

Signs and symptoms: Night waking and restlessness, intense itching around the anus or in the vagina, and the presence of thread-like one-centimetre-long worms that travel out of the rectum to deposit eggs around the anus or the vagina.

What you can do:
- Use a flashlight at night to try to detect worms coming out of your baby's anus (they're more visible in the dark) and/or place sticky tape around your baby's anus so that you can capture some eggs for your doctor to examine.
- Keep your baby's fingernails trimmed short to discourage scratching.

- Each member of the household will have to be treated with a medication to eradicate the parasite.

Condition: Tetanus (lockjaw)
Cause: Caused by bacteria in a deeply contaminated wound. The incubation period can be anywhere from 3 to 21 days.
Signs and symptoms: Muscle spasms, particularly in the jaw muscles; convulsions.
What you can do:
- Contact your doctor immediately. Your baby will need to be treated with antibiotics.

Condition: Urinary tract infections (UTIs)
Cause: Can be difficult to diagnose. If your child suffers from recurrent urinary tract infections, your doctor may order a kidney ultrasound or some other type of test to try to determine what's causing the infections to recur.
Signs and symptoms: Fever, painful and frequent urination, strong-smelling urine, and abdominal pain. In babies, a persistent fever with no obvious cause may be the only symptom of a urinary tract infection.
What you can do:
- Get in touch with your baby's doctor so that the urinary tract infection can be diagnosed, usually by obtaining a urine specimen, and so that antibiotic treatment can be started. Urine specimens are very difficult to obtain from babies. Often a clear plastic bag is taped to the infant's diaper area. To get the best urine specimen, a catheter is passed through the urethra and into the bladder.

---

baby talk Don't assume that your newborn baby has developed a urinary tract infection just because you happen to notice a reddish stain on his diaper. Chances are what you're seeing are urates—a substance that is commonly present in the urine of newborn babies. It's nothing to be concerned about and will disappear in a few days.

BABYPROOFING 101

As hard as it may be to believe, the sleepy newborn who keeps dozing off in your arms will soon be transformed into a curious baby or toddler on a mission to explore every possible inch of your home. The key to babyproofing your child's world is to learn how to see your home through your child's eyes. "It's a matter of developing a safety sense—of constantly asking yourself, 'What could happen in this situation, and what can I do to either prevent it from happening or minimize the injury?'" according to Valerie Lee, former president of the Kitchener, Ontario-based Infant and Toddler Safety Association.

While it's unrealistic to think that you can prevent every single accident from happening, there's much you can do to make your baby's world a safer and more secure place. Here's what you can do to minimize the major hazards in a typical home.

Every room

- Keep a set of emergency telephone numbers beside each telephone—not just your main telephone.
- Keep curtain and blind cords out of your baby's reach. Or, better yet, opt for curtains and blinds that are cord-free.
- Keep high chairs, cribs, and furniture away from windows, appliances, and other potential hazards.
- Ensure that all windows in your house are lockable and that the screens in each of your windows are secure and backed with screen guards (safety devices that are designed to catch the screen and your baby if your baby starts to fall out the window).
- Keep children away from baseboards and portable heaters as well as wood stoves and other sources of heat. Install baseboard heater covers and keep other heat sources safely barricaded away from baby.
- Use plastic safety covers and cord locks on electrical outlets and on door handles.
- Install babyproof latches on drawers and cupboard doors.
- Place window guards on all second-storey windows.
- Anchor bookcases and tall dressers to the wall to prevent tipping, and avoid placing heavy items on top of any piece of furniture that could be pulled over.

- Keep a fire extinguisher near each exit to your home.
- Store lighters and matches out of your baby's reach and insist that visitors do the same. (Remind them to put purses out of reach.)
- Change the batteries in your smoke detector at least twice a year (whenever you move your clock forward or back).
- Make sure that any space heaters, small appliances, and extension cords in use in your home are in good condition and meet current safety standards.
- Store medications and cleaners in their original containers so that you'll be able to identify which products your child has consumed in the event of a poisoning. (Medications are responsible for a large percentage of the poisonings that occur in the home.) Store medications in a cupboard that is out of reach of children and that is kept locked at all times. Medications should always be stored in containers with childproof lids.
- Wipe up spills promptly; and avoid decorating with area rugs, which can pose a tripping hazard to both adults (who may be carrying babies) and children (including babies and toddlers who are just learning to walk).
- Avoid leaving your baby and your pet alone in the same room.
- Keep coins, marbles, pen or marker caps, button-sized batteries, and other small items safely out of your baby's reach. This may mean clearing out the family junk drawer and/or locking the desk in your home office until your child is a lot older.
- Keep your cat's litter box in a part of the house that is off-limits to your child.
- Make sure that every plant in your home is baby-friendly. Call your local poison control centre if you're not sure which houseplants are and aren't dangerous if ingested. (You can find a list of provincial and territorial poison control centres at http://capcc.ca/provcentres/bc/bc.html.)

---

the baby department The Canadian Partnership for Children's Health anxd Environment (www.healthyenvironmentforkids.ca) is encouraging Canadian parents to think about "environmental childproofing" as well as traditional childproofing. Not only are babies and toddlers more vulnerable to environmental toxins than adults because their bodies are still developing; they come into contact with toxins more than adults do because they explore the world with their mouths and their hands and because they live their lives closer to the ground, where toxins tend to accumulate. Fortunately, there's a lot we can do to reduce the level of toxins in our homes, according to the CPCHE. They recommend that parents act on these five key tips.

1. **"Bust the dust."** Cleaning with a good-quality vacuum, a wet mop, or a damp mop will remove dust (one of the main sources of children's exposure to toxic chemicals) from the environment. Plan to vacuum or damp-mop twice a week if you have a child who is at the on-the-floor, crawling stage. And minimize the amount of dust in your environment by removing your shoes when at the door (use mats to trap dirt from outdoors), and eliminating clutter (store toys in closed containers).

2. **"Go green when you clean."** Use non-toxic cleaning products. Avoid antibacterial soap. Steer clear of air fresheners, dryer sheets, and scented laundry detergent. Avoid dry cleaning (or choose a dry cleaner who uses a non-toxic process).

3. **"Renovate right."** Choose less toxic paints, finishes, and glues (those labelled VOC-free (for volatile organic compounds free), zero-VOC, or low-VOC); and ensure proper ventilation while using these products. Use plastic sheeting and duct tape to seal off the portion of your house that is being renovated, and be sure to close off heating and cooling vents. Keep your work clothes separate from other household laundry. Keep pregnant women and young children away from the area being renovated.

4. **"Get drastic with plastic."** Don't use plastic wrap or plastic containers in the microwave, even if the products claim to be microwave-safe. Heat and store food in glass rather than plastic containers. Eat fresh or frozen foods as much as possible (to minimize exposure to BPA, a chemical used in the lining of most food and drink cans). Avoid products manufactured from PVC or vinyl. They may contain phthalates, harmful chemicals which were banned from children's toys in June 2011.

5. **"Dish safer fish."** Choose varieties of fish that are lower in mercury: Atlantic mackerel, herring, rainbow trout, wild or canned salmon, and tilapia. If you eat canned tuna, choose light rather than white. And follow provincial and territorial guidelines regarding sports fishing.

Halls and stairways

- Hang a shelf near the front door so that Grandma can keep her purse (and her heart medication) out of your toddler's reach while she's visiting.
- Install wall-mounted baby gates at the top (and, if necessary, the bottom) of each set of stairs. And make sure that the baby gate is latched securely. Stairs are responsible for a large number of falls requiring hospitalization in children under age one.
- Ensure that each set of stairs is equipped with a handrail that is firmly attached to the wall or the floor, and that the carpet on the stairs is tacked down securely to prevent tripping.
- Keep the stairs free of objects.
- Get rid of your dry cleaning bags as soon as you bring your dry cleaning into the house. Tie them in knots and toss them in the recycling.
- Install door alarms on all exterior doors.

Nursery

- Ensure that any crib, cradle, or bassinet that you are using meets the latest Canadian safety standards (updated on December 1, 2010). The new standards state, in part, that
    - any crib, cradle, or bassinet that rocks or swings must not swing beyond a 20-degree angle from the vertical; and
    - a mattress that is supplied with a crib, cradle, or bassinet must not be more than 150 millimetres thick (in the case of a crib) or 38 millimetres thick (in the case of a cradle or a bassinet).
- Remove mobiles that are strung across your baby's crib as soon as he learns how to push up with his hands and knees.
- Before your child learns how to stand in his crib, drop the mattress to the lowest setting. And continue to keep your child's crib free of bumper pads.
- Make sure your baby wears fire-retardant sleepwear rather than regular clothing at bedtime. And contact your local fire department to see if they recommend that you put a special decal on the lower part of your child's door to indicate that there's a child sleeping in this room. (You can obtain decals from child safety supply stores.)

- Check that the safety strap on your baby's change table is still working properly, and get in the habit of using it whenever you're changing his diaper.
- Remove any drawstrings or cords from your baby's clothing in order to reduce the risk of strangulation.
- Keep the diaper pail out of reach of your baby or purchase a model with a childproof latch.
- Don't use decorative plug covers in your baby's room. They'll only encourage him to touch the electrical outlets. Stick with plain plug covers instead.
- Move rocking chairs and gliders to another part of the house as soon as your baby becomes mobile. They can pinch fingers or otherwise injure a baby.
- Replace your baby's pacifier every two months (before it begins to show any signs of deterioration).
- Tie a small parts tester (a.k.a. "choke tube") to your baby's change table. That way, you'll know where to find the tube whenever you want to test whether a particular toy contains parts that are small enough to pose a choking hazard. (If you're away from home, you can use a toilet paper roll instead. It's slightly larger than a choke tube, but it's best to err on the side of caution anyway.)

---

mother wisdom "No matter how strongly the nesting urge tells you to sand and paint the baby's room, you should never do it yourself when you're pregnant. Sanding can disturb old lead paint, resulting in toxic dust that is hard to avoid ingesting. Not only can this give you lead poisoning, but since lead crosses the placenta, this can be very dangerous for your fetus as well. And it takes a much smaller amount to harm a fetus."

—MINDY PENNYBACKER AND AISHA IKRAMUDDIN,
NATURAL BABY CARE: NONTOXIC AND
*ENVIRONMENTALLY FRIENDLY WAYS TO
TAKE CARE OF YOUR NEW CHILD*

mom's the word "I found that changing the baby in the crib when she was small and on the floor when she was bigger was a lot easier and less anxiety-provoking than using a diaper change table where I was always afraid she'd roll off."

—TAMMY, 32, MOTHER OF ONE

Bedroom

- Never leave a baby alone on your bed.
- Never place a baby on a waterbed.
- Don't allow a child under the age of 6 to sleep on the top bunk of a bunk bed. The risk of falls and/or suffocation is simply too great.
- Do not place a television set on top of a dresser. Young children may climb the drawers of a dresser to get at the television, causing the dresser to tip over.

Bathroom

- Check the temperature on your hot water heater. According to Safe Kids Canada, most water heaters are set at 60 degrees Celsius (140 degrees Fahrenheit) or higher, rather than the 49 degrees Celsius (120 degrees Fahrenheit) that most safety experts recommend.
- Fill your baby's bath with a few inches of cold water and then add hot water until the bath has reached the appropriate temperature. Finish up with a bit of cold water so that the last water to come out of the tap is cold water. (That way, if your child manages to turn on the tap, the first splash of water will be cold, not hot.)
- Place your baby as far away as possible from the taps and faucet, both to prevent him from reaching for the taps and accidentally scalding himself and to reduce the likelihood that he will bang his head on the faucet.
- Use bath mats in the bathtub to reduce the risk of slipping.
- Never leave a young baby in the bath under the supervision of an older child. A baby in a bathtub requires the supervision of an adult.
- Keep your baby in sight and within arm's reach at all times. Do not rely on a baby bath seat or bath ring to ensure your baby's safety.

- Empty the tub as soon as you're finished bathing your baby to reduce the risk of an accidental drowning; babies may be able to climb into the tub earlier and faster than you realize.

- Lock all medications (including vitamins) in a lockable medicine cabinet or, even better, store them in a small cash box or medium-sized fishing-tackle box that can be locked and then stashed on the top shelf of your bedroom closet.

- Keep all medications in their original containers and ensure that the products you buy are equipped with child safety caps. Make a point of weeding out the expired and obsolete medications on a regular basis. (Call your local pharmacy to find out about disposal options in your community.)

- Keep mouthwash, shampoo, cosmetics, and other toiletries out of your baby's reach, along with scissors, razor blades, and other hazardous objects.

- Keep electrical appliances like blow-dryers and flat-irons out of your baby's reach.

- Equip the toilet seat with a childproof latch.

- Get in the habit of keeping your bathroom door closed. That'll buy you at least a year or two's peace of mind—until your toddler masters the art of opening doorknobs. (At that point, you'll want to buy a babyguard for your doorknob.)

Kitchen

- Check that the base of your baby's high chair is wide enough to be stable, and check that the chair's safety harness is still functional.

- If you choose to use the type of baby seat that clamps onto your kitchen table, ensure that the seat is securely attached, that you use all safety harnesses, and that anything hazardous at the dinner table is out of baby's reach.

- Use placemats rather than a tablecloth at your kitchen table. Otherwise, your baby could tug on the tablecloth, causing everything on the table to come tumbling down on his head.

- Don't hold a baby or toddler when you're eating or drinking anything that's scalding hot. Likewise, don't place scalding hot liquid in the cup holder on your baby's stroller.

baby talk — Baby bottles containing bisphenol A have been prohibited in Canada since March 31, 2010. And since June 10, 2011, the allowable concentrations of di(2-ethylhexyl) phthalate (DEHP), dibutyl phthalate (DBP), and benzyl butyl phthalate (BBP) have been restricted to no more than 1,000 mg/kg (0.1 per cent) in the soft vinyl of all children's toys and childcare articles. What's more, the allowable concentrations of diisononyl phthalate (DINP), diisodecyl phthalate (DIDP), and di-n-octyl phthalate (DNOP) are restricted to no more than 1,000 mg/kg (0.1 per cent) in the soft vinyl of children's toys and childcare articles in situations in which the product is likely be placed in the mouth of a child under 4 years (48 months) of age.

- Keep cords for kettles, toasters, and other electrical appliances out of the reach of children, and get in the habit of leaving appliances unplugged unless they're actually in use.
- Turn pot handles toward the back of the stove and only cook on the back burners.
- Keep stuffed animals and other flammable toys away from the cooking area.
- Be aware that some oven doors can get hot enough to burn children. Be sure to supervise your baby carefully the entire time he's in the kitchen and to turn off the oven immediately after you're finished using it to reduce the odds of his being burned.
- Consider installing a child safety lock on your oven door. Some curious tots open the oven door, crawl on the door, and use it as a means of reaching what's on the stove.
- Organize your kitchen cupboards so that the items of greatest interest to your child are the farthest distance from the stove.
- Keep knives, can openers, and other sharp items out of the reach of children.
- Learn which foods (for example, whole grapes, carrot sticks) pose a choking risk to babies, and either avoid them entirely until your child

- is older or learn how to prepare them so that they don't pose the same risk to your child.

- Be careful if you heat your baby's food in the microwave. Microwave cooking tends to produce hot spots in food. To avoid burning your baby, stir food thoroughly after warming and check its temperature carefully before serving it to your baby.

- Keep household cleaners—including dishwasher detergent—out of reach of children. Better yet, use non-toxic cleaners to reduce your child's exposure to toxins in the home.

- Be mindful of where you place your baby's high chair. You want to make sure that it's clear of walls or other objects that your baby could push against, potentially tipping the high chair, and far away from hazards such as stoves.

- Never leave your baby unattended when he's eating. Choking is responsible for a significant number of infant deaths each year.

- Since you're likely to be spending a lot of time in the kitchen, make sure that your baby has a safe play area. When he starts exploring the cupboards, give him his own cupboard full of plastic containers, measuring spoons, and other "treasures" that he can dump on the floor. These will soon become his favourite toys.

Family room

- Make sure that the toys you buy for your child are age-appropriate. (See Chapter 10 for more about babies and play.)

- Avoid buying toys that have sharp points or edges or that contain smaller pieces that could be removed and swallowed (for example, check to make sure that the eyes and noses on stuffed animals and the wheels on toy cars are attached securely).

- Steer clear of toys that feature drawstrings and other dangling strings that are any longer than 20 centimetres (7 inches). If your child inherits any such toys from an older cousin or friend, take scissors to any offending strings.

- Ensure that the packaging that came with the toy is disposed of appropriately to avoid any choking or suffocation hazards.

baby talk — Baby walkers were banned in Canada in 2004. Anyone who owns a baby walker is advised to destroy and discard it. It is illegal to sell or give away a baby walker. It is also illegal to import a baby walker from another country, even for your own use.

- Discard any broken toys that have developed sharp edges or that could present a choking hazard.
- Ensure that any toys that require batteries have child-safe battery compartments (ones that can only be opened with a screwdriver).
- Don't allow balloons into your house while you have young children. They pose a huge choking risk to babies, toddlers, and preschoolers.
- If you use a toy box, make sure that your toy box is safe (lid-free). If it has a lid, the lid should be lightweight and the toy box should have a safety hinge to prevent the lid from closing too quickly. (Heavy lids can fall on children's heads and fingers, causing serious injury.) The toy box should also have ventilation holes to ensure that your baby will be able to breathe if he happens to get trapped inside.
- Make sure that the mesh on your baby's playpen is fine enough to prevent a button from catching—something that could pose a strangulation risk.

mom's the word — "We took precautions with a glass coffee table we have downstairs. I was nervous when Cole started walking, envisioning him hurting himself on that table. Our solution was to buy some pipe foam covers that worked just great. We wrapped the edge with black pipe foam and used black tape to secure it. It doesn't look bad at all and it works just great."

—DIANA, 36, MOTHER OF ONE

Living room
- Use a fireplace pad on your fireplace hearth and keep your child far away from the fireplace while it's being used.

- Put your vacuum cleaner away when it's not being used so that your child won't accidentally hurt his fingers or toes with the beater bar.
- Position floor lamps so that they're out of your child's reach or pack them away entirely.
- Place table lamps toward the back of the table and wrap the cord around the table leg for added stability.

Laundry room
- Store laundry products out of your baby's reach.
- Never allow your baby to play in or around the washer or dryer, and ensure that the washer and dryer doors are kept closed at all times.

Basement
- Store paints, glues, and other harmful substances out of your baby's reach—ideally in a locked cabinet.
- Ensure that woodworking tools are kept in a locked room or cabinet.

Garage
- Store your baby's ride-on toys and other outdoor playthings somewhere other than the garage so that she learns that the garage is off-limits to children. (Unless, of course, you intend to use your garage only for children's things: in that case, plan to store tools and other items off-limits to children in a backyard shed or someplace else.)
- Ensure that the garage door is equipped with a safety feature that will cause it to go back up if it comes into contact with a person or object.
- Store tools, automotive parts, and other hazardous items out of your child's reach or in a backyard shed (and lock it).

Backyard
- Keep the barbecue away from your child's play area.
- Get in the habit of putting your garden hose away when you're finished using it; otherwise, the water in the hose may become hot enough to scald a curious baby or toddler.
- Ensure that your pool area is properly fenced (the fence should be at least 1.2 metres (4 feet) high and should surround the entire pool) and that the gate on the fence is both self-closing and self-locking.

- Check that any playground equipment is safe and well anchored.
- Empty your child's wading pool whenever it's not in use.
- Ensure that his sandbox has a lid to keep neighbourhood cats out. Cat feces is not only a nuisance, it can be highly toxic to babies, children, and pregnant women.

---

mother wisdom Remember to be extra vigilant when you are visiting other people: you have no way of knowing whether their house is babyproofed to the same degree as yours. (Unless they have a baby the same age, chances are it's not.)

- Keep your baby away from any poisonous plants or weeds that are growing in your yard—or, better yet, plant something else until your baby is a little older.
- Don't try to mow the lawn or use any electrical garden tools while your baby's underfoot. It's simply too risky.
- When you're choosing ride-on toys, keep your child's age, size, and abilities in mind. Use the toy in a safe area that is away from stairs, traffic, swimming pools, and other hazards.
- When you're choosing a stroller, choose a sturdy model with a stable base (one that won't tip over easily). Use the safety harness and lap belts; and avoid using pillows and blankets as padding as they pose a suffocation risk for your baby. Don't use a stroller on an escalator: look for an elevator or a ramp instead.

---

mom's the word "Make sure that the stroller model you choose is lightweight enough that you can carry it yourself if there's no other adult around to help you, and simple enough to open and close so that you won't have to drag the manual around with you!"

—LISA, 36, MOTHER OF THREE

Miscellaneous

- When your baby is old enough to sit up in a grocery cart, make sure that you use a child restraint belt or harness. Don't count on the grocery store to have one. Bring your own. (You can pick one up at a child safety store.)

- When you're choosing a baby wrap or baby carrier, choose one that is comfortable, safe, and appropriate for the age and size of your baby, and that comes with easy-to-follow instructions. You may want to ask a friend who has experience with the particular product to help you practise getting your baby in and out of the wrap or carrier. Given recent product recalls (and some infant deaths related to these types of products), you will want to pay careful attention to product design. This means looking for a product that allows you to see your baby's face at all times (your baby's face should be "visible and kissable"); and that provides adequate support for your baby's neck, hips, and legs (look for a carrier that supports your baby hammock-style as opposed to suspending him in a parachute-style vertical position).

- Keep up to date about recalls on juvenile products by visiting the Health Canada website on a regular basis: http://cpsr-rspc.hc-sc.gc.ca/PR-RP/home-accueil-eng.jsp.

SAFETY ON THE ROAD

While most parents assume that they've done their bit for safety by buckling their child into his car seat, studies have shown that the majority of car seats are installed incorrectly or improperly used. Here's what you need to know to prevent a needless tragedy.

Rear-facing infant car seats

Make sure that you're using your baby's infant car seat properly. That means ensuring that

- your baby is the appropriate weight (most rear-facing infant car seats are designed to be used for babies up to 22 pounds (10 kilograms), but a few models will accommodate children up to 45 pounds (20 kilograms);

- the harness straps are tightened snugly enough that only one of your fingers fits between the straps and your baby's shoulder;

- the harness straps pass through the slots in the back of the car seat at the appropriate level—at or just below your child's shoulder height

(Note: The top slots in some seats are designed to be used only in the forward-facing position, so make sure you find out which slots are designed to be used in the rear-facing position and which ones aren't);

- the chest clip is at the level of your baby's armpits;
- the harness is buckled between your baby's legs;
- your baby is free of bulky clothing and blankets (you want the restraining straps to fit your baby snugly, so any blankets should be placed on top of the straps, not between your baby and the straps);
- the infant car seat is facing backward rather than forward;
- the car seat is not in a passenger seat that has an airbag;
- a locking clip is used to hold the seat belt in place if you are using a shoulder belt/lap belt combination (Note: A locking clip is an H-shaped piece of metal that locks the lap and shoulder portion of a seat belt together to keep the car seat firmly in place) and;
- the car seat is placed at a 45-degree angle so that your baby's head is supported.

Note: You can install the car seat using the Universal Anchorage System (UAS), if you have it in your car. You can use a seat belt only if your seat belt has a built-in locking feature. If it doesn't have such a feature, you will need to use a seat belt with a locking clip. (Check the owner's manual that came with your car to find out which options are available to you.)

---

mother wisdom Don't be in a rush to switch your child from a rear-facing seat to a forward-facing seat. A rear-facing seat provides the greatest protection to a baby or toddler, so you should use this style of seat for as long as possible. If you'd like to be able to keep a better eye on your child while you're on the road, simply install a mirror in the back seat of your car and angle it appropriately. This will allow you to sneak peeks at your child while you're in transit.

Front-facing car seats

Front-facing car seats are designed to be used by older children with stronger back and neck muscles. Once your child reaches the weight limit for his rear-facing car seat, he will need to move up to a forward-facing car seat (or a rear-facing car seat that is designed for children his age or size). At that point, you'll need to make sure that

- you install the front-facing car seat in the back seat of your car (see the owner's manual that came with your car to find out whether you should be using the Universal Anchorage System (UAS), a seat belt only, or a seat belt with a locking clip;
- the harness straps pass through the slots in the back of the car seat at the appropriate level (at or just above your child's shoulder height);
- the seat is facing forward;
- only one finger can fit between the harness straps and your child's chest; and
- the chest clip is closed properly and at your child's armpit level.

---

mother wisdom Keep your child in his forward-facing car seat for as long as you can (as opposed to moving him up to a booster seat). While some provincial/territorial laws allow children to move into booster seats once they reach 40 pounds (18 kilograms), forward-facing car seats provide a safer alternative (by spreading the force of a collision or sudden stop over the strongest parts of your child's body). Some forward-facing car seats can be used until children reach 65 pounds (30 kilograms).

- Don't forget to send in the warranty card for the car seat you just purchased. That way, you'll automatically be notified of any product recalls for that particular make and model.

Note: Always use a tether strap with a forward-facing car seat. Your owner's manual will tell you where to find the tether anchors in your vehicle.

Other car safety tips

Here are some other important car safety tips.

- Always use a Canadian government–approved car seat (apparently our standards are a bit more rigorous than the standards of our neighbours to the south, so that means sticking to home-grown car seats rather

CHAPTER 8 — THE HEALTH AND SAFETY DEPARTMENT | 313

than trying to bring one across the border). And don't attempt to use any other sort of infant carrier as a substitute for a "real" car seat.

- Plan to buy car seats new. Car seats made before January 1, 2012, may not meet the latest standards as set out by Health Canada and Transport Canada. What's more, car seats aren't designed to last for more than five to nine years. (The number of years varies by make and model. See www.tc.gc.ca/eng/roadsafety/safedrivers-childsafety-notices-2011c01–1168.htm for full details.) After this period of time (assuming, of course, that a car seat hasn't been recalled in the meantime), car seats should be discarded because they may no longer offer the same protection to children. Plastic deteriorates due to exposure to sunlight; labels become difficult to read; parts may wear and stop working properly; safety standards and regulations may change; instruction manuals may be misplaced; and second and subsequent owners may not receive product safety recall notices, if problems arise.

---

baby talk All forward-facing car seats in Canada are fitted with a tether strap that is designed to hold the seat in place in the event of a collision or sudden stop. The tether anchorage hardware must be securely attached to the frame of the vehicle. If you're not sure where to find your car's tether anchors, consult the owner's manual that came with your vehicle or visit the dealership for further information.

- Never allow your baby to ride in your arms when the car is moving, no matter how unhappy your baby may be about being strapped in his car seat. (Hint: You're likely to have a happier baby if you're realistic about the length of the car trips you plan at this stage of your baby's life. It's a rare baby indeed who can stand spending more than a couple of hours in the car at a time. Some actually start wailing the moment their bodies make contact with their car seats.) If you have to make a longer trip because you're visiting far-flung friends and relatives, plan for frequent breaks. Baby will need them.

- Don't place groceries or other objects near your baby in case they end up becoming dangerous projectiles in the event of an accident. Store them in your trunk or luggage compartment instead. A soup can flying at 100 kilometres an hour will cause severe injury to a baby or young child.

PREPARED

It's a rare baby who manages to make it through the first year of life without some minor bumps and bruises. After all, it's pretty hard to master the basics of crawling and walking without falling flat on your face or taking a tumble every now and again. Sometimes more serious accidents occur in the home, which is why it's important to take an infant first-aid and cardiopulmonary resuscitation (CPR) course before or shortly after you become a parent. Organizations such as the Canadian Red Cross (www.redcross.ca) and St. John Ambulance (www.sja.ca) offer such training on a regular basis.

But even if you have taken appropriate training in emergency first aid, it can be easy to draw a blank when your child starts choking or gets a bad burn. That's why I decided to include a quick reference chart outlining some basic infant first-aid procedures (see Table 8.7). Please note that I was barely able to scratch the surface here, due to space constraints, so don't make the mistake of considering this chart to be a substitute for proper training (and regular recertification) in first aid and CPR.

TABLE 8.7

Emergency First-Aid Procedures

Type of Emergency	What to Do
Allergic reaction	• If your baby is exhibiting the symptoms of an allergic reaction (e.g., swollen hands and eyelids, wheezing, and a hive-like rash), take your baby to the hospital emergency ward immediately. • Talk to your doctor about how to handle future allergic reactions, which, by the way, are likely to be more severe. You might want to carry a kit with injectable adrenaline in order to buy your baby enough time to get to the hospital for emergency treatment.
Bleeding	• If your child starts bleeding and the cut appears to be fairly deep, place a clean piece of gauze or cloth over the site of the bleeding and apply firm pressure for two minutes. If that stops the bleeding, you should attempt to clean the wound by running it under cold water. If the bleeding continues, apply more gauze and wrap tape around the cut to keep pressure on the bleeding.

CHAPTER 8 —— THE HEALTH AND SAFETY DEPARTMENT | 315

- Position your baby so that the area that is bleeding is above the level of his heart. This will help to reduce the amount of bleeding.
- If the bleeding still won't stop, the wound is gaping, or the cut appears to be quite deep, you will need to take your baby to the hospital or your doctor's office for stitches. You will also need to seek medical attention for your baby if the cut has dirt in it that won't come out; the cut becomes inflamed; your child starts running a fever; the cut begins oozing a thick, creamy, greyish fluid; red streaks form near the wound; or the wound is caused by a human or animal bite.

Breathing, cessation of

- Call 9–1–1 or have someone else make the call for you immediately. Try to figure out why your baby isn't breathing if you discover that your baby is pale or turning blue. Look for any foreign objects in the mouth and clear out any vomit, mucus, or fluid that could be making it difficult for your baby to breathe by turning your baby on one side.
- Place your baby on his back. Push down on the back of his head and up on his chin in order to clear the tongue away from the back of his throat. Don't push his head too far back, however, or you may end up obstructing the airway. If you roll a small towel and slide it under your baby's neck, you'll probably end up with your baby in the correct position.
- Give your baby mouth-to-mouth resuscitation. With your mouth, make a seal around your baby's mouth and nose and give two quick breaths. If your baby's chest rises with each breath, the airway is clear and you should continue administering mouth-to-mouth resuscitation until help arrives or your child starts breathing on his own. If your baby still isn't breathing, follow the procedures outlined below for dealing with choking.
- Check your baby's pulse to see if his heart is beating. If it's not, you will need to begin chest compressions (rhythmic thrusts of two to three fingers on your baby's breastbone at a rate of at least 100 thrusts per minute), pausing to give the baby a puff of air through mouth-to-mouth resuscitation after every fifth heart compression.

(continued)

Type of Emergency	What to Do
Burns	• Assess the severity of the burn. First-degree burns (such as sunburns) cause redness and minor soreness and can be treated with cool water. Second-degree burns cause blistering, swelling, and peeling and are very painful and may require medical treatment. Third-degree burns damage the underlying layers of the skin and can lead to permanent damage; medical treatment is a must. • Submerge the burned area in cool water for at least 20 minutes (or, in the case of a burn to the face, apply a cool, water-soaked face cloth to the burn). Not only will this help to ease your baby's pain, it also lessens the amount of skin damage. Note: Do not apply ice to a burn as this can cause damage to the tissues. • If the skin becomes blistered, white, or charred, cover the wound before heading to your doctor's office or the hospital. Note: You'll also want to give your baby a dose of acetaminophen to help control the pain. • If your child gets a chemical burn as a result of coming into contact with a caustic substance, immerse the burned area under cool running water for 20 minutes. Gently wash the affected area with soap. (Vigorous scrubbing will cause more of the poison to be absorbed into the skin.) If the substance was also inhaled or swallowed, get in touch with your local poison control centre immediately. If a caustic substance was splashed into your baby's eyes, flush the area for 20 minutes. (Swaddle your baby in a towel to keep his arms out of the way and lay him on his side. Then pour water into his eye and onto a towel below. If your baby closes his eyes tightly, pull down on the lower lid or put your index finger on the upper lid just below the eyebrow and gently pry your baby's eyes open. Once you have finished flushing your baby's eyes, call for medical advice.)
Choking	• Quickly determine whether your baby is able to breathe. If your baby can cough, cry, or speak, the airway is not obstructed, and your baby's built-in gag and cough reflex will help to dislodge the object. In this case, your best bet is to do nothing other than to reassure your baby that he's going to be all right.

- If your baby does not appear to be breathing, he will likely be gasping for air or turning blue, losing consciousness, and/or looking panicked (eyes wide and mouth wide open). In this case, you should straddle the baby along your forearm so that his head is lower than his feet and his face is pointing toward the floor, and then apply four quick, forceful blows between your baby's shoulder blades using the heel of your hand. If you are in a public place, shout for help; if you're at home alone, run with the baby to the phone and dial 9–1–1 while you attempt to resuscitate your baby.
- If the back blows don't dislodge the object and your baby still isn't breathing, immediately flip your baby over and deal four quick, forceful chest thrusts to the baby's breastbone (about one finger's width below the level of the baby's nipples, in the middle of the chest). To administer a chest thrust, you quickly depress the breastbone to a depth of 1.5 to 2.5 centimetres (1/2 inch to 1 inch). You keep your fingers in the same position between thrusts but allow the breastbone to return to its normal position.
- If your baby is still not breathing, hold the baby's tongue down with your thumb and forefinger, lift the jaw open, and check if you can see the object that's causing the blockage. (The mere act of holding your baby's tongue away from the back of the throat may relieve the obstruction.) If you see the object, carefully sweep it out. If you can't see it, don't poke your finger down your baby's throat or you may accidentally cause an object that's out of sight to become further lodged in your child's throat.
- If the tongue-jaw lift doesn't work, begin mouth-to-mouth resuscitation on your baby. Make a seal around your baby's mouth and nose and give two quick breaths. If your baby's chest rises with each breath and the airway is clear, you should continue administering mouth-to-mouth resuscitation until help arrives or your child starts breathing on his own.
- If your baby still isn't breathing, repeat all of these steps until help arrives.

(continued)

Type of Emergency	What to Do
Convulsions (seizures)	• Assess the severity of the convulsion. Convulsions can range from localized muscle shakes to full-body shakes (grand mal seizures), which may involve falling and writhing on the ground, the rolling back of the eyes, frothing at the mouth, tongue biting, and a temporary loss of consciousness. • Place the baby safely on the floor, either face down or on his side to allow the tongue to come forward. This will also help to drain secretions from the mouth. • Keep your baby away from furniture so that he won't injure himself during the convulsion. • Don't give your baby any food or drink during or immediately after a convulsion. • If your baby's lips start to turn blue or he stops breathing, clear his airway and give mouth-to-mouth resuscitation. Make a seal around your baby's mouth and nose and give two quick breaths. If your baby's chest rises with each breath, the airway is clear and you should continue administering mouth-to-mouth resuscitation until help arrives or your child starts breathing on his own. • Have your baby seen by a doctor.
Head injury	• Try to assess the seriousness of the situation. If your baby is unconscious but is breathing and pink in colour rather than blue, lay him on a flat surface and call for emergency assistance. Note: Do not attempt to move him if you suspect that his neck may be injured. • If he's not breathing, follow the steps outlined above on dealing with a child who isn't breathing. • If your baby is acting like himself (e.g., he's alert and conscious and seems to be behaving normally), apply an ice pack (wrapped in a sock or a face cloth) or a bag of frozen vegetables to the cut or bump and monitor your baby closely over the next 24 hours—checking him every two hours around the clock to see if his colour is still normal (pink rather than pale or blue), that he's breathing normally (there may be cause for concern if your baby's breathing becomes shallow or irregular, he's gasping for air, or he periodically stops breathing altogether), and is rousable with gentle stimulation. If he seems well, you can let him continue sleeping. If you are concerned that there could be a problem, sit or stand your baby up and then lay him back down again. Normally this will cause the baby to react. If you don't get a suitable reaction, seek medical attention immediately.

- Seek medical attention immediately if you notice any signs of disorientation; crossed eyes; pupils that are unequal sizes; persistent vomiting (as opposed to just a one-time occurrence); oozing of blood or watery fluid from the ear canal or nose; convulsions; or any signs that your baby's sense of balance has been thrown off by the fall.

Poisoning	• Seek emergency medical attention if your baby seems to be exhibiting any signs of severe poisoning-related distress (e.g., severe throat pain, excessive drooling, difficulty breathing, convulsions, and/or excessive drowsiness). • Call your local poison control centre immediately. The person handling the call will want to know the name of the product that was ingested and what its ingredients are, so be sure to have this information handy. You'll also be asked the time of the poisoning and approximately how much of the poison your baby ingested, the age and weight of your baby, and whether your baby is exhibiting any symptoms (e.g., vomiting, coughing, behavioural changes, and so on). • Do not attempt to induce vomiting without specific medical instructions. Inducing vomiting under the wrong circumstances (e.g., if a caustic substance was ingested) can lead to severe tissue damage.

WELCOMING A PREMATURE BABY OR A BABY WITH HEALTH PROBLEMS

If your baby is born prematurely or with a lot of health problems, she'll likely spend her first weeks or months in the hospital—something that may be very upsetting to you and your partner. (After all, your dreams of the perfect birth didn't include watching your baby be whisked away to the neonatal intensive care unit or checking out of the hospital without your baby.) But even if you give birth to a healthy baby, there's always the chance that your baby could end up being hospitalized at some point due to an illness or an injury.

Here are some tips on surviving your baby's hospitalization:

- Find out as much as you can about your baby's specific medical condition, either by talking to the medical staff, by connecting with other parents who have walked this path before you, or by asking a friend or family member to do some research on your behalf. "Don't be afraid to ask a doctor to explain himself if you don't understand what he said,"

mother wisdom

"For most parents, delivering a baby prematurely is an emotionally traumatic experience. Not only are you afraid for your tiny baby who is transferred directly from the womb to the intensive care nursery, but many of your hopes and dreams are shattered. Instead of warm snuggles, you are separated from your baby. Instead of nursing, you are giving breast milk to a pump. Instead of learning how to take care of simple newborn needs, you are watching highly skilled professionals do what it takes to help your baby live. Instead of being filled with joy and pride, you are swamped with sorrow and fear. All of these circumstances can make you feel undermined and useless as a parent. Not feeling like a parent, feeling displaced by doctors and nurses, not feeling like this baby belongs to you, but instead belongs to the NICU, you may feel powerless to protect and nurture your newborn. Worst of all, you may feel unconnected to your baby. Where are those feelings of unabashed love and devotion that you expected to feel after delivery? To add insult to injury, you may feel isolated from friends and family who don't really understand the heartache, the worry, and the fears you're enduring. You are also not a member of that community of new parents who can show off their babies to admirers and compare notes on such mundane issues as sleep, appetite, diaper rash, and fussiness. Who can you turn to for support and understanding about apnea, bradycardia, gavage feeding, supplemental oxygen and appropriate pain control?"

—DEBORAH L. DAVIS, PH.D., CO-AUTHOR OF
THE EMOTIONAL JOURNEY OF PARENTING YOUR PREMATURE BABY: A BOOK OF HOPE AND HEALING

---

says Karen, a 33-year-old mother of three. "I always had a nurse with me when the doctor was talking to me so that if I still didn't understand what he was saying after the second explanation, I'd be able to ask the nurse to explain it again after the doctor left."

- Do your best to master the NICU lingo. (For the record, "NICU" stands for Neonatal Intensive Care Unit.) Ask a nurse or another parent to explain the terminology so that you won't feel quite so confused and overwhelmed.

- Keep your own records. "I kept a separate journal just for in the hospital and I recorded everything: when my baby ate and how much, how much she weighed, what meds she was given, when she slept," recalls Karen. "I wrote it all down. This allowed me to have my own record of what was going on."

- Let the hospital staff know that you would like to offer kangaroo care to your baby as soon as it is possible to do so. Researchers who have studied the benefits of kangaroo care (skin-to-skin contact between parent and baby) when practised with premature infants have found that it can stabilize the baby's heart rate, regulate the baby's breathing pattern, improve oxygen delivery to the baby's tissues and organs, help baby sleep better, improve weight gain, decrease crying, encourage breastfeeding, and result in earlier discharge from hospital. Kangaroo care also delivers significant benefits to the parents by increasing the mother's breast milk supply, encouraging infant-parent bonding, increasing parental confidence in their ability to care for their baby, reassuring parents that their babies are being well cared for, and providing parents with a measure of control in a situation in which they often feel they have none.

- Learn what types of support services are available to you while your baby is in the hospital. Is there a parent lounge where you can relax or grab a quick catnap if you need a break from the NICU or the pediatric ward? Is there a parent coordinator available to answer your questions and help you to navigate your new world? (Sunnybrook Health Sciences Centre in Toronto recently added such a position to its NICU team—the second Canadian hospital to do so.) Are there any subsidized (or free) accommodations for parents available in the area? Is it possible to purchase a parking pass at a discount if you'll be a regular at the hospital for a while?

---

mom's the word "Madeline had a fairly lengthy stay in hospital—11 weeks. People were constantly asking me why I didn't stay in the family housing that was available for parents with children in the hospital instead of commuting an hour and a half each way every day, but I felt that I really needed the sanity of home and to be with my 2-year-old son. He really kept me going for all those weeks."

—MONIQUE, 28, MOTHER OF TWO

- Play as active a role as you can in your baby's care, but don't put superhuman demands on yourself to do so. No one expects you to hang out at the hospital 24 hours a day, nor should you expect this of yourself. You should also not feel pressured to leave, if you prefer to stay close to your baby. Some hospitals have "care by parent" rooms near the NICU where parents can stay, or there may be a Ronald McDonald House near the hospital where you can sleep but still be able to see your baby frequently.

- Learn how to establish or maintain your milk production if your baby is too premature or too ill to feed at the breast. It's a good idea to line up some support from a lactation consultant or your local La Leche League leader. You'll also want to start pumping (with a hospital-grade double-horned breast pump) or expressing milk manually (via hand expression) within six hours of your baby's birth. Pump eight to ten times each day (including at least once during the night) during each 10-hour period. Pump for 15 minutes per session initially (before your milk is in). Then increase your pumping sessions to 30 minutes each (after your milk is in). For best results, massage your breasts before you start pumping; massage and compress your breasts during pumping; and keep pumping for two to five minutes after the last drops of milk have been removed from your breasts (to increase your milk supply). (To compress your breast, squeeze and hold your breast so that internal pressure within the breast increases, thereby increasing the flow of milk.)

- Look for ways to avoid having to update a million and one people about your baby's progress on a daily basis—something that can be tremendously draining, especially if the news you have to report isn't as positive as you'd like. Either post an update on Facebook, send out a group e-mail message, or have a supportive friend help spread the news via phone, passing along additional information about what specific types of hands-on help you could most use right now. (If she's smart, she'll quickly form a phone tree so that each person who receives a phone call is responsible in turn for calling a couple of other people. It's a great way to lighten the workload of any given person and get the word out fast.)

- Accept any and all offers of help—and if you're not getting enough offers, ask for help. This is one time in your life when you're expected to call in any and all favours. Ask people to drop off nutritious meals at the hospital at a particular time so that you can enjoy a healthy home-cooked meal while you're visiting your baby. Or if you're in need of a break, ask a trusted friend to stay with your baby so that you and your partner can grab a guilt-free bite to eat outside of the hospital.

- Start preparing for the day when you'll be able to bring your baby home. The more you participate in your baby's day-to-day care while he's in the hospital, the less intimidated you'll feel when it's time to bring him home. And before you check your baby out of the hospital, line up as much support as you can on the home front. Some insurance companies cover the services of a visiting nurse, particularly if you've given birth to multiples.

mother wisdom "As discharge and homecoming approach, you may have mixed feelings. Having your baby at home, enfolded in your family circle, is your most heartfelt desire. But you may also be consumed with anxiety. You may wonder, 'Will I know how to take care of my baby without the assistance of trained medical professionals? Will my baby continue to have extraordinary needs? Will an emergency situation arise and will I know how to handle it?' Rest assured that while homecoming feels like a huge step, you know more than you think you do.

But even as you step across the threshold of your house with your precious infant in your arms, parenting may still feel like an intense experience. Not only are you especially grateful and appreciative of your precious little one, but you may also feel on guard about germs, illness, growth, and development. Your heightened protectiveness and vigilance is a normal part of having a premature baby. Your continued grief about what you've missed is also natural. If your baby has persistent medical needs or developmental delays, you'll have even more to grieve for.

As part of becoming a special kind of parent to your special baby, it is important for you to acknowledge and deal with all of your feelings. By working through your painful emotions, you will free yourself to experience the pleasant emotions and to continue to form a deepening bond with your baby. Give yourself the time, space and nurturing you need to get through the painful stuff, so that you can have the energy and ability to devote yourself to your little one. You do deserve to feel the rewards of parental joy and love."

—DEBORAH L. DAVIS, PH.D., CO-AUTHOR OF
THE EMOTIONAL JOURNEY OF PARENTING YOUR PREMATURE BABY: A BOOK OF HOPE AND HEALING

REDUCING THE RISK OF SIDS

SIDS is the sudden and unexpected death of an apparently healthy infant under one year of age that remains unexplained after all known and possible causes have been ruled out through autopsy, death scene investigation, and review of the medical history. It is more common in boys than in girls, and the peak risk period occurs when a baby is 2 to 4 months of age. The incidence of SIDS increases during the winter months. Other risk factors for SIDS include

- the age of the mother (mothers age 20 or younger face the greatest risk of losing a baby to SIDS);
- the mother's lifestyle (mothers who smoke during or after pregnancy, who are exposed to second-hand smoke during pregnancy, who use drugs, or who do not receive adequate prenatal care face a higher-than-average risk of losing a baby to SIDS);
- the interval between the mother's pregnancy with this baby and her previous pregnancy (a short gap between pregnancy increases the risk of SIDS);
- the mother's socioeconomic status (the lower her socioeconomic status, the greater the risk);
- the baby's birth weight (low birth weight babies face a higher-than-average risk);
- the baby's gestational age (babies born prematurely face a greater risk than babies born at term);
- whether or not the baby was a twin or other multiple (multiples are at greater risk than singletons);

- having a brother or sister who succumbed to SIDS;
- the baby's sleeping position (sleeping on the stomach increases the risk of a SIDS-related death);
- the baby's sleeping environment (soft bedding, bumper pads, pillows, or other objects in the crib; bed-sharing with a parent, particularly if that adult has been drinking, is heavily medicated, or is extremely obese); and
- the baby's health immediately prior to death (approximately one-third of babies who succumb to SIDS are found to have had some sort of upper respiratory infection at the time of death).

While nothing can eliminate the risk of SIDS entirely, there's plenty that you can do to reduce your odds of experiencing this terrible heartbreak. The Canadian Paediatric Society has reached the following conclusions, based on the best SIDS-related research available to date.

- **Placing your baby to sleep on his back reduces the risk of SIDS.** Studies have shown that SIDS is less common in babies who sleep in this position than in those who sleep on their tummies or sides; and, contrary to popular belief, babies who sleep on their backs are no more likely to choke than babies who sleep in other positions. The SIDS risk skyrockets, however, if a baby who usually sleeps on his back is placed to sleep on his stomach. This doesn't mean that your baby should never spend any time on her tummy; regular tummy time each day is essential for your baby's development and will also help to avoid temporary flat spots that sometimes develop on the back of a baby's head (plagiocephaly) as a result of spending so much time lying on her back. Where the risk lies is in allowing your baby to lie in this position when you are not there to supervise her.

---

baby talk When babies fall asleep in the sitting position in strollers, swings, bouncers, and car seats, their heads can fall over, constricting their airway. It's important to move a baby to a crib, cradle, or bassinet to sleep as opposed to allowing a baby to nap unsupervised in a stroller, swing, bouncer, or car seat.

- **Room-sharing (as opposed to bed-sharing) reduces the risk of SIDS.** Having your baby sleep in the same room allows you to respond to her quickly and easily in the night, easing the fatigue and stress of nighttime parenting.

- **Bed-sharing increases the risk of SIDS.** If an adult rolls up against a baby, the baby can suffocate or the adult's body can function like a large pillow, causing large quantities of carbon dioxide to pool around the baby's head. Note: Sleeping with an infant on a sofa or recliner is associated with a particularly high risk of SIDS. Ditto for bed-sharing with anyone other than a parent.

---

baby talk Research by sleep anthropologist James McKenna and others suggests that breastfeeding mothers use different sleep positions when they sleep with their babies than formula-feeding mothers use. Breastfeeding mothers tend to face their babies and place an arm above their babies' heads; while formula-feeding mothers tend to sleep with their backs facing their babies (which reduces a mother's awareness of where her baby is while she is sleeping).

- **Using bedding, soft pillows, and other soft materials increases the risk of SIDS.** To create a safe sleeping environment for your baby, ensure that the crib mattress is firm and that your baby's crib is free of pillows, blankets, stuffed animals, crib bumpers, and other soft bedding that could increase the risk of suffocation or cause large quantities of carbon dioxide to pool around your baby's head. (Problems with the baby's ability to wake up and a failure to detect a buildup of carbon dioxide in the blood are believed to be two factors related to SIDS deaths.)

---

baby talk Don't worry if your baby ends up sleeping on his tummy once he's old enough to roll over from his back to his tummy on his own (something that typically happens at around age 5 months). If he rolls himself over, he can stay on his side or his tummy.

---

baby talk — Make sure that anyone else who cares for your baby is aware that it's important to put the baby to sleep on his back. Not only is it dangerous in and of itself, researchers at the Children's National Medical Center in Washington, D.C., found that infants who are unaccustomed to sleeping on their stomachs face a higher risk of SIDS if they are placed to sleep in this position.

Here are some strategies for reducing the risk of SIDS:

- **Don't use a sleep positioner.** Tempted to purchase a sleep positioner (a product that is designed to keep a baby on his back)? You might want to think twice. Not only is there no solid research to document the benefits of these products, the U.S.-based Consumer Product Safety Commission recently asked manufacturers of sleep positioners to stop marketing their products to parents—this in the wake of 13 infant deaths over a 13-year period. In an article in the *Globe and Mail,* Denis Leduc, past president of the Canadian Paediatric Society, called on Health Canada to introduce legislation limiting the kinds of claims manufacturers can make about juvenile products, including products that claim to prevent SIDS.

- **Keep your baby at a comfortable temperature.** Overheating is a risk factor for SIDS. Infants are safest when placed to sleep in fitted one-piece sleepwear. The easiest way to monitor your baby's temperature is by placing your hand on the back of your baby's neck. If she's sweating, she's too warm.

- **Breastfeed your baby.** According to Canada's *Joint Statement on Safe Sleep* (2011), "Any breastfeeding for any duration provides a protective effect for SIDS, and exclusive breastfeeding offers greater protection." Exclusive breastfeeding for the first six months—the period when the risk of SIDS is greatest—may reduce the SIDS risk by as much as 50 per cent.

- **Offer your baby a pacifier at bedtime.** (If your baby is breastfed, wait until breastfeeding is well-established before introducing a pacifier.) Pacifiers appear to provide a protective effect against SIDS, either by keeping the airway more open or by preventing a baby from falling into an overly deep sleep. A baby who arouses from sleep more easily is more likely to be able to get herself out of a dangerous sleep situation.

mother wisdom — Don't dip a pacifier in honey in an effort to make the pacifier more enticing to a baby. Honey can cause botulism in young children, increasing the risk of SIDS. If your baby doesn't want a pacifier, your baby doesn't want a pacifier. It's okay: there are plenty of other things you can do to reduce the risk of SIDS.

Coping with SIDS-related fears

While most worries are relatively easy to chase away once you've pulled out your baby books or made a quick call to your doctor's office, some of them are more deeply rooted, keeping you awake at 3 a.m. when you know you should be sleeping. At the top of the list for most parents is the fear that their baby will become a victim of sudden infant death syndrome (SIDS).

According to Deborah Davis, co-author of *The Emotional Journey of Parenting Your Premature Baby: A Book of Hope and Healing*, the key to learning to live with SIDS-related fears is to accept the fact that there are some aspects of parenting that are beyond your control: "With regard to feelings of vulnerability to tragedy, their intensity does fade as you are able to accept that life and death just happen. And when you realize that the death of your child has no bearing on your worth as a parent or as a person, then you can accept that you truly do have little control over many circumstances. Not everything is your fault or deserved. You just try to control the things you can, and let go of what you can't. Peace comes from experiencing that feeling of 'letting go.'"

EVERY PARENT'S WORST NIGHTMARE

Despite all the amazing advances in neonatal medicine we've witnessed over the past few decades, there are still a number of problems that medical science is unable to treat or prevent. As a result, approximately 5.1 out of every 1,000 live-born infants (or roughly one in every 200 babies) dies during the first year of life.

Approximately two-thirds of infant deaths occur during the first month of life—during the so-called neonatal period. The two leading causes of neonatal death are conditions originating in the perinatal period (for example, respiratory distress syndrome; problems associated with prematurity and/or low birth weight; maternal complications of pregnancy, such as gestational diabetes or pre-eclampsia; problems with the placenta, umbilical cord, and amniotic sac; complications of labour and delivery; slow fetal growth and fetal malnutrition; birth trauma; intrauterine hypoxia and birth hypoxia—when the baby is deprived of oxygen prior to or during birth; hemorrhage; and perinatal jaundice) and congenital anomalies (for example, neural tube defects such as anencephaly, spina bifida, and hydrocephalus; heart and other circulatory system defects; problems with the respiratory, digestive, genitourinary, and musculoskeletal systems; and chromosomal anomalies). The two leading causes of post-neonatal death (deaths occurring between one month and one year of age) are sudden infant death syndrome (SIDS) and congenital anomalies.

Surviving the unthinkable

If the unthinkable happens and you experience the death of your much-loved baby, you may feel shocked and overwhelmed that this has even happened. (*"How could this happen? Babies aren't supposed to die...."*) You may feel as though you're on autopilot, going through the motions of everyday life, even though your mind is endlessly processing—trying to make sense of something that makes no sense at all.

You may also find yourself denying that your baby has died or wishing desperately that he hadn't; blaming yourself or others for his death; and coping with feelings of depression and despair. You may find yourself having wonderful dreams—dreams in which you are still pregnant or your baby is still alive—only to wake up to a nightmarish reality in which your baby is really dead. You may wish you could slip back into that dream, that you never had to wake up.

You may find yourself experiencing the psychological and physical fallout of grief as you begin to process the fact of your baby's death: preoccupation with thoughts of the baby you lost, irritability, restlessness, anxiety, fear, yearning, hopelessness, confusion, shortness of breath, tightness in the throat, fatigue, crying spells, an empty feeling in your abdomen, sleeplessness, a change in appetite, heart palpitations, and other physical symptoms of anxiety. Some bereaved parents experience some additional symptoms: empty, aching arms and illusions about seeing, hearing, or feeling the presence of the baby.

Some parents who have experienced the death of a baby are afraid to work through their grief, believing that doing so will cause them to move on and forget about the baby they lost. Here are some reassuring words from Deborah Davis, Ph.D., author of *Empty Cradle, Broken Heart:* "You will never forget your baby. Many people mistakenly believe that resolution means you stop grieving, forget about the baby, and meekly abandon your baby to death. To the contrary, grief does not end. You will always feel some sadness and wish that things could have turned out better. But, with time, the denial, failure, guilt, and anger fade; the sadness becomes manageable . . . The peaceful feelings that come with resolution are a blessed change from the ravages of grief."

Here are some suggestions on surviving the first few days, weeks, and months after the death of your baby.

- Let the staff of the hospital or funeral home know if you would like to spend some time alone with your baby or if you would like to be involved in bathing or dressing your baby yourself. Some parents find it tremendously comforting to be able to do these things for their baby.

- If you decide to dress your baby in a special outfit or have your baby buried along with a toy or other memento, you might want to take photos of these items with your baby and/or to purchase duplicates so that you'll have something to hold on to in the months ahead when your arms are feeling painfully empty.

- Decide whether you would like other family members to have the chance to spend some time with your baby, too. You might, for example, want your other children to see and hold the baby, particularly if the baby died shortly after the birth and your other children never had the chance to meet their little brother or sister. Be prepared to provide your children with clear reasons about how and why the baby died; telling them that the baby has "gone to sleep" or has been "lost" may cause them to become unnecessarily fearful.

- Think about taking some photographs of your baby. While this may seem like a morbid idea at first, some parents find it helpful to have some photos to look back on during the difficult months and years ahead, if only because these photos are tangible proof that their baby existed. You might want to take some photographs of your baby in your arms, in your partner's arms, with other special people in your life (such as his grandparents), and, in the case of a twin pregnancy, with the surviving twin. These photos may become some of your most treasured mementoes of the time you spent with your baby.

mother wisdom — If you decide to take some photos of your baby, you might want to think about using black and white film for at least some of the photos. This is because the skin changes that happen after a baby dies are less apparent in black and white photos.

- Think about what other mementoes you might want to have of your baby: perhaps a lock of his hair or a set of his handprints or footprints. (Note: Many hospitals are offering to make handprints and footprints of babies who die, so don't worry that anyone will think you're strange if you inquire about whether this option is available.)
- Give some thoughts to your baby's funeral arrangements. Even though other relatives may offer to handle these details on your behalf to save you some pain, most parents find that they prefer to handle these details themselves because it's one of the last things they'll ever have the opportunity to do for their baby.
- Find out whether a post mortem is required in your province or territory (the rules vary across the country) or whether this is a decision that you and your partner need to make.
- If you're worried about the costs of burying your child, talk to your doctor or midwife about burial options for families with modest incomes. You may find that a local funeral home offers a significant discount or waives its fees entirely for families who have lost a child.
- Find ways of involving your living children in the funeral arrangements. They may wish to help pick out flowers for the funeral bouquet or to draw a picture for the baby who died. It's important to explain what has happened, even to very young children. They will pick up on your emotions and sense that something terrible has happened. They need to know that they are safe and that you and the family will be okay: you are just very sad about the baby who died. The way you handle this loss with them will begin to set the tone for the way loss is handled within your family.
- Think about ways you might want to honour your baby's memory. You might choose to make a donation to a charity or to buy a piece of equipment for your hospital's neonatal ward in your baby's name. Or

you might wish to participate in a community ceremony for bereaved parents or to come up with a ritual of remembrance that will hold particular meaning for your family. If you are breastfeeding, you may have stored milk or milk that you express as you gradually reduce your milk production, and this could be donated to help other babies.

- Understand that some children avoid expressing their feelings of grief openly, for fear of upsetting their parents. Others become very clingy, demonstrating their fear that something could happen to you. Some will react with attention-seeking behaviours, sensing (quite rightly) that your attention is elsewhere right now. Girls aged 7 to 12 years who had strongly identified with their mother's pregnancy are particularly likely to want to "fix" their mother's grief. They may feel the loss of the baby particularly acutely or they may fear for their own death. Children who may have expressed feelings that they regret now (such as negative feelings toward the pregnancy or the baby) need to be given the opportunity to work through any feelings of guilt they may be harbouring. Children who have lost a baby sibling suffer in other ways as well. At the very time they need their parents the most, their parents may be emotionally treading water themselves.

- Don't forget that grandparents grieve, too. They grieve the death of their grandchild and they hurt because their children are hurting. Sometimes a bereaved grandmother will try to shut down her daughter's grief—an indication of her own feelings about the power of grief.

- Let family and friends know how they can be helpful to you. Tell them that their phone calls and visits are important to you: grief is lonely. Let them know what you would appreciate most right now: personal visits, daily phone calls, someone to run errands for you (or with you), someone to help you with chores at home. And thank them for their patience and support.

---

mother wisdom Families need some time to grieve in privacy—some time to process their loss without a constant stampede of visitors. But this needs to be balanced with the need for care and support from the community.

- Make sure you understand the circumstances that led to your baby's death. You may have a difficult time grasping this information when you are dealing with the shock of your baby's death, so you might find it helpful to ask the hospital staff to write down this information for you or to have a support person accompany you and your partner to meetings with the doctor or the coroner so that your support person can absorb some of this information for you. Don't be afraid to set up a follow-up appointment with the health-care practitioners involved if you discover down the road that you still have many unanswered questions about your baby's death; or to ask the medical staff to repeat information a couple of different times if you're having difficulty making sense of what you're hearing. Include your partner in all such appointments so that he/she also benefits from this sharing of information and can also express his/her feelings of loss.

- Accept the fact that you'll probably always have questions about your baby's death. The one question that parents want answered most is the one that is generally the most difficult to answer: "Why did this happen to *my* baby?"

- Understand that the death of a baby is a life-shattering experience, as Deborah Davis, Ph.D., notes in her book *Empty Cradle, Broken Heart*: "While the death of a parent or friend represents a loss of your past, when your baby dies you lose part of your future. You grieve not only for your baby, but for your parenthood. Times you had looked forward to—maternity leave, family gatherings, and holidays—can seem worthless or trivial without your baby."

- Realize that you and your partner may grieve differently. Don't automatically assume that he's less affected by the loss just because he's less willing to express his emotions. Many bereaved fathers feel tremendous pressure to "hold it together" when their partners are falling apart. Because fathers tend to be less verbal about their grief, the extent of their grief has been underestimated in grief research. A 2002 study conducted by researchers at the University of Queensland in Australia found that grief in fathers tends to peak around 30 months after the death of a baby. Other research has shown that symptoms of trauma show up in fathers around the time those symptoms begin to ease in mothers. It's important to keep communicating with your partner as you begin to work through the potential minefield of emotions surrounding your baby's death. Shutting out your partner will only add to the loneliness of grief.

- Resist the temptation to bury your grief by turning to alcohol or prescription drugs or by throwing yourself into your work and refusing to face your feelings. You can't avoid working through your grief—you can only postpone it. Grief is patient. It will wait for you.

- Take care of your physical needs as well as your emotional needs. Get the sleep you need, exercise regularly, and make a point of eating nutritious, well-balanced meals. Your body has been through a lot. It deserves some loving care.

- Don't expect yourself to be able to carry as much responsibility at home and at work as you normally would. Grief takes energy—both mental and physical. While bereavement leaves vary from province to territory, unless you have a particularly understanding employer or the financial freedom to quit your job, you may find yourself forced to return to work before you feel that you are ready.

---

mother wisdom If your baby is stillborn or dies shortly after birth or after breastfeeding has already been established, you may also have to cope with breast engorgement (overly full and uncomfortable breasts). Having milk leaking from your breasts after your baby has died can be both physically and emotionally distressing. You may feel as though your entire body is mourning the loss of your baby—which, in fact, it is. The period of engorgement tends to last for about 48 hours. You can relieve your breast tenderness in the meantime by expressing a small amount of milk. (Don't express too much or your body will start producing more milk.) Binding your breasts tightly, applying ice packs to your breasts, and wearing a snug bra at all times can also help to reduce your discomfort. Note: If you notice red, warm, hard, or tender areas in your breasts, develop a fever of more than 37 degrees Celsius (100 degrees Fahrenheit), notice that the lymph nodes under your arm are becoming uncomfortable, or feel generally ill, it could be because you're developing a breast infection. Contact your doctor or midwife to talk about treatment options.

- Find out if there are support groups in your community for parents who have experienced the death of a baby. It can be tremendously helpful to talk to other parents who have been through this, too, both to validate what you're feeling and to reassure you that you will be able to find a reason to go on, even though you may find that hard to believe right now.
- Don't be afraid to reach out for professional help if you find your feelings of grief overwhelming, if you are struggling with anxiety and depression, or if you are exhibiting some of the symptoms of post-traumatic stress disorder in the wake of your baby's death.
- Understand that there's no statute of limitations on grief. Your grief doesn't magically disappear after a certain period of time.

---

mom's the word

"Nothing will ever take the pain away entirely, but time does heal, even though it can be hard to hear that at the time."

—MONIQUE, 28, MOTHER OF TWO LIVING CHILDREN AND ONE BABY WHO DIED DURING LABOUR

- Remind yourself that you have the strength to get through this—that as painful as it is to have to say goodbye to a baby you desperately wanted, you can survive this heartbreak. As hard as it may be for you to believe right now, you will find joy in your life again.

chapter 9

EATING AND SLEEPING REVISITED

"My first two babies ate like champs: anything and everything I put in front of them was gobbled up. My third baby, however, was very fussy. She never liked baby food from the first bite until I gave up trying to feed it to her. It was very frustrating to have meal after meal refused by her, and I racked my brains trying to think of tasty things I could feed her. I finally figured out that she did not want to be fed by me: she wanted to feed herself! As a result, my third baby ended up eating finger foods much earlier than my other two did!"

—CAROLIN, 35, MOTHER OF THREE

Babies spend a lot of time eating and sleeping during their first year of life. It's hardly surprising, then, that first-time parents have so many questions about these two issues.

The early chapters of this book focused on eating and sleeping from the vantage point of the newborn. Now we're going to return to these two topics and consider them from the perspective of an older baby—a baby who is about to start solid foods and who may be getting ready to sleep through the night sometime soon. (By age 9 months, 75 per cent of babies are sleeping through the night most of the time. That means that 25 per cent of babies are still waking up in the night on a regular basis. So don't feel like you have the only baby who is still getting up in the night: the statistics tell a very different story.)

INTRODUCING SOLID FOOD

Up until now, you haven't had to give much thought to what to feed your baby or when to feed your baby. You've been letting her tell you when she is hungry and sticking to a one-item menu. Now that your baby is approaching the six-month mark, things are about to change.

Health Canada and other pediatric health authorities here in Canada have chosen to follow the lead of the World Health Organization (WHO) in recommending exclusive breastfeeding until age 6 months. (That doesn't mean that breastfeeding should stop at age 6 months: the World Health Organization recommends that babies continue to be breastfed to age 2 and beyond, if mother and baby are willing.)

---

mother wisdom "Until the end of the seventeenth century, babies continued to be raised in traditional ways. At three or four months, they were given pap made with lard and cabbage, wine, and sometimes alcohol. In order to immunize them against certain illnesses, pious images of the protector saints reduced to powder were added to the broth."
—BÉATRICE FONTANEL AND CLAIR D'HARCOURT,
BABIES: HISTORY, ART, AND FOLKLORE

Six months of exclusive breastfeeding is recommended because most healthy full-term babies don't require any foods other than breast milk until they are at least 6 months of age, at which point iron-deficiency begins to become a possible concern. Introducing iron-fortified and vitamin-C fortified foods to babies, starting at age 6 months, reduces the risk of iron deficiency. (Some full-term babies who are small for gestational age or who were born to mothers who were iron-deficient may be at increased risk of iron deficiency. Their nutritional status will need to be monitored more closely by a healthcare professional.)

There are other compelling reasons for starting solid foods at around 6 months. Babies this age are physiologically and developmentally ready to deal with new foods, new textures, and new ways of eating.

Introducing solid foods to a baby before he or she is ready (something that is frequently done in the mistaken belief that offering a very young baby solid food will help that baby to sleep through the night sooner) can be harmful to a baby. Doing so

- increases the risk of choking because the baby doesn't have the necessary chewing and swallowing skills;

- may cause gastrointestinal discomfort (because the baby's gastrointestinal system isn't mature enough to handle foods other than breast milk);
- can reduce the amount of breast milk that is being consumed and produced, thereby depriving the baby of important nutrients and potentially bringing an end to breastfeeding;
- increases the risk of the baby developing food allergies (particularly in families in which there is a history of food allergies);
- reduces the amount of iron that the baby's body is capable of absorbing from human milk (iron absorption is affected when milk comes into contact with other foods in the proximal small bowel); and
- increases the baby's lifelong risk of becoming overweight or obese (infants who grow too rapidly during the first two years of life are more likely to become obese during childhood and adulthood).

Delaying the introduction of solid foods can lead to problems as well. Infant development experts believe that babies are particularly interested in learning how to eat solid foods before age 9 months. Babies who are not exposed to solid foods by that time tend to be more resistant to trying solid foods and may experience more difficulty acquiring eating-related skills, like how to chew, which can affect the development of speech skills later on.

---

mother wisdom If your baby was born four or more weeks ahead of his due date, your health-care provider may advise you to go with his corrected age (his chronological age in weeks less the number of weeks he was born early) rather than his chronological age when predicting the age at which he is likely to be ready to start solid food. Your baby's doctor will also use his corrected age to assess his overall growth and development.

A baby is born with roughly a six-month stockpile of iron—enough to carry him over until the age at which he can begin to eat solid foods. If he doesn't start to eat solid foods within a few months, he may become anemic (iron-deficient), something that can interfere with his overall health and development.

Note: A study by Pisacane (conducted in 1995) found that babies who were exclusively breastfed until age 7 months had higher hemoglobin (iron) levels at age one year than babies who started solid foods before age 7 months. So don't panic if your baby doesn't take to solid foods right away. But do touch base with your baby's doctor so the two of you can start discussing strategies for introducing solids sooner rather than later.

Baby, give me a sign

Of course, a baby has to be developmentally ready to start solids. Fortunately, your baby has that covered. She'll give you plenty of signs that she's ready to start dining with the rest of the family. Here's what to watch for.

Your baby

- can sit up well, so you know she's ready for a high chair or other feeding chair.
- has good control over her head and neck muscles when she's seated. (You want her to be able to turn her head toward you when she wants another spoonful or away from you when she's had enough to eat.)
- can move her tongue well. (In order to swallow solid food, she needs to be able to move food from the front of her mouth to the back.)
- is interested in food and the process of eating. (You notice that she's fascinated by what you're doing when you're eating, and that she tracks the path of your spoon as it moves from your bowl to your mouth.)
- opens her mouth when she sees food coming her way on a spoon—an indication that she understands the connection between food and eating.

---

mother wisdom Sometimes babies who are new to the world of solid foods push food out with their tongues or allow food to ooze out of their mouths when they are eating. In some cases, they don't like the taste of the food or the sensation of having solid foods in their mouths. In other cases, they simply do not know what to do with solid foods. In such a situation, you may want to reintroduce solids in a couple of days' time. By that time, they may be more open to trying new foods or they may have figured out how to move solid food around in their mouths. If your baby becomes upset at the sight of solid food, take a break for a week or two and then try again. A baby can do a lot of changing and growing over that period of time.

Baby's first feeding

Here are some tips that will help to ensure that baby's first experience with solid food is enjoyable for both of you.

---

mom's the word "We use a high chair for every feeding to help establish a routine. Elizabeth knows that it's feeding time whenever we put her in her chair."

—CYNTHIA, 31, MOTHER OF ONE

- **Decide which food to start with.** Dietitians recommend that you start with an iron-rich food because the iron supply that your baby was born with begins to dwindle after age 6 months. Examples of iron-rich foods that are suitable for babies include infant cereals (which are fortified with iron), chicken, pork, beef, wild meat, egg yolks, and legumes. Note: The aborption of both heme iron (iron from animal sources) and non-heme iron (iron from non-animal sources) can be increased if the food containing iron is consumed along with foods that are rich in vitamin C.

    Note: Some parents choose not to stress about the iron issue and opt instead for foods like bananas or sweet potato as Baby's first foods. Once their baby is used to the idea of eating solid food, they start introducing more iron-rich foods.

    Note: You should introduce one food at a time and wait a few days before introducing any additional new foods so that you can watch for any signs of food allergies or intolerances. (See the following section.)

---

mom's the word "Each time I introduced a new food, I wrote down the date. That way, if my baby showed signs of having a reaction to a food, I would know what the last food I'd introduced was."

—MARIA, 32, MOTHER OF TWO

- **Consider your timing.** Choose a time of day when your baby is likely to be happy and relaxed. And offer solids after he has been breastfed (so he won't be frustrated and distracted because he's totally famished and because you do not want the solid foods to replace the breast milk).

- **Get the texture right.** A first solid food for a baby around age 6 months is thick (like porridge) or soft and mashed. (See Table 9.1.) She is capable (and will be quite eager) to feed herself foods of this texture, if you let her. And you should let her. It may be messy, but it's important developmentally for her to master these early self-feeding skills.

- **Get the temperature right.** Your baby will be more willing to try solid food if it is warmed up to body temperature. If the food is too cold, she might not want anything to do with it.

---

baby talk Don't add infant cereal or other puréed foods to bottles containing breast milk or other liquids. It's important for your baby to master the art of eating from a spoon and to make the transition from ingesting liquids to eating more textured foods. Sucking thick liquids or food from a bottle may also increase the risk of choking or aspiration—reason enough to avoid going this route.

- **Offer tiny spoonfuls.** A little bit of food on the tip of a baby-sized spoon is all a beginner can handle until he's proven he's got the swing of things. And don't expect him to eat much more than 5 mL (a teaspoonful) at his first feeding—if he even manages to eat that much. Pretty soon he'll get the hang of this eating thing. He'll keep opening his mouth like a baby bird in search of a worm—waiting for that spoon to appear.

- **See if baby knows what to do with the food in his mouth.** Does he know how to close his lips over the spoon and to use his lips to remove food from the spoon? Is he capable of keeping the food in his mouth rather than allowing it to dribble out the front of his mouth? (He may not figure this out right away, but this is what you're trying to teach him.)

TABLE 9.1

Baby Food Textures Guide

As your baby's chewing and swallowing skills improve, she'll graduate from one texture to another. Here's how to create foods of increasingly complex textures and what you'll notice about your baby's eating habits as she masters one eating skill after another.

Baby food texture	How to create foods of this texture	What you'll notice about your baby's eating habits at this stage
Ground, grated, and mashed foods	Serve some of your baby's foods grated, mashed, or ground (using a baby food mill or small food chopper) as opposed to serving all of her foods puréed. Note: She will find it difficult to manage mixed textures (lumpy foods mixed in with smooth foods) until she's had a little more practice with solid foods.	Your baby is capable of moving food from side to side using her tongue.
Chopped foods (finger foods)	Offer your baby foods that are easy for her to pick up with her fingers and that she can chew easily. (Chop your baby's food into small, fine pieces to avoid any choking hazard.)	Your baby is becoming much more interested in feeding herself, and her chewing abilities are improving every day.
Table foods	Start introducing other tastes and textures, including crunchy and chewy foods. Continue to watch your child closely while she's eating and to cut her food into tiny, bite-sized pieces.	By the time your baby becomes a toddler, she should be capable of eating most of the foods that you enjoy. Just remember to steer clear of foods that pose a choking hazard; and bear in mind that the taste buds of young children are much more sensitive than those of adults. (If a certain vegetable tastes bitter to you, it may taste overpoweringly bitter to your child.)

- **Wait for a signal from your baby that she's ready for more food** (a look of interest or excitement when she sees the spoon coming; opening her mouth). Don't shove the spoon in her mouth before she's ready or you could end up with a thoroughly outraged baby.

mother wisdom — Pablum was invented in the 1920s by a team of doctors at the Hospital for Sick Children in Toronto. In 1931, they brought their product to market so that all Canadian babies would be able to benefit from it. Royalty income from sales of the product funded important pediatric research, including techniques for repairing congenital hip dislocation, lateral curvature of the spine, and a certain type of heart defect. Talk about the breakfast of champions!

And after that first feeding . . .

Once you've determined that your baby hasn't experienced a reaction to that first food (you'll know within a couple of days), you can begin to introduce other foods to her diet. Here are some tips on introducing new foods and keeping mealtimes stress-free for you and your newcomer to the world of solid foods.

- **Encourage your baby to taste new foods, but don't coax her to eat foods that she doesn't like.** If she seems less than thrilled with the veggie du jour, simply reintroduce it in a few weeks' time. Her taste buds may be a bit more adventurous by then. Research has shown that it can take 15 to 20 exposures to a new food for a baby or toddler to decide that she likes it.

- **Watch for the stop sign.** If you're trying to feed your baby with a spoon, pay attention to your baby's signals when he tries to tell you that he's had enough to eat. He'll turn his head away or close his mouth. You don't want to teach him to disregard his natural signals of fullness. Doing so can encourage unhealthy eating habits and can lead to weight or eating problems. If you let your baby feed himself, he can tune into those signals of fullness (something he has been doing the entire time he has been breastfed) and simply stop eating the moment he senses he's had enough.

- **Don't get frazzled if your baby doesn't eat as much as a single mouthful at a particular meal.** As Ellyn Satter notes in her book *Child of Mine: Feeding with Love and Good Sense*, "Adults are responsible for what, when, and where children are fed; children are responsible for how much and whether they eat." If you can master that concept right from day one, you'll save yourself a lot of worry.

mother wisdom — Don't worry if your baby doesn't eat much when he's first learning how to eat solid food. He's trying to master a new skill—learning how to move food around in his mouth and how to swallow it. He's also learning to become comfortable with a new method of eating and a new type of food. You don't have to worry about how much he is—or isn't eating—because breast milk will continue to be the mainstay of his diet while he is making the transition to solid foods.

Added tastes and textures

You can encourage your baby to develop self-feeding skills by offering her a variety of finger foods. Choose foods that she's able to chew and swallow on her own: for example, easy-to-digest and easy-to-chew cereals, salt-free crackers, tiny pieces of toast, pieces of rice cakes, soft fresh fruit (cut into small pieces), cooked vegetables (cut into small pieces), well-cooked pasta (cut into small pieces), and hard cheese (cut into small pieces or grated).

When she gets a little older (age 9 months and up), you can provide her with opportunities to practise using a spoon. Just realize that learning to use a spoon is tougher than it looks. Baby may become frustrated, ditch her spoon(s), and use her hands to move food from her bowl to her mouth. (Don't worry. You'll have many years to help her polish her table manners before her first job interview.)

mother wisdom — Forget about using those super-cutesy cotton bibs that are designed more for catching dainty little drools than dealing with the fallout from self-feeding. Think maximum coverage.

mother wisdom — Place finger foods on the high chair tray rather than in a bowl. It'll take baby longer to get the food on the floor and some may even make it into her mouth first.

mother wisdom Give your baby a spoon for each hand while you continue to offer her food from another spoon. That way, she won't be as likely to try to grab the spoon from your hands. (If she decides she wants the spoon you're using to feed her, simply trade spoons.)

MAKING YOUR OWN BABY FOOD

If you decide to start with baby food pureés (perhaps because your baby has difficulty tolerating foods of a mashed, porridge-like texture), you may appreciate having some quick-and-easy recipes for whipping up your own baby food at home. It's easy and it can save you a lot of money (as compared to the cost of purchasing commercially manufactured baby food). Here are the main things you need to know to start making nutritious, baby-pleasing foods.

mom's the word "Making baby food is so simple you'll be amazed. All you need is some fruit, veggies, or meat, a way to cook them, and a blender or food processor. I could make enough food to last a month in a couple of hours. I found the best way to do it was to make big batches of food, pour the food into ice cube trays, freeze the trays, and then pop out the frozen cubes and put them into labelled freezer bags. Just be sure to label the bags: all those orange fruits and veggies look amazingly the same in a freezer bag! When your baby is a little bit older, you can even purée soups and stews to the desired consistency and freeze them in the same manner. By making your own baby food, you will save yourself a ton of money and feel secure in the knowledge that you know exactly what your baby is eating and how it was prepared."
—CAROLIN, 35, MOTHER OF THREE

- Start with the freshest ingredients you can find. Frozen or canned will do as a backup, but fresh means more flavour. And give yourself bonus marks if you manage to pull off local, too. You're doing your bit to sustain your local agricultural economy. (If you can afford to eat organic produce, that's even better. All-natural is always the best way to go.)

---

mom's the word "My son was born in September, so there was limited fresh produce in season by the time he was ready to start solids. I used frozen vegetables and canned fruit, no sugar added."

—HELENA, 32, MOTHER OF ONE

- Cut the produce into small, similarly sized pieces to reduce the amount of time you have to spend blending or processing the food after the produce has been steamed or cooked, and to allow you to achieve a uniform consistency in your purée.
- Follow the cooking instructions on Table 9.2 to make various types of baby food purées. Set aside some of the water that you used to steam your fruit or vegetables and use this liquid when you're making your purées (to capture additional nutrients). If you decide to add breast milk rather than water to your baby's fruit or vegetable purées, you need to do this *right before you serve the food to your baby* (as opposed to adding breast milk to a large batch of baby food that is destined for the freezer, which will remove some of the nutrients from the breast milk).
- If you use a blender or food processor to make baby food, keep the amount of blending time to a minimum. This will help to reduce the amount of oxygen exposure, thereby limiting the number of nutrients that are destroyed while the food is being processed.
- If you're planning to use your baby food within the next few days, store the food in single-serving portions in sealed containers in your refrigerator.
- If your baby won't be able to eat all of this food within the next few days, freeze your baby food in ice cube trays or mini-muffin tins. Then transfer the frozen portions into a freezer bag. Be sure to label and date it.
- Thaw your frozen baby food in the refrigerator, in a small bowl inside a larger bowl of hot water, or in a double-boiler. Thawing baby food at room temperature can allow bacteria to form. And reheating baby food in the microwave can allow hot spots to develop in the food.

Note: Never refreeze baby food that has been thawed and don't save any partially eaten servings of food.

- Once your baby has become accustomed to eating a variety of foods, you can create the baby-world equivalent of casseroles by combining purées. See Table 9.3 for some advice on which flavours blend well together.

TABLE 9.2

Basic Baby Food Recipes

Fruit

Wash, peel, core, and remove seeds. Cut into small cubes or slices to reduce cooking time. Cook until soft enough to run through a blender, food mill, ricer, or food processor; or to force through a sieve.

Apples: 4 cups of apples, peeled, cored, and sliced; ½ cup water. Cover and cook over medium heat until fruit is tender (15 to 20 minutes). Purée.

Apricots (fresh): 4 cups apricots, peeled, pitted, and chopped; ½ cup water. Cover and cook in a steamer basket until fruit is tender (7 to 9 minutes). Purée.

Bananas: 4 very ripe bananas, broken into small chunks. No cooking necessary. Purée.

Cantaloupe: 4 cups cantaloupe, peeled and chopped into little pieces. No cooking necessary. Purée.

Honeydew: 4 cups cantaloupe, peeled and chopped into little pieces. No cooking necessary. Purée.

Mangoes: 4 cups mangoes, peeled and sliced; 1/3 cup water. No cooking necessary. Purée.

Nectarines: 4 medium-sized nectarines. Cover and cook in a steamer basket in a pot over low heat until fruit is tender (2 to 4 minutes). Purée.

Papaya: 4 cups papaya, peeled and sliced; 1/3 cup water. No cooking necessary. Purée.

Peaches: 4 cups fresh peaches, peeled (or frozen or unsweetened canned peaches with liquid); ½ cup water (or liquid from canned peaches). Cover and cook in a steamer basket in a pot over low heat until fruit is tender (2 to 4 minutes). Purée.

Pears: 4 cups pears, chopped, and peeled (or unsweetened canned pears with liquid); ½ cup water (or liquid from canned pears). No cooking necessary. Purée.

Pineapple: 1 pineapple, peeled and chopped (or unsweetened canned pineapple). No cooking necessary. Purée and then force mixture through a mesh sieve using a spatula.

Plums: 4 cups plums, peeled and chopped. Cover and cook in a steamer basket in a pot over low heat until fruit is tender (2 to 4 minutes). Purée.

Prunes: 2 cups prunes; 2/3 cup water. Cover and cook over low heat or steam until fruit is tender (15 to 20 minutes). Purée.

Watermelon: 4 cups watermelon, chopped and seeded. No cooking necessary. Purée.

Vegetables

Wash, peel, core, and remove seeds. Cut into small cubes or slices to reduce cooking time. Cook until soft enough to run through a blender, food mill, ricer, or food processor; or to force through a sieve. Note: Resist the temptation to add salt, margarine, butter, or spices to your child's vegetables: it's best to encourage her to develop a taste for them "au naturel."

Asparagus: 1 bunch asparagus; ½ cup water. Cook over medium-low heat until water comes to a boil, then simmer for 15 to 20 minutes or until tender. Purée.

Avocado:* 1 avocado, chopped and peeled. No cooking necessary. Purée.

Beans, green or yellow: 4 cups beans; ½ cup water. Cook over medium-low heat until beans come to a boil, then simmer for 15 minutes or until tender. Purée and then run through a sieve to achieve a smoother texture.

Beets: 2 cups beets; ½ cup water. Cook in a steamer basket over a pot of boiling water for 45 to 60 minutes or until tender. Purée.

Broccoli: 4 cups broccoli; ½ cup water. Steam for 10 minutes or until tender. Purée.

Carrots: 4 cups carrots, peeled and sliced; ½ cup water. Cook over medium-low heat until carrots come to a boil, then simmer for 20 minutes or until tender. Purée.

Cauliflower: 4 cups carrots, peeled and sliced; ½ cup water. Cook over medium-low heat until carrots come to a boil, then simmer for 20 minutes or until tender. Purée.

Lima beans: 2 cups lima beans; ¼ cup water. Cook over medium-low heat until lima beans come to a boil, then simmer for 20 minutes or until tender. Purée.

Peas: 3 cups peas; 2 cups water. Cook over medium-low heat until peas come to a boil, then simmer for 5 minutes or until tender. Purée.

Potatoes: 1 cup potatoes; ¼ cup water. Cook over medium-low heat until potatoes come to a boil, then simmer for 15 to 20 minutes or until tender. For best results, use a food mill or sieve rather than a blender or food processor to purée. Note: Potatoes do not freeze well.

(continued)

Pumpkin:* 8 cups pumpkin, peeled. Steam for 20 to 30 minutes or until tender. Purée.

Spinach: 2 packages fresh spinach, washed and cleaned, or 1 package frozen; ½ cup water. Cook over medium-low heat, until leaves start to wilt (about 3 minutes). Purée.

Squash: 4 cups squash; ½ cup water. Cook over medium-low heat until squash comes to a boil, then simmer for 20 minutes or until tender. Purée.

Sweet potatoes: 4 cups sweet potatoes; ½ cup water. Microwave on high for 7 to 9 minutes, or until tender. For best results, use a food mill or sieve rather than a blender or food processor. Purée.

Yams: 4 cups yams; ½ cup water. Microwave on high for 7 to 9 minutes or until tender. For best results, use a food mill or sieve rather than a blender or food processor. Purée.

Meats and beans

Beans, red kidney, black, or white: 1 large can of beans (low salt or salt-free; drained and well-rinsed). Purée.

Beef: 1 cup cooked beef, chopped into small pieces; ½ cup water or vegetable stock. Purée. Variation: To achieve a less grainy texture, purée beef and liquid with cooked potatoes and cooked carrots.

Chicken: 1 cup cooked chicken, chopped into small pieces; ½ cup water or vegetable stock. Purée. Variation: To achieve a less grainy texture, purée chicken and liquid with cooked potatoes and cooked carrots.

Chickpeas (also known as garbanzo beans or ceci): 1 large can of chickpeas (look for low-salt or salt-free varieties), drained and well-rinsed. Purée. If texture is too thick, add a small amount of water or vegetable stock.

Lentils: 7 ounces small red lentils; ½ cup water. Bring lentils and water to boil over medium-high heat. Simmer until the lentils are thoroughly cooked (about 14 minutes). Purée.

*Avocados and pumpkins are fruits, but because most of us tend to treat them like vegetables when we're cooking, I've listed them under vegetables.

Adapted from a chart that originally appeared in *Mealtime Solutions for Your Baby, Toddler, and Preschooler* by Ann Douglas (Wiley, 2006).

---

the baby department Babies and toddlers need to be supervised whenever they're eating. And both parents and caregivers need to know how to handle an incident of choking if it occurs.

TABLE 9.3

Mix and Match Baby Food Purées

Once you have introduced a variety of purées to your baby's diet, you can start combining purées to add variety to your baby's diet and to maximize both nutrients and taste. You may need to add a bit of liquid (vegetable stock, fruit juice, breast milk, or water) to achieve the desired consistency. And you'll want to ensure that your baby has demonstrated that she can tolerate each of the individual foods before you start combining foods. All that said, these are some flavour combinations that babies love.

Base Purée	Add One or More of These Other Purées
Fruit	
Apple	Apricot, Blueberry, Carrot, Chicken, Raspberry, Squash, Strawberry, Sweet Potato
Banana	Avocado, Blueberry, Cottage Cheese, Mango, Nectarine, Papaya, Peach, Pineapple, Prune, Raspberry, Squash, Sweet Potato, Tofu, Yam, Yogurt
Pear	Apple, Apricot, Banana, Blueberry, Carrot, Cauliflower, Cottage Cheese, Peach, Peas, Plum, Prune, Squash, Sweet Potato, Yam
Prune	Apple, Banana, Carrot, Cottage Cheese, Pear, Sweet Potato, Yogurt
Vegetable	
Avocado	Banana, Papaya
Carrot	Pear, Pineapple, Squash, Yogurt
Potato	Apple, Broccoli, Peas, Sweet Potato
Sweet Potato	Cauliflower
Squash	Apple, Carrot, Peach, Pear
Meat and Legumes	
Beef	Asparagus, Bean, Carrot, Cauliflower, Pea, Pineapple, Potato, Sweet Potato
Chicken	Apple, Bean, Broccoli, Carrot, Nectarine, Pea, Pineapple, Potatoes, Rice
Chickpeas	Black Bean, Carrot, Chicken
Beans and Legumes	Red Kidney Bean, Black Bean, White Bean, Lentils
Infant Cereals	
Infant Cereals, iron-fortified	Fruit Purées, Vegetable Purées, Yogurt, Cottage Cheese

Note: While it's possible to make your own cereals at home, homemade cereals should not be considered a substitute for iron-fortified infant cereals, which play an important role in your baby's diet into the toddler years.

Adapted from a chart that originally appeared in *Mealtime Solutions for Your Baby, Toddler, and Preschooler* by Ann Douglas (Wiley, 2006).

the baby department Don't feed your baby in the car because it may be difficult for you to safely and quickly pull over if she begins to choke. What's more, a sudden car stop could cause food to become lodged in your baby's throat.

SIPPY CUP SKILLS

A baby is capable of learning how to drink out of a sippy cup by the age of 6 months. (At this point you'll be holding the sippy cup for your baby as opposed to expecting her to go solo.)

Then, sometime between 9 and 12 months of age, she'll begin to show an interest in holding her cup for herself. In fact, she may insist on holding her own cup.

At first, she'll go a little crazy with her new-found cup freedom. She'll play with it, shake it, turn it upside down, and bang it on her high chair tray (or turn it upside down in the bathtub), watching with fascination as liquid spurts upward—all important first steps in figuring out how to make the cup work when there's no grownup in charge.

If you've chosen a sippy cup with a no-spill valve, you won't have to worry about the spills that usually accompany such experimentation, but your baby may have a bit of difficulty getting liquid to flow from the cup. (Tip: Breastfed babies tend to have greater success using cups with built-in straws. Their well-honed sucking skills come in handy.)

If you've chosen a cup without a no-spill valve, your baby will be able to get the liquid out easily (and she'll be fascinated by the puddles she can create on her high chair tray), but she may not get around to drinking any of the liquid. A good compromise is to put water in a cup without a no-spill valve. This way, the water comes out easily and you won't be stressed out if you have to keep refilling the cup. You can keep showing her how to put the cup in her mouth (so she can take a drink). Just make sure the water doesn't come out too quickly. You don't want her to choke or she might be put off this whole drinking-from-a-cup thing.

Most babies can be weaned from a bottle to a cup at around 12 months of age. Parents should wean a baby to a cup as soon as possible after the first birthday and by no later than 15 months of age, due to dental concerns.

If you're wondering what other types of liquids you can offer your baby in a sippy cup (or a bottle, if you choose to go that route), here's what Health Canada has to say:

- **Breast milk:** Breastfeeding continues to be the best method of feeding babies, ages 6 months and up.

- **Infant formulas:** Follow-up formulas offer an alternative to cow's milk for babies who are no longer breastfeeding and who are already eating solid foods. According to Health Canada, follow-up formulas provide more appropriate quantities and forms of nutrients as compared to cow's milk for infants from 6 months to one year. Follow-up formulas have not been proven to be better than regular infant formulas—and, of course, no infant formula has proven to be superior to breast milk. Infants who are unable to consume cow's milk products and who are not being breastfed should continue to consume commercial soy formula until the age of 2. Soy-based formulas should only be consumed by those infants who cannot consume dairy-based products for health, cultural, or religious reasons.

- **Cow's milk:** Pasteurized whole cow's milk may be introduced at 9 to 12 months of age and continued throughout the second year of life. It is not recommended before that point because cow's milk is lower in iron than breast milk and formula. Unpasteurized milk is not recommended due to the increased risk of infection.

- **Goat's milk:** Goat's milk is not appropriate for infants before 9 to 12 months of age because it is lower in iron and, depending on the brand, it may or may not be fortified with vitamin D. What's more, many infants who are allergic to cow's milk protein are also allergic to goat's milk protein. After 9 months of age, full-fat goat's milk may be used as an alternative to cow's milk.

- **Soy and rice beverages that are intended for adults** (as opposed to soy-based infant formula): These beverages are not suitable for babies because these beverages tend to be lower in fat and protein than breast milk and infant formulas.

- **Fruit juice:** If you decide to offer your baby fruit juice (a source of vitamin C), limit your baby's consumption to a maximum of 125 millilitres (4 ounces) per day. Excessive juice consumption can lead to diarrhea, poor weight gain, and dental caries, and it can interfere with the intake of breast milk. Note: Juice should always be given in a cup, never in a bottle.

FOOD ALLERGIES AND FOOD INTOLERANCES

Food intolerances are much more common in infants than food allergies. Only 8 per cent of babies have full-blown food allergies, and half of them will outgrow these allergies by the time they reach 3 years of age.

- *A food intolerance* occurs when the body has difficulty tolerating a particular food or an additive such as an artificial flavour or colour. The body responds with such symptoms as cramps, vomiting, and diarrhea. Food intolerances are the most common type of food reaction experienced by babies.

- *A food allergy* poses a much greater health threat. Symptoms—which usually occur within minutes but may take up to 72 hours to appear—can range from vomiting and diarrhea, to wheezing, a skin rash. Fortunately, full-blown anaphylactic shock (when a child's mouth or throat swells, the child has difficulty breathing, and the child begins to go into shock) is rare, but requires immediate medical treatment.

Here are some key facts about food allergies in children:

- A few foods are responsible for 90 per cent of food allergies in children: peanuts, wheat, cow's milk, soy, eggs, and shellfish. Refer back to Table 9.4 for more details about some of these foods.

- Certain types of food allergies tend to run in families. If this is the case for your baby, your health-care provider may recommend that you hold off on introducing certain foods during baby's first year—or perhaps even longer—just to play it safe.

- If you suspect that your baby is allergic to a particular food, it is important to have your suspicions confirmed by your health-care provider. She will likely recommend avoiding the food for a couple of years and then bringing your child in for a challenge test, in which your child is re-exposed to the food in a medically supervised environment. The purpose of the challenge test is to determine whether your child has outgrown the allergy (in which case, he or she will be able to eat the food again) or whether your child will need to continue to avoid that food.

- Milk, wheat, and egg allergies are commonly outgrown by 2 years of age. Children are much less likely to outgrow peanut and shellfish allergies.

TABLE 9.4

Foods That Aren't Suitable for Babies

Not every food is suitable for a baby. It's important for both parents and caregivers to know which foods are off-limits to babies and why.

Foods that should be avoided for food allergy reasons

Nuts and nut products: Avoid peanuts and tree nuts (hazelnuts, walnuts, almonds, cashews) as well as nut products (peanut butter) and any products that may have come into contact with these products during baby's first year.

Egg whites: Avoid egg whites during baby's first year. You can give your baby well-cooked scrambled egg yolks, starting at age 9 months, unless your baby is at high risk of an egg allergy. In this case, you should talk to your baby's health-care provider and plan to avoid offering your baby egg yolks, all egg substitutes, and foods containing albumin, flobulin, ovomucin, and vetellin.

Shellfish: Avoid until after age 18 months.

Citrus fruits (including kiwi): Avoid until after age one year.

Foods that pose a choking risk for babies and young children

Berries: Slice into tiny strips or wedges (as opposed to penny- or marble-shaped pieces). Avoid strawberries until after age one year.

Celery: Choking hazard can't be eliminated, so avoid.

Grapes: Cut into tiny strips or wedges (as opposed to penny- or marble-shaped pieces).

Candies, hard as well as soft and jellied, and chewing gum: Choking hazard can't be eliminated, so avoid.

Carrots, raw: Cook and serve puréed. Then move on to mashed or finely chopped cooked carrots, as baby adjusts to more complex food textures.

Corn: Hold off on offering to your baby until after age one year.

Nuts: Choking hazard can't be eliminated, so avoid.

Olives: Remove pit and slice into tiny pieces.

Popcorn: Choking hazard can't be eliminated, so avoid.

Raisins: Choking hazard can't be eliminated, so avoid.

Tomatoes, cherry: Cut into tiny strips or wedges (as opposed to penny- or marble-shaped pieces).

Sausages: Slice into thin strips lengthwise and then chop into bite-sized pieces crosswise. Do not cut into penny-shaped pieces. Not recommended until baby is older and should only be offered in limited amounts due to high salt content.

Unpeeled fruits: Peel from fruits such as apples and pears can cause a baby to choke. Peel the fruit and cook, if necessary, to create a softer texture.

(continued)

Foods and beverages that should be avoided for other reasons

Honey: Honey can contain botulism spores. Avoid honey until after baby is one year of age.

Cow's milk: Cow's milk is difficult for babies to digest because cow's milk is biologically different from breast milk (which is designed for human babies) or infant formula (which has been altered to make it more digestible). Your baby can start drinking cow's milk (homogenized, because baby's brain needs the added fat) between 9 and 12 months of age, according to the Canadian Paediatric Society. You can introduce other dairy products (whole-milk versions of cottage cheese, grated cheese, yogurt, and other dairy products, as opposed to lower-fat versions) as your baby is making the transition to solid foods.

Herbal teas: Some types of herbal teas are toxic to babies.

Caffeinated beverages: In addition to containing caffeine (which is not recommended for babies), many also contain theobromine (a caffeine-related substance which acts as a stimulant and which is also not recommended for babies).

Sodas, fruit punches, and sports drinks: These beverages are high in sugar but low in nutrients other than carbohydrates. They may also contribute to dental caries (tooth decay).

Foods and beverages containing artificial sweeteners: They may interfere with the intake of more nutrient-rich foods.

Luncheon meat, lox, raw milk and raw milk cheese, soft cheeses, unpasteurized apple juice, bean sprouts, alfalfa sprouts: These foods are at risk of being contaminated with harmful bacteria and should be avoided by babies, toddlers, and preschoolers as well as pregnant and breastfeeding women.

Adapted from a chart that originally appeared in *Mealtime Solutions for Your Baby, Toddler, and Preschooler* by Ann Douglas (Wiley, 2006).

---

mom's the word "Find out all the names food manufacturers use for the food your baby is allergic to. I discovered that there are about 20 ways to say 'milk' on an ingredient list."
—CAROLIN, 35, MOTHER OF THREE, WHOSE THIRD CHILD IS ALLERGIC TO MILK

SLEEPING THROUGH THE NIGHT

Once your baby gets to be about 3 months of age, the pressure to start sleep training your baby becomes pretty intense (unless, of course, you've been experiencing this pressure since the day your baby arrived). These not-so-subtle messages (that you're an indulgent parent and that you're causing your baby long-term harm by not getting this sleep "problem" under control) can erode your confidence as a new parent.

Fortunately, there are ways to handle this all-too-common situation.

Learning a few facts about sleep (what's normal for older babies) can help to ease the pressure to do something about a baby sleep problem that, developmentally speaking, may not be a problem at all.

---

mom's the word "A sleep issue is only a problem if it bothers you. It doesn't bother me to get up at night with my children, so I don't consider their nightwaking to be a problem."

—COLLEEN, 38, MOTHER OF FOUR

---

mom's the word "Every child and every parent is different, and therefore every family needs to experiment with what works for them. That being said, I am not comfortable with the 'cry it out' approach, although I do recognize that there are often tears as we try to teach our children to sleep on their own and fall back to sleep on their own. On the other hand, it is not fair to parents to have them believe that they need to rush in at every squeak to get babies settled back to sleep. The best path for most families may be somewhere between these two schools of thought.

"I also think that many of these philosophies worry parents into thinking their child has a sleep 'problem' or 'disorder,' and words like that undermine parents' confidence. My daughter is what some people might call a 'problem sleeper,' but I try to spin it more positively: she simply hasn't mastered sleeping through the night on her own yet. I know she will. Of course, that doesn't mean I'm any less frustrated when I'm trying to get her back to sleep at 3 a.m."

—SARAH, 32, MOTHER OF ONE

The facts about older babies and sleep

Your baby's sleep patterns have changed a great deal since he was a newborn—and they'll continue to evolve during the months ahead.

Your 6- to 9-month-old

By the time babies reach 6 months of age, their sleep patterns are a lot more predictable than when they were younger. They may have settled into a routine which includes two to four daytime naps that may range from 30 minutes to 2 hours in duration. And they are likely to be doing most of their sleeping at night.

Some babies who slept through the night when they were younger may start waking through the night at around 6 months of age. This can be the result of physical discomfort (teething, for example) or increased cognitive abilities (you find your baby practising a new skill in the middle of the night: his busy brain doesn't want to take a break!).

Sometimes babies who wake up in the middle of the night are doing so because they are overtired. They are so wired that, when they wake up briefly in the night, they can't get back to sleep. (Sometimes this happens to adults, too.) If you are putting your baby to bed between 8 and 9 p.m. and she's consistently experiencing middle-of-the-night waking problems that don't have any other apparent cause (see Checklist 9.1), you may want to try putting her to bed half an hour to an hour earlier to see if that helps to solve the problem.

CHECKLIST 9.1

Reasons for Nightwaking in Babies

Baby is hungry
Your baby may still wake up looking for the occasional middle-of-the-night feeding, even after she's been sleeping through the night on a fairly regular basis. These feedings can help to maintain your milk production. (Prolactin levels are higher during the night feedings.) And they may be providing your baby with some food she missed out on during the day. (If your baby is a real go-getter during the day, she may miss out on the odd meal or snack and wake up hungry in the night.)

Baby is overtired
Soothe her back to sleep and try to ensure that she gets her naps tomorrow.

Baby has a wet diaper
Add an insert to your baby's diaper (to increase its absorbency). Or try a different make of diaper.

Baby has a soiled diaper

If your baby tends to soil his diapers a short time after you put him to bed, try moving his pre-bedtime feeding up a bit in the hope that he'll have his bowel movement before he goes to bed.

Baby has a painful diaper rash

If your baby is prone to diaper rashes, change her diapers as often as possible during the day (at least every two hours for wet diapers and right away when you notice that a diaper is soiled). Use wet washcloths to clean baby's skin and then add a protective barrier of zinc oxide to protect baby's skin until the next diaper change. Tip: Adding a half-cup of vinegar to the rinse cycle when you are washing cloth diapers helps to remove the alkaline buildup that can be irritating to baby's skin.

Baby is teething

If your baby is up in the night pulling on her teeth and gums, suspect teething pain (even though the experts continue to debate whether teething pain results in disrupted sleep or not).

Baby's sleep environment is preventing her from getting a good night's sleep

If baby is too warm, too cold, or wearing sleepwear with a tag that keeps poking her neck, she'll have a difficult time sleeping. Try to figure out what's bothering her and then do your best to resolve the problem.

Baby hasn't learned how to get back to sleep on her own

Babies with extra-sensitive temperaments and/or less developed self-soothing skills are more likely to wake up when they pass through periods of light sleep (something that happens about once every 60 minutes). This issue will resolve itself over time. All that's needed in the meantime is love and patience on your part.

Baby needs some extra comfort or reassurance

Baby has learned to turn to you for comfort and reassurance when she needs it in the daytime. Is it surprising that she sometimes uses this strategy during the nighttime as well?

Baby is struggling with separation anxiety

Not wanting to be separated from the people they love most in the world, even in the middle of the night, is a common cause of sleep disruptions during baby's first year. Remember your baby isn't able to think to herself, "Oh, Mom is just in that room down the hall." If she can't see or hear or touch you, you've fallen off the planet. That's scary for a baby who feels very vulnerable when she's alone.

Baby is in the process of mastering a new skill and wants to practise it day and night

Your baby is so excited by what she's learning that she can't sleep—literally. If she's learning to stand up on her own, she wants to do that in her crib at 3 a.m. (And sometimes she gets stuck in a standing-up position. That leaves her with little alternative than to holler for help from you.)

(continued)

> **Baby's routine has changed**
> Baby was sleeping through the night until she started teething. Or until she got a bad cold. Or until you took that out-of-town trip and all stayed in one hotel room. The good news is that if she slept through the night before, she will probably do it again, with some patience and encouragement from you.
>
> **Baby is ill, is in pain, or has a medical condition that is interfering with sleep**
> If your baby only sleeps for a short time (just long enough to take the edge off her exhaustion) or if she's only able to sleep in a particular position (sitting up in your arms, for example), it's possible that she's experiencing pain related to an illness. Medical conditions that can interfere with sleep include gastroesophageal reflux, ear infections, eczema, pinworms, asthma, food intolerances, and sleep disorders.

Other babies who wake up in the night at around this age may be doing so because they are struggling with separation anxiety (it has suddenly occurred to them that the two of you are separate human beings and they feel an urgent need—even in the middle of the night—to check that you are still there) or dealing with a major change in their lives (a move to a new house, for example).

Your 9- to 12-month-old

Seventy to 80 per cent of babies between the ages of 9 months and one year are sleeping through the night *most* (but *not all*) of the time. The myth that all babies are sleeping through the night by age 6 months (or younger) is just that—*a myth*.

At around 10 months of age, your baby may start waking up and going to sleep at a predictable time each day.

By the time your baby celebrates his first birthday, he may be sleeping approximately eight to nine hours each night and taking two daytime naps as well (with the two daytime naps totalling about two and a half hours).

Sleep training versus sleep learning

The idea of sleep training babies is talked about so much in our culture that we sometimes forget that there's an alternative: allowing babies to learn about sleep and start sleeping through the night on their own (what some parents refer to as "sleep learning").

Sleep scientists have identified a number of ways that parents can encourage babies' sleep learning without forcing the process (think "baby-led" rather than "parent-led"). They take into account such factors as developmental readiness and temperament (the ultimate wild card when it comes to sleep).

mom's the word "I do believe children need sleep training, but when they're older. When my daughter was so new, and needed to suckle often and nurse through the night, it was easier and more comforting for both of us for me to be right there. For almost the first year, her cries at night never escalated to the point of waking her up entirely because I was so close by. Then, at the point when she could go through the night without needing to nurse, I was right there to soothe her back down quickly as we dropped feedings one at a time. Then, when it was time to put her down in the crib to sleep, it was only a few nights of having to get up to soothe and pat her back down to sleep. But at this point, just after a year old, she was able to understand what 'sleepy time' meant. She may not have liked it, but she understood. Before then, it was just upsetting screams. Even now, at almost 16 months, I understand that she's a little person who might need comfort during the night—not 'training.' But it was my need to sleep more and my understanding that we were keeping her from sleeping better that hardened my heart enough to see it through—before that, my hormones and tender emotions just made me want to keep her close to me."

—MARLA, 36, MOTHER OF ONE

- **Tune into your baby's sleep cues.** There's a window of opportunity when it comes to babies and sleep—a time when babies are tired, but not so tired that they are no longer able to relax and succumb to sleep. If you can learn to spot the signs that your baby is becoming sleepy (your baby is calmer and less active; your baby is less tuned into her surroundings; your baby is becoming quieter and less chatty; your baby is nursing more slowly; your baby is yawning) and get your baby down for a nap or off to bed right away, you'll (generally) find that your baby is easier to settle.
- **Make baby's daytime sleep a priority.** Babies who nap during the day sleep better and longer at night. While it's not a huge deal if your baby misses out on some daytime naps (because Thursday afternoons are the day of your yoga class), if nap times are sacrificed on a daily basis, both you and baby will pay the price. (You'll end up with a grumpy baby who has a limited attention span during the day, and

who is too wired to sleep well at night. And that is unlikely to result in a very happy you.) And while some babies are able to nap on the go, others aren't able to settle into a truly restful sleep.

- **Help your baby to learn that daytime is daytime and nighttime is nighttime.** With an older baby, this means accentuating the rhythms of your household. You want your baby to learn that daytime is for playing and nighttime is for sleeping. You can accomplish this by dimming the lights and keeping the noise level lower in the evening, a time of day when your baby is making the transition between daytime and nighttime. Tip: Getting your baby out of doors first thing in the morning helps to set his circadian rhythm, which, in turn, helps to improve the quality of his nighttime sleep.

- **Help your baby to anticipate bedtime by creating a predictable bedtime routine.** If your baby finds bathtime soothing, you may want to work that into his bedtime routine. If he gets revved up during bathtime, you may want to shift bathtime to earlier in the day, substituting storytime or cuddle time in the evening instead.

- **Learn how to interpret your baby's nighttime noises.** As you've no doubt noticed by now, babies have an entire repertoire of sounds they make in the night. Some sounds mean, without question, "I need you right now!" Others are a little more subtle: they may require your intervention—or they may simply be noises your baby makes while she's still sound asleep. Sometimes a baby wakes up for a minute, talks or fusses for a moment, and then drifts back to sleep. Other times, a baby wakes up and, if you don't go in to offer assistance right away, she'll become so upset that it will take what feels like forever to soothe her back to sleep.

    Your job, as a parent sleep detective, is to learn to differentiate between these various sleep sounds. You want to give your baby the opportunity to learn how to get back to sleep, if she can. Likewise, you *don't* want to wake up a sleeping baby by rushing in and picking her up each time she makes a peep in her sleep. On the other hand, you want to be responsive to her needs in the night when she needs you. Parenting a baby is a 24-hour-a-day commitment, after all.

- **Provide your baby with opportunities to learn how to fall asleep in other ways than being nursed to sleep.** Most of us play an active role in helping our babies fall asleep during the early months. But once babies become capable of forming sleep associations at around 4 months of age (associating falling asleep with being nursed, for example), you may want to start using some other ways of soothing him to sleep, such as patting him or rocking him or talking to him in a soothing voice, for example. You're not expecting him to fall asleep on his own quite yet (although some babies manage to do this, starting quite early). You're simply trying to expose him to different ways of falling asleep so that he won't think that the only way to fall asleep (or to get back to sleep) is to have someone nurse him to sleep.

If he isn't ready to learn this skill quite yet (he protests vehemently when you try to encourage him to fall asleep in any other way than by being nursed), try again when he is a little older. He may have a few more self-soothing skills to rely on by then—something that makes a world of difference. And remember that it's normal for baby mammals, including baby humans, to want to nurse to sleep, and that all babies outgrow this need eventually. It's part of Mother Nature's master plan.

---

the baby department Researchers at the University of Reading, UK, have confirmed what parents have long suspected: temperament has a major impact on infant sleep. The researchers discovered that high-needs or spirited children benefit from consistent bedtime rituals, consistent bedtimes, consistent wake times, and parental help in learning self-soothing behaviours.

- **Recognize that it takes some babies longer than others to start sleeping through the night.** (Just a reminder: "Sleeping through the night" means sleeping for a five-and-a-half hour stretch at some point between dusk and dawn. If you're holding out for a 12-hour stretch of sleep, you could be waiting for a very long time.) "I'm 33 years old and I still fight going to sleep," says Marcelle, a mother of two. "I pretty much have to have my husband drag me away from a project, housekeeping activity, book, or TV show and point me in the direction of the bedroom or I'll stay up until the wee hours of the morning and then complain the next day about how tired I am. Should it surprise me that I've got a child who does the same thing?"

mom's the word "For a long time, we gravitated toward methods that had worked for our friends, as well as 'sleep solutions' that were backed by reassuring research. The biggest factor—which we ignored—was our child's personality."

—KARA, 33, MOTHER OF TWO

COMMON SLEEP CONCERNS ABOUT OLDER BABIES

When parents get together and start talking about the sleep issues that concern them most about babies aged 6 to 12 months, the following issues tend to top the list.

Nightwaking

It's one thing to know that becoming a parent means sacrificing sleep. It's quite another to get out of bed, night after night, to meet your baby's needs. Is it any wonder that new parents are more than a little obsessed about babies and nightwaking?

Babies, for their part, have plenty of good reasons for waking in the night. A long list of reasons, in fact. You may find it helpful to run through the reasons in Checklist 9.1 if your baby is waking frequently during the night and you're trying to figure out why.

mother wisdom Just when you think your baby has settled into something resembling a predictable daily routine, he decides to drop one of his naps. That can lead to a major outbreak of the grumpies over the short run, as he adjusts to making due with one less nap than he's used to.

You can expect the first of these scheduling shifts to occur at around age 6 months (when baby makes the shift from three naps a day to two naps a day). If you time these two naps so that they fall earlier in the day (a mid-morning nap and an early afternoon nap), you won't have to worry about your baby's naps interfering with his bedtime. A nap that ends after 4:30 p.m. can make it difficult for a baby to fall asleep in the evening.

Difficulty settling down at bedtime

Settling your baby at bedtime has become a two-hour marathon. And, by the time the marathon is finished, you're finished, too. Here are some questions you might want to ask yourself as you try to figure out how to deal with the situation:

- Does your baby need more daytime naps?
- Does the timing of his daytime naps need to be adjusted?
- Would he benefit from an earlier bedtime?
- Would he benefit from a later bedtime?

Note: Review the list of items in Checklist 9.1, too. Many of the issues that contribute to nightwaking in babies can also make it difficult for a baby to fall asleep in the first place.

Early rising

Your baby goes to bed early in the evening and sleeps all night. But he wants to start his day at 4:30 a.m. (You don't.)

This situation is surprisingly common and the root cause is—you guessed it—an overtired baby. Try putting your baby to bed a half-hour earlier and ensuring that he gets his daytime naps (even if you have to stay with him while he naps, as a means of easing him back into a daytime sleep routine). And, when he wakes in the morning, treat any feeding before 6 a.m. as a nighttime feeding. (In other words, put your baby back to bed and go back to sleep yourself.)

Just a few final words as we wrap up this section about sleep. Parenting isn't a competition, and having a baby who sleeps through the night sooner rather than later doesn't make you a better parent—or your baby a better baby. It just makes you a slightly more rested parent *right now*.

And, despite what some too-smug parents of babies who have been sleeping through the night practically since birth might have you believe, past sleep good fortune—at least as far as young babies is concerned—is no guarantee of future sleep good fortune. It may tilt the sleep roulette wheel slightly in your favour for the foreseeable future, but that's about it.

chapter 10

THE INCREDIBLE GROWING BABY

"I loved all the firsts, especially with my firstborn. It's so exciting to see your baby learning new skills and to witness the joy on their face when they discover their feet or figure out how to clap their hands."

—MARIA, 32, MOTHER OF TWO

It's one of the greatest joys of becoming a parent—witnessing your baby's exciting "firsts."

In this chapter, we talk about the smorgasbord of marvellous firsts that await you and your baby during his amazing first year. We'll start out by considering what developmental milestones can and can't tell you about your baby. (Contrary to what most people think, the fact that your baby was the first baby in your prenatal class to start babbling doesn't necessarily mean that she is a shoe-in for class valedictorian 18 years from now.) Then, once we've talked about the limitations of developmental milestones in predicting your baby's future abilities, we'll zero in on the specific developmental milestones that you can expect your baby to achieve at various points during his first year of life—give or take a couple of months, of course. Finally, we'll wrap up the chapter by considering the joys and challenges of parenting babies of various ages and considering just how much growing and developing you will have done yourself by the time the first year of parenthood draws to a close. Your baby isn't the only one who will undergo a major metamorphosis between now and then, after all.

BABY GENIUSES

There's bound to be at least one baby genius in your prenatal class—a baby who achieves key developmental milestones weeks, if not months, ahead of the other babies, and whose parents have got him pegged as McGill scholarship material. (I mean, if he's smiling at 3 weeks of age and crawling by the time he's 5 months old, it's only a matter of time before those scholarship offers start rolling in.)

As you've no doubt noticed by now, new parents seem to like nothing more than to compare notes on their babies with other parents, eagerly looking for evidence that their resident genius is either miles ahead of the other babies or at least holding his own. As Joyce, a 42-year-old mother of two, notes, rolling her eyes, "If your baby is excelling, you must be a super parent, and who wants to be judged as anything less?"

What you need to know right from the get-go is that no two babies follow the exact same timeline when it comes to growth and development. While it can be helpful to look at charts outlining the approximate date by which your baby should have mastered a particular developmental task (see Table 10.1), it's crucial to keep in mind that what you're looking at is a rough timeline rather than a rigid blueprint for development. So take heart: the fact that your baby crawled, talked, and walked a good month or two behind the other babies in your prenatal class doesn't mean that your baby is sentenced to a lifetime of being an "also ran"; it simply means that he took his time rather than heading straight over to the baby fast lane. Do yourself (and your baby) a favour: treat infant development as a journey to be enjoyed at any pace, not a winner-takes-all sprint event.

That's not to say that charts outlining the key developmental milestones for babies of various ages are entirely without merit. If they were, I would hardly have chosen to include such a detailed one in this book. What these charts can do is give you an indication of the rough order in which babies tend to master particular skills (for example, uttering vowel sounds before they move on to consonants) and a rough idea of when these milestones are achieved on average by a typical baby (although I must admit I've yet to meet that mythical typical baby). While most babies will deviate in minor ways from the developmental blueprint—some babies go from sitting to walking without ever mastering the art of crawling, for example—if a baby is consistently missing milestones, it could be an indication that his development is lagging behind that of his age mates for some reason—and that might warrant further investigation by your baby's doctor or an infant development specialist, so that a treatment plan can be mapped out.

CHAPTER 10 — THE INCREDIBLE GROWING BABY

TABLE 10.1

Developmental Highlights of Your Baby's First Year

The first year of your baby's life is a time of amazing firsts. Every time you turn around, your baby has mastered another new skill. Here's what to expect each month in terms of physical, cognitive, and social development from your incredible growing baby.

Your Newborn	
Physical and motor development	• Your newborn's movements are generally uncontrolled and not deliberate. Most of his movements happen automatically without any conscious intention on his part. It will take time for him to learn how to control his movements. • While your baby can move his head from side to side when he's lying on his stomach, and he can raise his head an inch or two off the ground when he's lying on his back, his neck and shoulder muscles will need to develop further before he can support his head on his own. • Your newborn is quite near-sighted. Even when he looks at objects that are within his ideal focal length (roughly 20 to 25 centimetres (8 to 10 inches), which is the distance of your face when you are nursing him), those objects look quite fuzzy to him. Your baby's eyes should not be crossed, however. If they are, you should have his eyes checked by a doctor as soon as possible. You should never wait for a baby to "just grow out of" an eye problem. Always have your baby or child checked if you have any concern about your child's eyes or his vision. • When your baby looks at something, he focuses on particular details rather than looking at the whole object. For example, when he looks at your face, he only takes in your eyes or your mouth, not your face as a whole. • Your baby's eyes are only able to track objects within a 90-degree range of vision, and his eye movements are short and jerky. He has not yet figured out that he can move his head to follow objects beyond this range.

Your Newborn (*continued*)

	- Your baby's hearing is not yet as acute as the hearing of an adult. He can't hear very soft sounds like whispers. He's more attracted to high-pitched sounds than low-pitched sounds, something that helps to explain why parents around the world lapse into "parentese" (exaggerated speech patterns) when they start communicating with a baby.
- Your baby is born with a reflex that encourages him to turn his head in the direction of a sound. It will be another month, however, before he is able to identify the source of a particular sound.
- Your newborn instinctively grasps any object that is placed in his palm. He can't intentionally hold onto objects quite yet.
Cognitive and language development	- Your baby experiences brief periods of quiet alertness but spends most of his time sleeping (although he'll wake up frequently to eat). As the length and frequency of these periods of alertness increase, he will become increasingly tuned into the world around him.
Social and emotional development	- Your baby is fascinated by human faces and human voices right from birth. He quickly learns how to pick up his mother's scent, to recognize the sound of her voice, and to recognize her face. In fact, he started getting used to his mother's scent and voice long before birth.

Your 1-Month-Old

Physical and motor development	- Your baby's neck and shoulder muscles are much stronger than they were a month ago, which has resulted in significantly improved head control. While his head still lags when you pull him from a lying to a sitting position and you still need to support his head while you're walking around with him, he may be able to support his head for short periods of time when you're sitting or standing still. He can also lift his chin off the ground when he's lying on his stomach—a manoeuvre he couldn't have mastered a few short weeks ago.
- Your baby still spends a lot of time looking blankly around the room, but he's spending a greater proportion of his time taking in his surroundings. While he isn't able to take in much when you're walking around (just think of how hard it is for you to enjoy

- the scenery when you're taking a bus ride down a bumpy road!), he's able to process visual information quite readily when you're sitting or standing still.
- Your baby is increasingly fascinated by human faces and high-contrast patterns like black-and-white checkerboards, bull's-eyes, and polka dots, while he'll barely give his growing collection of pastel-coloured stuffed animals the time of day. The reason is simple: the higher the contrast, the easier it is for him to see the object in question.
- Your baby is very interested in listening to human voices—your voice in particular. He's also starting to develop an ear for music: he will often stop mid-squall to listen intently if you start playing music or singing to him.
- Now that his larynx is more flexible and mobile, your baby is starting to experiment with making some language-like sounds. Originally, these sounds will resemble throat-clearing sounds. Then, at around age 6 weeks, he'll start making sounds like "ah," "eh," and "uh." He'll initially make these sounds by accident, but once he figures out how to make them, he'll amuse himself—and others around him—by cooing and gurgling over and over.
- Your baby's hand is generally held in a closed position. If you open his fingers he is able to grasp an object for a couple of seconds before dropping it.

Cognitive and language development

- Your baby's brain is working overtime these days—something that can easily result in overstimulation. Even though your baby may be tired of looking at a particular object, he does not know how to look away. It's hard to imagine your baby getting burned out from spending too much time staring at his baby mobile, but, believe it or not, it can happen! In fact, if you find that your baby tends to get crabby by late afternoon (a classic pattern for young babies), it could be overstimulation that's to blame. He may not know how to tell you what he needs, but odds are what he's craving is a brief time-out rather than more stimulation.
- Your baby has already learned how to tell the difference between nipples that deliver food and nipples that don't—a skill he'll be only too happy to demonstrate if you make the mistake of offering him a pacifier when he's looking for a breast.

Your 1-Month-Old (*continued*)

Social and emotional development

- Your baby is more socially responsive than he was as a newborn. He may become excited and breathe more rapidly when you pick him up.
- At around 2 weeks of age, your baby may become fussier or more irritable than he has was during the early days of life—the result of sensory overload. (He is increasingly tuned into the world around him, but he does not yet possess the coping skills to handle all that stimulation.) The result may be periods of what is known as PURPLE crying. PURPLE stands for Peak of crying, Unexpected, Resists soothing, Pain-like face (even though the baby is not in pain), Long-lasting (crying that lasts for as long as five hours per day), and Evening (crying that is most likely to occur during late afternoon and evening). The best ways to cope with PURPLE crying are by lining up support and by understanding that what you are going through is normal, very common, and relatively short-lived (although it may feel like it is going to last forever). PURPLE crying starts at age 2 weeks, peaks at age 6 weeks, and ends by age 3 to 4 months.

Your 2-Month-Old

Physical and motor development

- Your baby's head control continues to improve. He can now lift his head and shoulders several inches above the mattress and support himself with his arms when he's lying on his stomach. And he can support his own head briefly when he's braced against your shoulder.
- When your baby lies on his back, he raises his hands above his head in a U. The symmetrical positioning of his arms is a very significant milestone: it indicates that it is only a matter of time until he learns how to use two hands at once to accomplish a particular task.
- Your baby is starting to seem more like a baby and less like a newborn. The stepping reflex (Baby "walks" when supported in an upright position on a solid surface) has started to fade. And your baby's grasp reflex isn't as strong as it once was. His fingers open if an object is placed in his palm and he then tries to bring that object to his mouth.

	• Your baby's eyes are starting to work together and his overall vision has improved, giving him a much more alert look. He is now capable of tracking objects that are moving vertically as well as objects that are moving horizontally, and he is particularly drawn to objects that are in motion. He is now able to recognize familiar people and toys. • Your baby's hearing has improved since he was a newborn. He is now able to hear sounds of a variety of different pitches, intensities, and intonations.
Cognitive and language development	• Your baby is exhibiting clear signals that he's able to process information. For example, he may stop crying when he is placed in the breastfeeding position because he knows he's going to be fed. • Your baby has developed an entire repertoire of sounds and cries to express various emotions. • Your baby is starting to understand how conversations work: that people take turns talking and listening. He makes sounds and smiles to indicate that he's ready to "talk" to you and then eagerly awaits your response. He's so fascinated by conversations, in fact, that you can sometimes convince him to stop crying simply by talking to him—a great ace card to have up your sleeve if he begins wailing when you're zooming down the highway at 100 kilometres an hour.
Social and emotional development	• Your baby looks at you and studies your face. He imitates your facial expressions. He smiles when you smile. • Your baby calms down when you try to comfort him. He enjoys being cuddled and touched.

Your 3-Month-Old

Physical and motor development	• Your baby's neck and shoulder muscles are even stronger than they were a month ago, but your baby is still not able to support his own head for long periods of time. • When your baby reaches for an object, he takes a two-handed approach. He hasn't learned how to use one hand at a time. • Your baby's arm movements are more deliberate and coordinated. • Your baby's leg muscles are getting quite a workout in preparation for rolling over, crawling, and walking; he makes a point of kicking his legs vigorously whenever he's on his tummy or back.

Your 3-Month-Old (*continued*)		
		• Your baby will open his hand when an object is offered to him, but he will then proceed to drop the object almost immediately.
• Your baby uses his palm and fingers when he's holding an object, but he has not yet figured out that his thumb could be useful as well.
• Your baby is able to see objects more clearly than he could in the past. He can now tell the difference between smiling and frowning faces and will rarely smile at someone who is frowning.
• Your baby now turns his head when he hears a sound from a nearby object (e.g., the ringing of a telephone).
	Cognitive and language development	• Your baby's spatial perception skills improve. He is beginning to understand that he can't reach that toy across the room unless someone else is willing to play courier.
• Your baby is always up for a game of "vocal tennis" (you imitate your baby and your baby imitates you). He loves making vowel sounds (ohs and ahs) and is most likely to be found practising his vocalizations when he's feeling happy or amused. While baby may be babbling to you, you can talk to him with real words. He may not be able to speak yet, but he's soaking up language like a sponge. When he becomes capable of forming words (which comes later than understanding words), he'll be able to draw upon the vocabulary he has been learning all along.
	Social and emotional development	• If it hasn't already happened, this is likely to be the month when your baby masters the long-awaited first social smile. His self-soothing skills are also improving. You'll find he's a much happier baby because he's better able to soothe himself when he becomes distressed.
Your 4-Month-Old		
	Physical and motor development	• Your baby's back muscles are much stronger than they were and his arms and legs are capable of much more deliberate movements—skills that allow him to master the art of rolling from his stomach onto his back. Unfortunately, once he gets over on his back, he's stranded. He doesn't have sufficient strength to roll from his back to his stomach just yet—the cause of endless frustration

- to him. (Expect to be called to "rescue" him countless times each day until he masters the other half of the rolling-over equation.)
- While your baby now enjoys being held in a sitting position, he can't support himself in this position yet because he lacks the necessary strength in his lower back.
- Your baby is now able to visually detect subtle differences in the texture of objects and has developed a marked preference for objects that are red or blue.
- Your baby is starting to discover all the amazing things his hands can do for him. If you watch closely, you'll catch him looking at his hands while he guides them toward a toy. (Eventually, he'll just look at the toy, but right now he is still trying to figure out how to make his hands and eyes work together.) His thumb still doesn't move independently of his fingers or his hand, however, so his efforts to reach for toys are still rather clumsy.
- He enjoys batting at objects that are within his reach.
- He grasps and shakes toys that are easy for him to hold, such as rattles, but he'll only hold them briefly.
- He will play with a toy if it is placed in his hands, but he won't be able to pick it up if he drops it.
- He can now make a conscious choice whether or not to hold on to a toy. (When he was a newborn, he held on to any object that was placed in his hands.)
- Your baby's hearing continues to improve. He is able to hear much softer sounds than he was capable of hearing in the past.

Cognitive and language development	• Your baby has developed the ability to anticipate and remember important events (the cues that indicate he's about to be fed). • He is starting to become aware of the patterns and routines that provide structure to his day. • He uses different cries to express different needs. He's getting better at letting you know what he needs—and you're getting better at decoding the various cries in his repertoire—which makes for a happier baby and a happier parent! • He uses facial expressions, gestures, and sounds to communicate with others and to respond to others' communications.

Your 4-Month-Old (*continued*)	
	• He throws his arms up in the air when you approach him—a sure sign that he wants you to pick him up.
	• He is now chatting up a storm. He's mastered certain types of consonant sounds (m, k, g, p, and b) and he sometimes manages to pair up these consonants with a vowel sound (e.g., "gaa").
Social and emotional development	• This is the month when you can expect to hear your baby's first laugh—one of the most magical sounds in the world. You'll no doubt find yourself doing all kinds of crazy things to make him laugh again and again.
	• Your baby is beginning to tune in more to the world of people, with particular attention being focused on the people he knows best.
	• Your baby has learned to tell the difference between familiar people and unfamiliar people and may protest when a stranger tries to pick him up—or comes too close.
	• Your baby is beginning to express emotional reactions spontaneously, like smiling and frowning and fussing.
	• Your baby may start exhibiting the odd sign of jealousy. A group of researchers at the University of Portsmouth in England observed the reactions of 24 babies as young as four months when their mothers started showing love to another baby. They discovered that all but one baby became jealous.
Your 5-Month-Old	
Physical and motor development	• Your baby is having a great time exploring his body from head to toe—literally! Now that he's thoroughly taste-tested his fingers, he's moved on to his toes. Fortunately, his body is still flexible enough to allow him to guide his toes into his mouth—a feat you're unlikely to be able to match!
	• Your baby's neck, shoulder, and chest muscles are very strong, his back is almost fully straight, and his abdominal muscles are firm to the touch. Now that he has improved muscle tone throughout his torso, he is better able to support his upper body. He can also roll in both directions—from his stomach onto his back and from his back onto his stomach—and momentarily sit unassisted before toppling over. He's even started experimenting

	with crawling motions, but it will be a while before he actually takes off.
	- When your baby reaches for toys, he cups his hand to try to adjust the shape of his hand to the shape of the toy. Because his finger movements are still relatively uncoordinated, he finds it difficult to pick up small objects. He's much more adept at picking up slightly larger objects. Once he manages to get a toy in his hand, he explores it with his fingers and his mouth and passes it from hand to hand. Your baby enjoys mouthing toys because his lips and tongue have very sensitive nerve endings that allow him to explore objects in great detail. Your baby isn't capable of holding onto more than one toy at a time, however; if you place a toy in each hand, he'll invariably drop one.
	- Your baby's depth perception is improving by leaps and bounds: he can now tell the difference between a real face and a picture of a face. His understanding of language is also improving: he's beginning to react to the speaker's tone and he's starting to become familiar with the unique patterns of his native language.
Cognitive and language development	- Your baby now understands that it's possible to follow an object if it moves out of his line of vision. If he drops an object, he moves his head so that he can watch it fall.
	- Your baby is trying his best to see the world through your eyes—literally. If you look at an object, he'll follow your gaze to try to figure out what you're looking at, which allows him to learn more about the world around him and to start to make a link between the objects he sees you looking at and the words you use to describe them.
Social and emotional development	- Although your baby can now differentiate between familiar and unfamiliar people, he doesn't usually cry when a stranger arrives on the scene—at least, not yet!—but he may become quiet and sombre when someone he doesn't know approaches him. Over time, his wariness of strangers will evolve into full-blown anxiety, but for now he's willing to quietly tolerate them.
	- Your baby is starting to signal his likes and dislikes. He's also quite willing to let you know how frustrated he feels if he wants to do something but can't—a common state of affairs at this stage of his development.

Your 6-Month-Old	
Physical and motor development	• Your baby is on the move. He can roll over easily and may also inch his way across the room on his belly (a common precursor to crawling). He can also support himself in a sitting position and may even be able to propel himself backwards by pushing on his hands. You can encourage your baby to be active by placing toys just out of his reach and encouraging him to roll, crawl, or creep toward them. • Your baby's legs are strong enough to support him in a standing position for a minute or two, provided you're holding him under his arms. • He can pick up an object that has been dropped (provided it's within his reach). • He uses a raking grasp (as opposed to a thumb and index finger pincer grip) to pick up objects.
Cognitive and language development	• Your baby has become accustomed to his regular routine and will react to changes to it (e.g., if you bath him in the morning rather than at night one day). • He enjoys games like peek-a-boo and can find an object when it is partially hidden under a blanket. • He spends a lot of time studying toys and other objects, trying to figure out what to do with them. • He is mastering the concept of object permanence (the idea that objects still exist even when we can't see them). • Your baby has already learned how to distinguish between male and female voices and will react with surprise if a male voice seems to be coming from a female's mouth. • Your baby's babbling is sounding more and more like speech. The practice he's getting in making sounds now will prove invaluable when he starts saying his first real words in a couple of months' time. • Your baby is becoming quite the conversationalist. He is fascinated by the sound of his own voice. He responds to his own name. And he recognizes certain words. • He makes sounds while you are talking, an attempt to carry on his side of the conversation. The sounds he makes sound like single syllable words (ma, ba, da). He also imitates your cough and other sounds you make.

CHAPTER 10 — THE INCREDIBLE GROWING BABY | . 379

Social and emotional development	• Your baby smiles and babbles when he has your attention.
• Your baby enjoys looking at himself in the mirror.
• Your baby is starting to imitate your actions: you bang a toy and he bangs a toy; you cough, he coughs.
• He's also starting to imitate your emotions—putting on a sad face if he happens to catch you frowning, or breaking into a grin if you greet him with a big smile.
• He tries to soothe himself if he is upset.

Your 7-Month-Old

Physical and motor development	• Your baby is now able to sit on his own for prolonged periods of time, although he sometimes leans forward on his hands for support and stability. He can't get himself into a sitting position yet—you'll have to help him.
• Your baby can stand and bounce up and down with great enthusiasm—provided, of course, that you're holding on to him. It's the ultimate workout for his legs and your back.
• Your baby may have mastered the art of crawling by now. Approximately 50 per cent of babies are crawling by age 7 months. (Don't be alarmed if he hasn't, however; some babies go straight from sitting to walking, skipping the crawling stage entirely, or they invent other ways to get around, like sliding around on their bellies or bums.)
• Your baby is starting to reach for objects with a single hand rather than two hands, and he's now an old pro at transferring objects from one hand to the other.
Cognitive and language development	• If your baby doesn't think he's getting enough attention, he'll make a fake coughing noise or some other sound to get your attention.
• Your baby is capable of remembering someone's face for as long as a week—good news if he only sees his grandparents on Sundays.
• Your baby seems to have grasped the cause-and-effect relationship between dropping a toy and hearing the satisfying bang that it makes.
Social and emotional development	• Your baby thoroughly enjoys social games like peek-a-boo and pat-a-cake.

Your 8-Month-Old	
Physical and motor development	• Your baby can now sit without support and get himself into a sitting position without any help.
• Your baby is now capable of picking up objects using his thumb and index finger only, without having to press the object into the palm of his hand in order to get a good grip.
• Your baby's eyesight is finally as good as that of an adult. Now that he can see objects that are farther away, you'll find him staring off into the distance more often, taking in the scenery across the room.
Cognitive and language development	• Your baby is beginning to understand the link between words and gestures (e.g., saying goodbye and waving goodbye).
Social and emotional development	• Your baby is becoming a master at reading people's faces to determine how they are feeling.
• Your baby is now showing a marked preference for people he knows well and increased discomfort with strangers. You can help your baby to cope with his stranger anxiety by giving him time to get used to the stranger and indicating your own comfort with that person before you allow the other person to get too close.
Your 9-Month-Old	
Physical and motor development	• Your baby is now able to poke at objects with his index finger, something that makes it easier for him to explore objects in his hands. He has also figured out how to let go of objects voluntarily when he's finished playing with them, thereby eliminating a major cause of frustration.
Cognitive and language development.	• Your baby now understands that the baby in the mirror is, in fact, himself—a giant step forward in cognitive processing.
• Your baby is starting to learn how to solve problems on his own (e.g., he'll keep experimenting until he finds a way to get a block inside a bucket rather than give up in frustration right away). And, even more important, he's able to draw upon past solutions to problems rather than reinventing the wheel every time.
• Your baby will work away at a problem he is trying to solve—like how to pull himself up to a standing position on his own—until he figures it out. Then he'll practise that skill over and over until he has it mastered. The repetition helps to strengthen

	- the brain connections that are associated with that particular task
- Your baby now understands that objects still exist even if you can't see them—another major cognitive breakthrough.
- Your baby may start experiencing some sleep disruptions—the result, according to some scientists, of the onset of dreaming.
- Your baby responds to sounds such as a telephone ringing or a knock on the door.
- Your baby understands short instructions.
- Your baby uses sounds and gestures to communicate; and may be communicating via sign language if he has been taught how to sign. (See section on Baby Sign Language later in this chapter.)
- Your baby recognizes his own name and simple words.
- Your baby is beginning to understand that communication can be used to solve problems. You can help him to make this connection. Example: Before you hand him a toy, ask him if he wants it and then wait for him to respond with a sound or a gesture.
Social and emotional development	- Your baby is showing increased affection for the people who mean the most to him. He's not quite as liberal about sharing his smiles with strangers: he prefers to save them all for you.
- Your baby may become anxious or upset when a stranger approaches (stranger anxiety).
- Your baby is learning what to expect from others, based on his experiences with them.
- Your baby is developing a sense of self, based on his interactions with other people.
- Your baby is becoming a very social creature. He's likely to protest if left alone.
- Your baby enjoys interactive games such as peek-a-boo.
Your 10-Month-Old	
Physical and motor development	- Your baby can pull himself up to a standing position but may have difficulty getting back down. He may be capable of taking a few tentative steps while holding your hand.
- He can pass a toy from one hand to the other. He can also hold a toy in each hand and bang two toys together.

Your 10-Month-Old (*continued*)

Cognitive and language development	- Your baby now recognizes his own name.
- Your baby is becoming increasingly adept at repeating a sequence of actions: picking up a block with one hand, passing it to the other hand, and depositing it in the bucket beside him.
- Your baby is now the ultimate copycat—a master at imitating the gestures of other people.
- If your baby is struggling with a particular task, make a suggestion, but don't take over. Show him that a peg might fit better in a different hole, but then let him place the peg in the hole. He'll be so proud when he does it himself.
Social and emotional development	- Your baby is crystal clear about whom he likes and doesn't like—and you're at the top of the list of people he adores.
- Separation anxiety tends to occur at this age. Your baby has figured out that you still exist when you leave the room. This leads to protests—to prevent you from leaving. Playing hide-and-seek games like peek-a-boo can help baby to understand that a person can disappear and come back. If he wakes up in the middle of the night in a panic because he needs to know that you're still there, provide him with the reassurance he needs. (You eventually want to get to the point where verbal reassurance will be enough—as opposed to having to be picked up every time. You'll have to experiment to see what type of reassurance your baby requires in order to get back to sleep, while encouraging him to develop self-soothing skills.)
- Your baby is starting to look to you for information and guidance—a process that psychologists refer to as "social referencing." If he's not sure about a particular situation, he'll look to you for a reassuring smile or nod of the head.

Your 11-Month-Old

Physical and motor development	- Your baby can stand unsupported for a couple of seconds at a time—a feat that will no doubt have you bursting into thunderous applause. (Hey, it's moments like this that we parents live for!)
- Your baby can get himself from a standing position to a sitting position, so you'll no longer have to rush to his side to "rescue" him each time he decides he's tired of standing up.

Cognitive and language development	• Your baby is beginning to understand the meanings of an increasing number of words, but he still relies heavily on other "clues" that help him understand what you're saying: gestures, body language, speech intonation, and so on. One study showed that babies this age understand fewer than 25 per cent of the simple nouns and verbs that their parents use while they are playing with them. • Your baby is beginning to recognize the names for his various body parts.
Social and emotional development	• Your baby will likely utter his first words this month—another exciting milestone for you and your baby, and the beginning of an exciting dialogue that will last a lifetime. • Chances are your baby's favourite games these days involve some sort of motion, such as flying like an airplane or being bounced on your knee. • Your baby is becoming increasingly friendly with people he knows and trusts. • Your baby is increasingly capable of finding ways to manage his emotions (turning to you for comfort when he is afraid).

Your 12-Month-Old

Physical and motor development	• Your baby is either walking or is about to take his exciting first step. His wide-legged gait makes it very clear why one-year-olds are known as toddlers. (From a design perspective, that wide-legged stride actually makes a lot of sense: it lowers his centre of gravity and helps to improve his stability.) You'll also notice that these first efforts at walking require a tremendous amount of concentration; during the weeks ahead, your toddler will constantly be checking where his feet are in relation to objects around him. • Your baby is capable of stacking blocks and working with very simple frame-style puzzles (e.g., the kind where a piece with a handle fits into a wooden or plastic frame of the same shape). He's also becoming a pro at placing objects inside one another (e.g., toys like nesting cubes that stack inside one another). • Your baby may be starting to show a preference for one hand as opposed to the other. • Your baby may start to climb stairs or onto furniture. • Your baby enjoys putting objects into and out of containers (dump and fill play).

Your 12-Month-Old (*continued*)	
Cognitive and language development	• Your baby is able to use some very basic methods of sorting toys (e.g., grouping them by colour or shape). • Your baby uses common household objects correctly (drinking from a cup, brushing his teeth with a toothbrush). • Your baby is fascinated by cause and effect and will design his own experiments (throwing food on the floor) to see if the laws of gravity apply day after day. • Your baby has developed an attachment to a favourite toy or other object (blanket, pillow, book, etc.). • Your baby may understand as few as three words or as many as 100 words, but it's unlikely that he's able to say more than a dozen words at this stage of the game—and his pronunciation may still be quite garbled. • Your baby points to the correct picture in a book when an object is named ("Where is the bear?"). • Your baby repeats sounds and gestures in order to attract your attention. • Your baby understands simple requests ("Go get your boots."). • Your baby understands how to use gestures (e.g., pointing to objects, waving goodbye). • Your baby tries to imitate words that he hears other people using and may even be trying to combine words into rudimentary phrases. • Your baby uses expressions like "oh oh!" and "No!" (That "no" can mean anything from "no" to "I need a break" to "I am baby, hear me roar!") • Your baby is interested in simple picture books.
Social and emotional development	• Your baby is becoming increasingly independent—insisting on feeding and attempting to dress or undress himself. His catch phrase will soon become an indignant "Me do it!" Ready or not, your baby has become a toddler.

In some cases, the reason for the delay may be apparent. If your baby was born prematurely, for example, your baby's doctor will encourage you to focus on his corrected age rather than his gestational age when you're trying to figure out where he should be in terms of his development. (If your baby was born two months early, for example, you'd only expect him to be achieving the 10-month developmental milestones by the time his first birthday rolls around.) The same thing applies if your baby has been identified as having some sort of recognized medical condition, such as Down syndrome; in this case, you should forget about fixating on his chronological age and consider his corrected age instead. (Your baby's doctor will be able to give you an indication of where your baby should be in terms of his development given any medical conditions or developmental challenges he's dealing with.)

Regardless of when your baby achieves a particular developmental milestone—whether it's sooner rather than later or vice versa—you can expect to experience tremendous pride and joy. As Karen, a 33-year-old mother of three, notes, when you witness one of your baby's firsts, "you get to be an eye-witness to the true wonders this life has to offer."

Here are some other key points to keep in mind when you're trying to make sense of the developmental milestones in Table 10.1.

- **Each area of development (social, emotional, cognitive, language, motor skills, physical development) affects all other areas of development.** You can't look at a single area of development in isolation. If your baby is acquiring language quickly and easily, that will allow her to express her needs more clearly, leading to additional breakthroughs on the social and emotional fronts. Likewise, if she's struggling with her fine motor skills, that is likely to cause her a great deal of emotional distress.

- **A child's development doesn't proceed at a predictable rate.** There are periods when he achieves a number of developmental breakthroughs in rapid succession and periods when his development seems to plateau. What matters is the big picture—whether his development is on track over time.

- **Love the one you're with.** Loving your baby for who he is and where he is in terms of his developmental milestones will allow you to enjoy your baby and celebrate him for the unique little person he is.

baby talk

Baby signing (which involves teaching babies selected signs from American Sign Language) takes advantage of the fact that babies are able to use gestures long before they are able to speak. You introduce a sign to your baby while saying the word at the same time. According to Sara Bingham, author of *The Baby Signing Book*, the sooner you start introducing signs to your baby, the sooner your baby will start understanding the meaning of those signs.

When you're introducing signs, it's important to choose signs for words that have a lot of meaning for your baby. The signs for food items, his favourite toys, and the word "more" are all useful signs for a baby to know. Repeat these signs often, so that baby can learn to associate the sign with the word. And, when baby starts to sign (something that will happen at around eight to ten months, although the exact timing varies with each baby), be sure to confirm the sign by signing back so that he'll know you've understood him.

By the way, you don't have to worry about signing causing any delays to your baby's speech. Babies who are signed to tend to start talking earlier than other babies. What's more, they also tend to have larger vocabularies.

mom's the word

"Every time Maddy reaches a milestone, it is a great source of joy for us. Even more so, I think, than it was with Josh, perhaps because we always expected Josh to achieve those milestones. It can also be extremely frustrating, however, when she levels off and stays there for a long time. It's like she's never actually going to reach that milestone; it's taking so long. But then she'll master two or three things all at the same time. I would tell parents who are welcoming new babies with special needs to love their children for who they are, not who you hope they'll be."

—MONIQUE, 28, MOTHER OF TWO

TABLE 10.2

When There May Be Cause for Concern

It's a rare baby who manages to achieve each and every development milestone right on target. While there's generally little cause for concern if your baby is a little bit late achieving the odd milestone, there could be cause for concern (and you will want to talk to your baby's doctor) if...

your baby is one month of age and

... he doesn't react to loud noises by exhibiting the Moro reflex (startle reflex);

... he isn't able to suck and swallow with ease;

... he has a stronger grasp in one hand than the other;

... he doesn't make eye-to-eye contact when he is awake and being held;

... he doesn't stop crying when he is picked up and held;

... he doesn't roll his head from side to side when he is placed on his stomach.

your baby is four months of age and

... he isn't lifting his head at all;

... he isn't able to bring his hands together in front of his chest;

... he doesn't respond to social interactions;

... he has yet to smile or make other facial expressions;

... he doesn't appear to have any interest in people or objects;

... he doesn't respond to sounds.

your baby is eight months of age and

... he is still exhibiting the tonic neck reflex (the fencer's position—see Chapter 1);

... he isn't able to sit up on his own;

... he isn't smiling or showing any signs of pleasure;

... he still isn't interested in people or objects;

... he doesn't make any effort to reach for or grasp objects;

... he doesn't explore objects that are placed in his hand;

... he doesn't react to sounds or try to determine where those sounds are coming from;

... he isn't babbling, cooing, or otherwise experimenting with sounds;

... he hasn't learned to differentiate between night and day in terms of his sleeping patterns.

your baby is 13 months of age and (*continued*)

. . . he still doesn't have the ability to grasp objects or transfer objects from one hand to the other;

. . . he isn't creeping or crawling;

. . . he doesn't differentiate between people he knows well and complete strangers;

. . . he doesn't pay any attention to gestures;

. . . he is unable to follow simple directions;

. . . he is totally uninterested in social games;

. . . he has yet to start making any vowel or consonant sounds;

. . . he doesn't blink when fast-moving objects approach his eye.

BABY LOVE

It all begins with love—that powerful bond between you and your baby. A healthy attachment sets the stage for your baby's healthy development. Such an attachment helps to shape your baby's brain pathways. And the confidence he gains from this loving connection gives him the confidence he needs to try new things and acquire new skills. (He knows that he can return to the safety of your arms at any time, so he is willing to give in to his hard-wired curiosity and explore the world around him.)

Just as it takes two to tango, it takes two to become attached. And, once that process begins, it takes on a life of its own.

- Your baby becomes more and more attached to you as you become more and more attached to her.

- Your baby learns to trust you, to communicate her feelings, and to trust in the world around her. She begins to learn about herself and to make sense of the give-and-take of relationships as a result of her interactions with you.

- Bonding with your baby gives you a biological boost, too, triggering the release of energizing, feel-good endorphins that make it easier for you to cope with the sleep deprivation of the early weeks and months.

the baby department Babies' cries are almost impossible to ignore—and for good reason. Their very survival depends on convincing other people to care for them. And there's a considerable payoff for parents who give in to their hard-wired instincts to meet their babies' needs: researchers at the University of Iowa have discovered that preschoolers whose needs were met on a consistent basis by their parents back when they were infants tend to be well-behaved and to have highly developed self-regulation (self-control) skills.

The power of play

Just as you have an important role to play in ensuring that your baby's body gets the nutrients it needs to grow up strong and healthy, you play a critical role in ensuring that your baby's brain receives the stimulation it needs to develop in a healthy way. That means developing a loving relationship with your baby and providing him with plenty of opportunities for play and learning.

baby talk University of Illinois professor Anne Haas Dyson, an expert in early childhood learning and literacy development, blames the "baby genius edutainment complex" for convincing anxious parents that brain-boosting should take precedence over play.

Now before you turn your home into an infant education emporium, sticking flash cards on every surface and filling your home with thousands of dollars' worth of educational toys, allow me to explain. A more sensible (and less stressful) approach to providing your baby with the stimulation he needs to thrive is to take advantage of the opportunities for play and learning that naturally arise as you and your baby go about your day.

Here are some points to keep in mind.

- Create a safe environment. That way, you'll be able to encourage your baby to explore as opposed to trying to steer her clear of hazards or objects that are off-limits. (That creates frustration for her and more work for you.) See Chapter 8 for advice on babyproofing.

- Talk or sing to your baby, varying the tone and rhythm of your speech to keep your baby's interest. (Make exaggerated facial expressions or stick out your tongue. Your baby may surprise you by imitating you or bursting into coos of glee.) As he gets older, read him simple, repetitive storybooks and introduce games like peek-a-boo and pat-a-cake. (See Table 10.4 for suggestions for simple games babies enjoy at various ages.)

- When your baby starts responding with vocalizations and starts making faces at you, make a game out of imitating the sounds and the expressions he is making. Not only will the two of you be having fun, but you'll also be teaching him the basics of conversation. (People take turns talking when they are having a conversation.)

- Provide your baby with plenty of visual stimulation—ideally, toys and mobiles that are of very simple design. (See Table 10.4.) If your baby is too young to hold a toy by herself, hold it for her. Babies as young as 2 months of age enjoy batting at toys even though they have yet to develop the skills needed to hold on to a toy themselves.

- Educational programming for babies may have come a long way, but nothing can take the place of a parent. Researchers from Temple University and the University of Delaware have discovered that children under the age of 3 aren't capable of learning verbs (action words) from television or video. They need an actual human being to help them understand the meaning of these words.

- And speaking of television, there's a reason why the Canadian Paediatric Society recommends that parents hold off on introducing babies and toddlers under the age of 2 to any form of screen time: babies need to be doing their learning and exploring in the real world. Leaving the TV on in the background interferes with the quality of play babies enjoy, even if they aren't actively tuned in. Researchers at the University of Massachusetts discovered that babies as young as one played for shorter periods of time when the TV was on in the background. And, what's more, their parents communicated with their babies 20 per cent less often, and the quality of parent-child interactions declined, with parents being less active, attentive, and responsive to their children.

CHAPTER 10 — THE INCREDIBLE GROWING BABY

baby talk — Researchers at Temple University's Infant Lab have discovered that playing with blocks helps young children to learn the language required to think about spatial concepts (over, under, through). Spatial concepts are important for careers in the so-called STEM disciplines (science, technology, engineering, mathematics), but they are also important for everyday living.

The following toys are the best bets for babies under one year of age. Many of these toys will grow with your baby and be used well into the toddler years, too.

TABLE 10.3

Inside the Toy Box

- Rattles (including sock-style rattles that can be put on feet)
- Shatterproof mirror
- Mobiles (homemade or commercially made)
- Washable dolls and stuffed animals (with embroidered eyes)
- Brightly coloured cloth balls and textured balls
- Exercise balls or beach balls (for bouncing on, sitting on, leaning on)
- Soft stacking blocks
- Soft dolls
- Puppets
- Teething toys
- Nesting toys (toys that stack or nest inside one another)
- Dump and fill toys (e.g., a box of blocks, a shape-sorting toy)
- Ring stack sets
- Squeaky toys (with non-removable squeakers) and other toys that make noise (shakers)
- Water toys (especially toys that can be used for pouring)
- Books (cloth or board) and audiobooks
- Musical instruments (homemade or commercially made)
- Push and pull toys

- Dance with your baby to music. The rhythm of music isn't merely soothing to his soul: it helps him to tune into the sound beats in language. (Yes, Mama, grooving with your baby *is* an educational activity. So dance on!)
- Follow your baby's lead when he decides to initiate play. As he gets older, he'll love tossing toys off his high chair and watching you pick them up. It's his way of testing to see if the laws of gravity work each and every time and of seeing just how many times he can get you to reach down and pick up that toy.
- Watch for signs that your baby has had enough stimulation for now. Too much stimulation can make a baby just as unhappy as too little stimulation. If he begins to fuss or turn away, he may need to switch into relaxation mode for a while. (Babies can get stressed out, too.)

---

baby talk Babies need to be able to move their bodies freely in order to learn how their bodies work and to explore their worlds. You'll want to ensure that your baby has plenty of time for active play (on the floor, on your lap).

Games don't have to be complicated to be highly entertaining to a baby. As long as you are part of the game, it's bound to be fun. Remember, you are the most fascinating toy that was ever invented—or at least that's how your baby sees it.

Reading to your baby

Reading to your baby isn't all about fostering a life-long love of reading (although, of course, that's important, too): it's also about connecting with your baby and sharing the joy of reading together. If you're an avid reader yourself, most of this will come naturally to you. If you're not a life-long reader, relax: the most important thing to focus on is enjoying spending time with your baby. Here are a few practical tips to help you get started.

- **Choose age-appropriate books.** When babies are very young, they respond to bold patterns (think black-and-white checkerboards and swirls) and books featuring human faces. They also enjoy books that

TABLE 10.4

Simple Games Babies Love

Activity	Instructions	Why Baby Loves It / What Baby Learns
Birth to Three Months		
Over here, Baby	Hold your face about 12 inches away from your baby's face when he is lying on the floor. Slowly move your face to the right. Slowly move your face to the left. See if he can track your movements with his eyes.	Your baby is fascinated with your face. You can encourage him to practise tracking objects with his eyes by using your face as the incentive to play this very basic baby game.
Talk to the hand puppet	This is a simple variation on the activity above. Encourage your baby to track the movement of a hand puppet. (If you don't have a hand puppet, draw a face on an oven mitt or a sock. It will work just as well.)	The more bold and stark the design of your puppet, the more likely your puppet will capture your baby's attention. Simple works best with young babies. You can also have fun making funny voices—something that will also help to capture and maintain your baby's interest.
Talk to me, Baby	Alter the sound of your voice. Make your voice sound deep and then squeaky high (but without scaring your baby, of course). Talk in "parentese"—that exaggerated sing-song voice that parents have been using forever to soothe and entertain babies. See if you can get your baby to make some sounds in response.	Your baby loves listening to your voice. She's also fascinated by the sounds and rhythms of human speech. Your conversations with her will encourage her to engage in conversations with you one of these days.
Baby charades	Give your baby the basic vocabulary he needs to put his thoughts and feelings into words. That way, when he becomes capable of stringing sounds together to make words, he'll be able to draw upon the words he's been learning all along. Say, "You don't like having your clothes taken off" or "You just want someone to hold you." Or express things from his viewpoint, "I don't want to be naked, Mom!" "I just want someone to hold me, Mom!"	While your baby is learning new words, you'll be reminding yourself to tune into his body language so that you can read his cues and figure out what he wants and needs. It's kind of like a game of charades, but, in this case, everybody wins.

(continued)

Activity	Instructions	Why Baby Loves It / What Baby Learns
Tummy time	Tummy time (time spent on their tummies rather than on their backs) is more important than ever for babies, given the "back to sleep" safe sleeping guidelines. Babies need a chance to develop neck and upper-body strength (which they do when they push their arms and chests up off the ground) when they are lying on their tummies. Your baby may enjoy tummy time more if you place him on a colourful playmat, on top of a half-inflated beach ball, or on your chest while you are on your back. That way, when he works hard to raise his head, he'll be rewarded by the sight of your face. Or get down on the floor so that you are directly facing him. That way, you can sing to him, talk to him, or make funny faces at him. Start with just a few minutes of tummy time and try to work up to 15 minutes or longer at a stretch—whatever your baby can tolerate.	If babies spend all of their waking hours in the back-lying position, they are at increased risk of developing a condition known as placiocephaly (when one side of the head or the back of the head is flattened, often with little hair growing in that area). That is why tummy time is recommended. Your baby may not enjoy tummy time until she builds up some strength in her upper body but, with some gentle encouragement from you, she'll soon acquire the necessary strength to be able to play with toys in this position. Reminder: Supervise your baby during tummy time.
Jumping jacks	Lay your baby on a blanket or mat on the floor. Then help him to do "jumping jacks" while he is lying flat on the floor. Gently stretch out one arm so that it is pointing slightly upward (at roughly a 45-degree angle to his body). Gently extend the opposite leg so that it is pointing slightly outward (at roughly the same angle). Then switch arms and legs. Repeat while baby is enjoying it.	Your baby will find this activity relaxing and enjoyable. It feels good to stretch at any age.
Just for kicks	Encourage your baby to practise kicking his feet by giving him something to kick against that will make an interesting noise. Try holding up a tinfoil pie plate, for example.	This activity helps your baby learn how to coordinate the movement of his feet.

Reach for it	Dangle a toy from a set of plastic links. Slowly move the toy from side to side so that it is within grasping distance for baby.	Reaching for a moving object gives your baby a chance to work on her hand-eye coordination skills and to coordinate the movements of both sides of her body.
Four to Six Months		
Texture time	Gather together objects that are safe for Baby and that represent a variety of different textures: soft, hard, bumpy, tickly, crinkly. Hand the objects, one by one, to your baby and wait for his reaction.	Baby is in explorer mode. He's learning about different types of objects, and you're getting a sense of what he likes and dislikes. Put this activity on hold until another day if he shows signs of becoming overwhelmed. He may be hitting sensory overload.
Shake it, Baby, shake it	Place a small amount of macaroni into an empty plastic spice jar. Seal the lid with glue or duct tape.	Your baby will enjoy being able to control the noise the shaker makes. For added fun, partially fill a second shaker with a different type of material (rice or sand work well) and then seal the lid with glue or duct tape. Your baby will be fascinated by the fact that each shaker makes a different sound.
Baby airplane	Parents have been playing this game with their babies ever since there were airplanes. Someone probably played it with you. Hold your baby by his waist and gently fly him through the air, carefully watching his reaction.	Physical play is good for babies. It gives them a chance to move their bodies, to develop muscle tone, and to experience a variety of different sensations. Just pay attention to your baby's cues and to park the airplane for the rest of the day if he's had enough.

(continued)

Activity	Instructions	Why Baby Loves It / What Baby Learns
Bag of smiles	Cut six to twelve one-inch circles out of kitchen sponges of various colours. Draw happy faces on both sides of the sponges using a laundry pen or permanent marker. Allow the ink to dry. Place the happy faces in an extra-large zipper-seal plastic bag. Fill the bag about two-thirds of the way full with warm (but not hot) water. (Variation: Add a drop or two of dish soap as well.) Seal the bag and place the bag on your baby's high chair tray so that she can touch and squeeze it. (Place the open end of the bag away from Baby, just in case the zipper seal unzips. You can always hedge your bets by adding a layer of duct tape, too.)	Your baby will enjoy squishing the bag and watching the happy faces move around. With the bubble variation, the more she moves the bag around, the more bubbles she'll create. Note: Never leave a baby unsupervised with a plastic bag—even a zipper-seal plastic bag.
Baby face	Help your baby learn to read people's facial expressions by taking snapshots of family members hamming it up for the camera. Exaggerate various emotions—happy, sad, scared, angry, sleepy—and name the emotions for your baby when you read the book. Don't forget to include some photos of your baby modeling her full range of emotions, too.	Continue to add to this book as your baby grows. Include photos depicting more complex emotions and more subtle expressions. As your child heads into the toddler and preschool years, you'll want to encourage him to pay attention to how his body feels when he is experiencing powerful emotions. You'll also want to teach him strategies for working with those emotions.

Seven to Nine Months

Follow the leader	Copy your baby's actions. If he makes a sound, you copy that sound. If he shakes a toy, you shake a toy. If there's a lull in the action, make a funny face or a funny noise and see if your baby will try to copy you. When Baby starts crawling, you can take turns crawling after one another, too.	This game teaches your baby about the give and take of conversation. It also teaches him that he can influence the reactions of other people—a pretty exciting discovery for a baby.

Peek-a-boo	The beauty of this game is that it can be played anywhere, anytime (including when you're in line at the grocery store). You simply cover your face with your hands, gradually uncover your face, and say "peek-a-boo." Or, you can put a towel (or whatever else you have handy) over your head. Baby will want to join in, too. For a while, she'll think she's invisible while her face is covered. Too cute. Variation: Cover up a toy with a towel and show your baby how to look under the towel to find the toy. Repeat with other types of objects.	Parents have been playing this game with babies for generations—and for good reason. It helps to teach babies that objects (and people) continue to exist, even when you can't see them. This helps Baby to panic a little less when Mom leaves the room or when Baby wakes up in the middle of the night and can't figure out where Mom is.
The baby in the mirror	Give her a chance to study and play with the baby in the mirror. (Be sure to use an unbreakable mirror.)	It takes Baby a while to figure out that the gorgeous baby in the mirror is, in fact, herself. You can help the process along by using Baby's name and pointing to Baby's various body parts: e.g., "Julie's nose."
How big is the baby?	Ask your baby, "How big is the baby?" Then spread your arms out wide and exclaim, "So big!"	Your baby will find this game hilarious and will enjoy imitating your voice and your hand motions.
One-baby band	Gather up objects that make very different types of noises: a baby rattle, a set of measuring spoons, a ball of waxed paper (or some other type of paper that crinkles) tucked inside a sock, a toy that squeaks, etc.	Your baby will be fascinated by the different noises made by each object. While she plays, she'll be working on her tactile awareness (her awareness of the feel of objects) and her listening skills.
Dump and fill play	All you need for this activity is something for your baby to dump (blocks or other similar-sized toys) and something to put them back into (a bowl or other container that is safe for a baby). Show her how to dump the blocks and how to fill the container up again. Variation: Dump and fill play works well in the bathtub, too. Give your baby a small container and show her how she can fill it up with water and dump it again.	This activity teaches her about cause and effect and shows her that she can have an impact on her environment. She will enjoy repeating this activity over and over again to see if she gets the same result. Yes, your baby is a natural-born scientist.

(continued)

Activity	Instructions	Why Baby Loves It / What Baby Learns
Ten to Twelve Months		
Baby playdate	Invite a friend with a baby to come over, or connect with a playgroup in your area. Sit the babies down across from one another so that they can have a chance to get to know one another.	As your baby heads into the toddler years, she's ready to start making friends. (When she was younger, she was more likely to stare over the head of another baby than to look that baby in the eye.) The more opportunity your baby has to play with babies and other children, the more opportunity she'll have to work on her social skills.
Texture time	Make a series of texture swatches for your baby to touch and explore. Cut small squares of fabric and paper of various textures and glue these fabric swatches to individual canvas panels (available in postcard size or smaller from your local art store). Let your baby touch the cards so that she can become familiar with the different textures.	Your baby may want to hold some of the cards for herself—an indication that she likes certain textures. She may shy away from other textures that she doesn't find quite as appealing. She's expressing her own individuality and taking control of her world through play.
Walk in the park	Let Baby experience nature up close by visiting your neighbourhood park. Give her the opportunity to touch the trees, see and smell the flowers, and listen to the sounds the birds are making.	Being in nature isn't just incredibly stimulating for young children; it's also incredibly soothing. And that trip to the park will lower your stress level, too. Important: Tuck your cell phone away during this walk. You can't tune into nature while you're tuning into text messages.
Everything old is new again	Teach some familiar objects some new tricks. Pull a scarf through a paper towel roll—or use it as a prop for peek-a-boo. Bang two pot lids together.	Your baby will learn about the functions and properties of everyday objects—and you'll save a small fortune on so-called educational toys.

Great explorer	Create a tunnel for your baby using a large cardboard box. (Flatten both ends of the box and sit at the opposite side to your baby. Encourage your baby to crawl through.) Variation: Duct-tape two receiving blankets to the top end of the box, leaving a slight gap in the middle to produce a curtain effect. Show your baby that she can crawl through the curtains, too. Ta da! A star is born.	Your baby will have fun crawling through the box. You'll be helping her to understand spatial concepts and to learn how her body relates to other objects. (She can't go through solid objects: only objects with a big enough hole.)
Let's play ball	There are all kinds of ways to enjoy playing ball with a baby. You can roll a ball to a baby. You can bounce a baby on top of a large ball (like an exercise ball). Or you can drop balls into other objects, like laundry baskets. And that's just for starters. If you let your imagination go wild, you'll come up with your own baby-world variations on soccer, basketball, and, of course, hockey.	Playing ball with your baby teaches her about taking turns and encourages her to be active in a way that is both fun and social.
Pat-a-cake	Teach your baby the words and motions to the nursery rhyme *Pat-a-cake*. At first, you will need to make the motions with her while repeating the words. Gradually, she will start making the motions while you say the words. Then she'll start saying some of the words, too.	This is a fun way to reinforce the idea that words have meaning. In this case, the actions that accompany the nursery rhyme help to illustrate the meaning of the words (pat-a-cake, roll it, put it in the oven, etc.).

play with language (rhyming books and lullaby books) and word books that help them to learn the names of familiar objects in their world. During the second half of their first year of life, they enjoy an even wider variety of books. Best bets for babies this age include books that are highly tactile, books that feature moving parts (lift-the-flap and peek-a-boo books), books about bedtime and other daily routines in the life of a baby, alphabet books, and Sandra Boynton books ("Mother Goose rhymes for our era," according to Eleanor LeFave, owner of Toronto children's bookstore Mabel's Fables).

- **Choose the right time and the right place for story time.** You want to read to your baby when he is calm and relaxed (as opposed to hungry and overtired). And you want to choose a comfortable spot, where the two of you can cuddle up and get lost in books.

- **Accept the fact that your baby might only want to read a page or two of each book.** Your baby may have a favourite page in the story—one that he likes to return to again and again. Maybe he likes the picture. Maybe he likes the way you read the words in a funny, over-the-top voice. Or maybe—like many babies—he is simply entranced by the joy of repetition. Don't try to force him to read the book your way. Let him read it his way. You'll maximize his enjoyment by letting him take the lead.

- **Don't freak out if a book gets damaged.** Much-loved books will inevitably show some signs of wear and tear. The alternative—keeping your baby's books out of his reach for fear that something might happen to them—doesn't make any sense. Whose books are they anyway? Yours or your baby's?

Pink versus Blue

Forget nature. It's all about nurture. Or, as Rosalind C. Barnett and Caryl Rivers argue in their book *The Truth About Girls and Boys: Challenging Toxic Stereotypes About Our Children,* any noteworthy differences in behaviour between boys and girls that become obvious as children grow older are the result of how children are socialized rather than any characteristics with which they were born.

Beliefs about gender differences affect how we parent from babyhood on up. It's not unusual, for example, for parents to believe that baby girls are more fragile than baby boys—and to limit the amount of risk they expose their daughters to as compared to their sons as a result. In their book, Barnett and Rivers report on a study involving 11-month-old babies. Mothers were asked to adjust the angle of a carpeted ramp to reflect the angle their babies would be capable of crawling down. Mothers consistently underestimated baby girls' abilities even though, when the baby girls were given the chance to crawl down the ramp, they proved to be more daring than the baby boys.

We limit our children's opportunities for growth when we can't conceive of them being able to achieve beyond stereotypical ideas about what it means to be a boy or a girl. "Parents and teachers need to help children to understand that there are many different ways to be a boy or a girl," says Barnett. "That they are a boy or a girl, but they can do anything they want to do."

THE CHILDCARE CRUNCH

Planning to return to work in the near future? Shocked by how difficult it is to find a childcare space for your child in your community? Hundreds of thousands of other Canadian parents are dealing with the same problem. According to the YWCA Canada study "Educated, Employed, and Equal: The Economic Prosperity Case for National Child Care" (2011), 66.5 per cent of Canadian mothers with children under the age of 5 belong to the paid labour market, but there are only licensed childcare spaces for approximately one in five Canadian children under the age of 5 (*Early Childhood Education and Care in Canada*, Childcare Resource and Research Unit, 2008).

And even if you do manage to find a licensed childcare space, there's a world of difference between a childcare program that provides custodial care (keeping children safe and meeting their basic needs) and one that offers the type of nurturing, play-based learning experience that parents want for their children and that children deserve.

If none of the options available in your community are acceptable to you as a parent, let the politicians who represent you know that your child's needs are not being met and that the community is missing out on an important opportunity to invest in its own infrastructure. (Investing in childcare creates four times as many jobs as investing in construction. And, what's more, investments in childcare quickly pay for themselves in terms of taxes returned to various levels of government.)

Returning to work: The first week survival guide

After months of preparation, the moment of truth has finally arrived: you're about to go back to work. Here are some tips on weathering that challenging first week back on the job.

- Talk to your employer ahead of time to see what arrangements can be made to make your first week back at work as stress-free as possible. See if it would be possible to work part-time hours (half days or every other day) or to work only half a week (for example, start back to work on a Wednesday or Thursday so that you only have to work for two or three days before the weekend rolls around).

- Invite a co-worker to lunch the week before you return to work so that she can quickly bring you up to speed on what's been happening while you were on maternity leave. That way, you won't feel quite so overwhelmed during your first day on the job.

- Test-drive your childcare arrangements before you go back to work so that both you and your baby can get used to the routine. And use this opportunity to give your baby's childcare provider the information she will need in order to provide the best quality of care to your baby: details about her routine, her likes and dislikes, her food preferences, her sleep rituals, and so on. Provide this information in writing.

- Establish a rapport with your baby's childcare provider. The better you get to know her, the more comfortable you will feel about leaving your child in her care, and the easier it will be for the two of you to talk through concerns related to your child.

---

mother wisdom Try not to panic if your milk supply seems to drop during your first few days on the job. It could be the result of the stress and exhaustion of returning to work or because you've been so busy that you haven't been consuming your usual volume of fluids. The best way to deal with this particular problem is to hit the couch with your baby the moment you get home so that she can nurse and you can catch up on your rest. You'll also want to use whichever relaxation methods are most effective in bringing down your stress level (meditation, a warm bath, and/or talking to a friend) and ensure that you're drinking at least eight glasses of water each day.

- Look for ways to minimize your workload on the home front during your first week back on the job. If friends or family members ask what they can do to help, suggest that they show up on your doorstep bearing healthy, homemade meals—a much more appealing alternative to the takeout pizza or frozen leftovers that might otherwise find their way onto the dinner table that first week.

- Keep your evenings and weekends free so that you can spend as much of your non-working time as possible with your baby. You'll want to be with her every bit as much as she wants to be with you.

- If your baby is having a hard time settling into her new childcare arrangement, send along a comfort object or two—perhaps her favourite blanket and a stuffed toy or a sweatshirt that smells like you. (If your baby is under one year of age when you return to work, make sure your childcare provider understands that babies shouldn't sleep with blankets or stuffed animals, and that they should always be put to sleep on their backs.)

- Factor in a generous amount of time for the morning drop-off schedule. You and your baby will find it easier to part ways if your goodbyes don't have to be hurried.

- Resist the temptation to sneak out the door when your baby isn't looking. You might get away with it the first time, but you'll pay a pretty high price for that one-time escape: your baby will always be wondering if you're about to sneak away again, so she may insist on being in physical contact with you every minute when you're not at work.

- When it's time to leave for work, hand your child to the caregiver rather than having the caregiver take your baby from you. This will be more reassuring to your baby. And make sure that your body language is reassuring, even if you're feeling a little weepy inside. Otherwise, your baby will pick up on how you're feeling and become frightened and upset herself. An Academy Award–winning performance may be required. Fortunately, you only have to hold it together long enough to get out the door.

- Don't drag out your goodbyes any longer than necessary. Prolonging the goodbye will only make things more difficult for all concerned. If you want to know how well your baby settles for the caregiver, give the childcare provider a phone call once you get to work.

- Be prepared for some tears when you show up at the end of the day. Research has shown that babies are fussier when their parents return to pick them up than they are when their parents are at work. This is because babies feel most free to express their emotions when they're with the people they're most comfortable with— so consider it a compliment if your baby bursts into tears at the sight of you.

- If you're finding the transition back to work rough, talk to other parents who've been there about how you are feeling. They will reassure you that it's normal to miss your baby when you return to work, that your emotions won't always be this raw, and that things will get easier over time.

The Great Canadian Maternity-Leave Cash Crunch

It doesn't take much to derail a family financially—not in an era of mostly stagnant or declining wages (during the period from 1980 to 2005, wages rose for the wealthiest Canadians, were stagnant for the middle class, and declined for the lowest-earning Canadians, according to the Vanier Institute of the Family), record-breaking student debt levels, and the need for two full-time wage earners to pay the bills. This doesn't allow much room for families to set aside that much-lauded three- to six-month cushion of savings for emergencies. A study released in 2011 by the Canadian Payroll Association revealed that 75 per cent of Canadians are living from paycheque to paycheque.

And to add to the financial woes of Canadian families, a significant number of Canadian women—up to one-third—aren't even eligible for maternity benefits, often because they are hired as contractors rather than employees. "You have to be able to produce a record of employment to demonstrate that all of those hours of employment were EI-insurable," explains Armine Yalnizyan, senior economist with the Canadian Centre for Policy Alternatives. "Otherwise they don't count."

And even if a maternity leave is paid, it is paid at the rate of 55 per cent to a maximum of $39,000 per year (unless the employer offers a top-up in wages), something that can mean a significant loss of wages if the mother was the higher income earner in a family.

To attempt to sidestep the financial pitfalls that an underfinanced maternity leave can pose for your family, you'll want to know what you're spending and how much money a month you need to live on; understand what benefits you are entitled to from the government and from your employer; try to set aside a bit of a nest egg before you head off on maternity leave; and come up with a plan for repaying any debt you incur while you are on maternity leave.

---

baby talk A study of 6-month-old infants whose fathers work outside the home has revealed that low levels of support for dads in the workplace can make parenting harder. Researchers from Pennsylvania State University found that fathers who are under a lot of pressure at work may find it more difficult to connect with their babies and that these dads are more likely to exhibit negative emotions toward their babies than dads who aren't under as much stress. Those who work long hours and who are under a lot of pressure at work find it the most difficult to let go of their work-related worries and simply enjoy their babies, the researchers found.

THE SECRETS OF LESS-STRESSED-OUT PARENTS

As you've no doubt noticed by now, some parents are perpetually stressed out, while others take a much more laissez-faire approach to raising their offspring. Yes, temperament factors into the equation (the parent's temperament as well as the baby's) as does circumstance (you can't dodge all the parenting curveballs that are likely to come your way over the next 18 years or so), but there *are* things you can do to bring your overall stress level down at least a little, no matter what you're dealing with at any given time.

All that said, some of the points below will apply some of the time. Some of them may apply all of the time. And some of them may never apply to your situation at all. Use whichever bits of advice you find helpful and set aside the rest.

- **Find your new village.** Becoming a parent changes the entire landscape of your life. You're going to need to be able to reach out to an entirely new set of people who speak your new language (the language of parenting) and who understand the joys and challenges that you are living with right now. These people will become your support network for at least the foreseeable future—say, the next 15 to 20 years.

- **Continue to nurture your other relationships while you're busy raising your kids.** You may have to keep in touch with pre-kid friends and far-flung relatives by phone or Internet, or during once-a-year visits, but don't let the priority relationships fall off your radar screen.
- **Participate in the life of your community.** Shop at your local farmer's market. Purchase tickets to your community children's theatre. Take advantage of family resource programs and "Y" programs in your community. Make friends with other families with young children and eat dinner at one another's houses. You will feel so much more rooted and so much less alone. (Isolation breeds stress. Isolation is the enemy.)
- **Rethink the way you use the space in your home.** Is it family-friendly? How could you use each room differently so that the space supports your family's needs at this stage of child rearing? (It is so stressful to feel like you are constantly at war with your own living environment.)
- **Be clear about what matters most to your family and be a family that lives by what it believes** (giving back to the community, spending time together, making your home a welcoming space for family and friends). Living in sync with your values brings you a sense of peace.
- **Have realistic expectations of your children as they move through each age and stage.** If you know what types of behaviour are age-appropriate, you'll be a more empathetic and less stressed-out parent.
- **Recognize that parenting is an ongoing opportunity for personal growth.** That way, you won't expect yourself to have all the answers upfront. (No parent does.) Learn what you can about a particular parenting challenge, talk to your friends about how they handled similar situations, and make the best possible decision, given what you know about your child. And forgive yourself if Plan A doesn't quite work out the way you had hoped. (That's why Plan B was invented.)
- **Nurture yourself—mind, body, and soul—as often as you can.** And don't forget that there is more to you than your parenting self. Make a date to reconnect with that part of yourself that was passionate about such-and-such before you had kids. Spend some time doing that thing.

- **Have a picture in your head about your hopes and dreams for your child, your family, and yourself; and think about what it will take to create that kind of life.** You're in a wonderful place to be musing over these possibilities. You're at the very beginning of this journey.

GROWING WITH YOUR BABY

As you help your baby to blow out the candles on his birthday cake, you'll no doubt be struck by just how much he's grown. One year ago, he was a tiny, helpless newborn. Now he's a walking and talking toddler who's able to make a big hunk of chocolate cake disappear right before your very eyes!

What you might not stop to consider is just how much you yourself have changed during your baby's amazing first year of life—how much you've grown as a person and how much confidence you've gained as a parent. Remember those butterflies you experienced the first day you found yourself alone with your new baby? Now you don't even think twice about venturing here and there with your toddler in tow.

---

mom's the word "Now that my baby is older, he seems less fragile. He is obviously more independent and is, in fact, a very robust little person. I feel a great sense of relief not to have this delicate being in my midst. While he's still dependent, he's not dependent in the same way as a newborn. There is so much more feedback. We can play interactive games like rolling a ball back and forth, and his babble enchants me. I like to think that my early efforts to nurture his most basic needs have allowed him to develop into this happy baby on the brink of toddlerhood."

—JENNIFER, 35, MOTHER OF ONE

The challenges you faced as a parent changed remarkably over the course of the year. The early months of parenthood were basically an endurance test—an attempt to meet your baby's day-to-day needs while surviving on next to no sleep. And just when you thought you'd collapse from exhaustion, the reward period of parenting kicked in: suddenly there were perks, like your baby's smiles, to make this whole parenthood thing worthwhile. That's not to say that parenthood suddenly became a cakewalk, of course. There are challenges involved in parenting a child of any age. As Elisa, a 27-year-old mother of two, puts it: "Just when you think you have something under control, a new situation arises to keep you on your toes. That is the one thing about parenting: you always have to be prepared for something new and to constantly find creative ways to handle the situation. What worked one day or one week won't necessarily work the next."

But then again, it's the ever-changing landscape that makes the journey so exciting. Your role as a parent changes as the needs of your baby evolve. "You start out by being just a provider of food, shelter, love, and warmth," explains Karen, a 33-year-old mother of three. "Your role then expands to that of a teacher: you get to introduce your child to the world and the world to your child. And by showing your child the wonder of the world, you get to experience it yourself as if for the first time."

Enjoy the wonder of that journey.

Appendix A
GLOSSARY

Apgar test: A test that assesses a baby's overall health at birth by scoring the baby on five different attributes: heart rate, respiration, muscle tone, reflex responsiveness, and skin tone (e.g., whether the baby is "pinking up" or is still a little bit blue). The test is performed twice: at one minute after birth, and at five minutes after birth.

Amniotic fluid: The protective liquid consisting mostly of water that surrounds the baby inside the amniotic sac.

Anencephaly: A birth defect involving a malformed brain and skull. Anencephaly leads to stillbirth or death soon after birth.

Anomaly: A malformation or abnormality in any part of the body. Some anomalies are relatively minor; others can be serious, even fatal.

Areola: The flat pigmented area encircling the nipple of the breast.

Asthma: A lung condition that causes the air passages to become narrowed as a result of muscular spasms and swelling of the air passage walls.

Axillary temperature: A temperature reading that is taken by placing a thermometer in the armpit.

Balanoposthitis: Inflammation of the foreskin of the penis caused either by trauma or poor hygiene.

Bilirubin: A substance that is released as a newborn baby's body attempts to get rid of some of the excess red blood cells that he was born with.

Boils: Raised, red, tender, warm swellings on the skin that are most often found on the buttocks.

Breast abscess: A condition in which pus accumulates in one area of the breast.

Breast engorgement: When the breasts become swollen and full of milk.

Bronchiolitis: A viral infection of the small breathing tubes of the lungs.

Bronchitis: An infection of the central and larger airways of the lungs.

Caesarean section: A surgical procedure used to deliver a baby via an incision made in the mother's abdomen and uterus.

Café au lait marks: Permanent tan-coloured patches that can appear at birth or at any point during the first two years of life.

Campylobacter: A common bacterial cause of intestinal infections.

Capillary hemangioma: See strawberry hemangioma.

Cavernous hemangioma: A reddish or bluish-red birthmark that has a lumpy texture.

Cellulitis: Swollen, red, tender, warm areas of skin that are typically found on the extremities or the buttocks and that often start out as a boil or puncture wound prior to becoming infected.

Chromosomal abnormalities: Problems that result from errors in the duplication of the chromosomes—the thread-like structures in the nucleus of a cell that transmit genetic information.

Circumcision: Surgical removal of the foreskin of the penis.

Cleft lip: A condition in which there is a separation of the upper lip that can extend into the nose.

Cleft palate: A condition in which the roof of the mouth is incompletely formed.

Clubfoot: A condition in which the baby is born with the sole of one or both feet facing either down and inward or up and outward.

Colostrum: The first substance secreted from the breasts following childbirth. Colostrum is high in protein and antibodies.

Congenital anomaly: An abnormality that is present at birth. A congenital anomaly is acquired during pregnancy but is not necessarily genetic in origin.

Congenital pigmented nevi: The common mole.

Co-sleeping: Sharing sleep with your baby. If you share a bed, this is known as bed-sharing. If you share a room, this is known as room-sharing.

Cradle cap: A relatively common skin condition in the newborn that involves a yellowish, scaly buildup on the baby's head that may also be accompanied by redness in the creases of the skin.

Croup: A respiratory condition in which your baby's breathing becomes very noisy. In some cases, his windpipe may become obstructed.

Cytomegalovirus (CMV): A group of viruses from the herpes virus family.

Diastasis recti abdominis: The separation of the longitudinal abdominal muscles during pregnancy.

Diphtheria: A disease that attacks the throat and heart and that can lead to heart failure or death.

Dislocated hip: A condition that occurs when the ball at the head of the thigh bone doesn't fit snugly enough into its socket in the hip bone.

Doula: A childbirth or postpartum professional who provides support to a birthing woman or new mother and her family.

Down syndrome: A chromosomal abnormality that results in intellectual disability and a variety of medical conditions.

Early neonatal death: When a live-born infant dies before the seventh day following birth, this death is classified as an early neonatal death.

Eclampsia: A serious but rare condition that can affect pregnant or labouring women. It is a severe form of pre-eclampsia. Symptoms of eclampsia include hypertension, edema, and protein in the urine. An emergency delivery may be necessary if the eclampsia is severe enough.

Eczema: Extreme itchiness that results in a rash in areas that are scratched. Eczema can be caused by environmental irritants.

Encephalitis: An infection of the brain.

Engrossment: The term that is used to describe a new father's fascination with his new baby.

Epidural: A local anesthetic that is injected into the epidural space at the level of the spinal cord that you wish to numb. The most common form of pharmacological pain relief during labour. Used for Caesarean sections as well.

Epiglottitis: A life-threatening infection that causes swelling in the back of the throat.

Episiotomy: An incision made into the skin and the perineal muscle at the time of delivery to enlarge the vaginal opening and make it easier for the baby's head or body to emerge or to insert birthing instruments such as forceps.

Epispadias: A condition in which a baby is born with the urethral opening on the upper surface of the penis rather than the tip of the penis. The penis may curve upward.

Erythema infectiosum: See fifth disease.

Erythema toxicum neonatorum: Red splotches on the skin with yellowish-white bumps in the centre.

Erythromycin ointment: Ointment that is applied to a newborn baby's eyes within a couple of hours of the birth.

Febrile convulsions: Seizures that may occur when a baby's temperature shoots up very suddenly.

Fifth disease: A common childhood disease that is characterized by a fever and a bright red rash on the cheeks plus a red rash on the trunk and extremities. Also called erythema infectiosum.

Fontanelles: The two so-called soft spots that can be found in the centre and toward the back of a newborn baby's head.

Forceps: A tong-like instrument that may be placed around a baby's head to help guide the baby out of the birth canal during an instrumental vaginal delivery. Today, forceps are used less often than vacuum extraction (suction).

Foremilk: The milk that your breasts produce at the beginning of a feeding.

Frenulum: The piece of tissue that joins the bottom of the tongue to the floor of the mouth.

Gastroesophageal reflux: The movement of stomach contents up the esophagus.

German measles: See rubella.

Gestational diabetes: Diabetes that is triggered by pregnancy.

Giardia: A parasite in the stool that causes bowel infections.

Group B streptococcus: Bacteria found in the vagina and rectum of approximately 15 per cent of pregnant women. Women who test positive for group B strep may require antibiotics during labour to protect their babies from picking up this potentially life-threatening infection.

Haemophilus influenzae type b (Hib): A disease that can lead to meningitis, pneumonia, and a severe throat infection that can cause choking (epiglottitis).

Hand, foot, and mouth disease: A common childhood disease that is characterized by tiny blister-like sores in the mouth, on the palms of the hands, and on the soles of the feet. The sores are accompanied by a mild fever, a sore throat, and painful swallowing.

Hemorrhoids: Swollen blood vessels around the anus or in the rectal canal which may bleed and cause pain, especially after childbirth.

Herpangina: An inflammation of the inside of the mouth.

Hindmilk: The milk that your breasts produce toward the end of a feeding.

Hydrocephalus: An excessive increase in the fluid that cushions the brain—something that can result in brain damage.

Hypertension: High blood pressure.

Hypoglycemia: Low blood sugar.

Hypospadias: A condition in which a baby is born with the urethral opening on the underside of the glans of the penis. The penis may curve downward.

Hypothyroidism: A condition caused by an inadequate thyroid gland. If undetected or untreated, it can lead to intellectual disability.

Imperforate anus: When the anus is sealed, either because there is a tiny membrane of skin over the opening to the anus or because the anal canal failed to develop properly.

Impetigo: An infection of the skin that is characterized by yellow pustules or wide, honey-coloured scabs.

Intrauterine growth restriction (IUGR): When the baby's growth is less than what would normally be expected for a baby of that gestational age. It can be symmetric (e.g., both the head and the body are small) or asymmetric (e.g., just the body is small).

Kangaroo care: Skin-to-skin contact between parent and baby.

Kegels: Exercises that are designed to work the muscles of the pelvic floor, including those of the urethra, vagina, and rectum.

Lactation consultant: A health-care professional who is an expert on breastfeeding.

Lactiferous ducts: The canals in your breasts that transport the milk to your nipples.

Lactiferous sinuses: The milk pools in your breasts.

Lanugo: Soft, downy hair that covers parts of the body of a newborn baby.

Late neonatal death: A live-born infant who dies on or after the seventh day following birth, but before the twenty-eighth day following birth.

Lochia: The discharge of blood, mucus, and tissue from the uterus following childbirth. Lochia can last anywhere from a few weeks to six weeks or longer. It tends to be heaviest right after the birth and may contain large clots—some as large as a small lemon.

Low birth weight: Babies who weigh less than 5 pounds 8 ounces (2,500 grams) at birth. A baby who weighs less than 3 pounds (1,500 grams) at birth is considered to be a very low birth weight baby.

Mastitis: A painful infection of the breast characterized by fever, soreness, and swelling.

Meconium: The greenish-black tar-like substance that fills a baby's intestines before birth.

Meningitis: An inflammation of the membranes covering the brain and the spinal cord.

Milia: Tiny white bumps that resemble whiteheads. They appear to be raised, but they are actually flat and smooth to the touch, and are typically found on a baby's nose, forehead, and cheeks.

Miliaria: A raised rash that consists of small, fluid-filled blisters.

Milk-ejection reflex: A reflex triggered by the hormone oxytocin that causes the band-like muscles around the milk-production cells in your breast to contract, forcing the milk through your inner canal system and into your nipples, where it can be obtained by your baby. Also called the let-down reflex.

Mongolian spots: Greenish or bluish birthmarks that are caused by temporary accumulations of pigment under the skin.

Moro reflex (startle reflex): A newborn baby's instinctive reaction to any loud noise or sudden movement. He arches his back, throws open his arms and his legs, and may start to cry before pulling back his arms again.

Moulding: Temporary changes to the shape of a baby's head caused by pressure on the baby's skull during a vertex (head-first) vaginal delivery.

Mumps: An illness that is characterized by flu-like symptoms and an upset stomach followed by tender swollen glands beneath the earlobes two or three days later.

Nasogastric tube: A tube that extends through the baby's nose or mouth and into the baby's stomach.

Necrotizing enterocolitis (NEC): A disease in which intestinal tissue dies.

Neonatal death: The death of a live-born infant between birth and four weeks of age.

Neonatal intensive care unit (NICU): An intensive care unit that specializes in the care of premature, low birth-weight babies and seriously ill infants.

Neonatal urticaria: Red spots on the skin with yellowish centres that form because a baby's skin and pores are not yet working efficiently. More commonly known as newborn acne.

Neural-tube defects: Abnormalities in the development of the spinal cord and brain in a fetus, including anencephaly, hydrocephalus, and spina bifida.

Newborn jaundice: The yellowish tinge of a newborn's skin caused by too much bilirubin in the blood. Jaundice typically develops on the second or third day of life and lasts until the baby is seven to ten days old. Newborn jaundice can usually be corrected by special light treatment.

NICU: See neonatal intensive care unit.

Nursing strike: A breastfed baby's sudden refusal to nurse.

Oral pseudomembranous candidiasis: See thrush.

Otitis media: An ear infection.

Oxytocin: The naturally occurring hormone that causes uterine contractions and is responsible for triggering the milk-ejection reflex.

Paraphimosis: An emergency situation that can occur if the foreskin gets stuck when it's first retracted.

Parentese: A form of speech that parents around the world use when communicating with their babies. It involves exaggerated speech and high-pitched voices.

Pathological jaundice: A serious form of jaundice that occurs within 24 hours of the birth and that may have to be treated with a blood transfusion. It is usually the result of Rh-incompatibility between mother and baby.

Pelvic floor muscles: The group of muscles at the base of the pelvis that helps support the bladder, uterus, urethra, vagina, and rectum.

Perineum: The name given to the muscle and tissue located between the vagina and the rectum.

Pertussis: See whooping cough.

Phenylketonuria (PKU): A recessive genetic disorder in which a liver enzyme is defective, making it impossible for an individual to digest an amino acid known as phenylalanine. PKU is detected through a blood test done at birth and may be controlled by a special diet. If untreated, PKU results in intellectual disability.

Phimosis: A condition in which the foreskin and the penis are fused together.

Phototherapy: A method of treating jaundice that involves exposing the baby's skin to a special type of light that helps his body dissolve the extra pigment in the skin.

Physiological jaundice: A form of jaundice that typically occurs in three- to five-day-old babies and that disappears as the baby's liver matures.

Pinworms: Intestinal worms.

Placenta: The organ that develops in the uterus during pregnancy, providing nutrients for the fetus and eliminating its waste products.

Pneumonia: An infection of the lungs.

Polio: A disease that can result in muscle pain and paralysis and/or death.

Port wine stains: Large, flat, irregularly shaped red or purple areas that are caused by a surplus of blood vessels under the skin.

Postpartum blues: The hormone-driven wave of emotion that tends to come crashing down on about 80 per cent of new mothers three to five days after giving birth, leading to temporary, mild depression. This type of depression tends to last only a few days. If the feelings of depression last longer than this or are particularly severe, a mother may be suffering from postpartum depression.

Postpartum depression (PPD): Clinical depression that can occur at any point during the year following the delivery. Postpartum depression is characterized by sadness, impatience, restlessness, and—in particularly severe cases—an inability to care for the baby. Severe cases in which the mother suffers hallucinations or a desire to hurt the baby are classified as postpartum psychosis.

Postpartum doula: A caregiver who provides hands-on assistance to new parents during the early days postpartum.

Postpartum hemorrhage: The loss of more than 450 millilitres (15 ounces) of blood during a vaginal delivery or 1 litre (4 cups) during a Caesarean section.

Pre-eclampsia: A serious medical condition during pregnancy that is characterized by sudden edema, high blood pressure, and protein in the urine.

Pregnancy-induced hypertension (PIH): A pregnancy-related condition in which a woman's blood pressure is temporarily elevated. Her blood pressure returns to normal shortly after she gives birth.

Premature baby: A baby born before 37 completed weeks of pregnancy.

Preterm birth: A birth that occurs two weeks before the baby was due and that results in an infant who weighs less than 5 pounds 8 ounces (2,500 grams).

Primary lactation failure: A rare condition that is typically diagnosed if you fail to experience any breast changes during pregnancy.

Projectile vomiting: A condition in which a large amount of food is forcibly ejected from a baby's stomach.

Prolactin: The hormone responsible for milk production and for suppressing ovulation in a nursing mother. Prolactin is released following the delivery of the placenta and the membranes.

Pustular melanosis: Small blisters that quickly dry up and peel away, leaving dark, freckle-like spots underneath.

Pyloric stenosis: A partial blockage of the passage leading from the stomach to the small intestine. It is characterized by projectile vomiting, constipation, and/or dehydration.

Renal disease: Kidney disease.

Respiratory syncytial virus (RSV): A respiratory infection that results in a raspy cough, rapid breathing, and wheezing.

Rheumatic fever: A serious disease that can result in heart damage and/or joint swelling.

Ringworm: An itchy and flaky rash that may be ring-shaped with a raised edge.

Rooting reflex: A newborn baby's instinctive ability to root for a nipple to latch on to if her mouth is touched or her cheek is stroked on one side.

Roseola: A common childhood illness that is characterized by a high fever followed by the appearance of a faint pink rash on the trunk and the extremities. Lasts for one day.

Rotavirus: A virus in the stool that is spread through person-to-person contact.

Rubella: A disease that is characterized by a low-grade fever, flu-like symptoms, a slight cold, and a pinkish-red spotted rash that starts on the face, spreads rapidly to the trunk, and then disappears by the third day. Rubella can be harmful—even fatal—to a developing fetus. Also known as German measles.

Scarlet fever: See strep throat.

Scrotum: The pouch of skin and thin muscle tissue that holds the testes.

Seborrhoeic dermatitis: See cradle cap.

Separation anxiety: A baby's fear of being separated from the person or persons he cares most about.

Sepsis: A serious infection caused by bacteria that has entered a wound or body tissue. Commonly known as "blood poisoning."

Shigella: An illness that is caused by a virus in the stool that can be spread from person to person.

Shingles: A disease that is characterized by a rash with small blisters that begin to crust over, resulting in itching and intense and prolonged pain.

Single gene abnormalities: Genetic problems that are inherited from one or both parents.

Skin tags: Small, soft, flesh-coloured or pigmented growths of skin.

Social referencing: When a baby looks to his parents for information and guidance.

Soft spot: See fontanelles.

Spider nevi: Thin, dilated blood vessels that are spider-like in shape and that radiate outward from a central red spot.

Spina bifida: A condition in which the spinal column fails to close properly during the early weeks of embryonic development. It can result in hydrocephalus, muscle weakness or paralysis, and bowel and bladder problems.

Stale air: Air that has been previously breathed in. A key reason for removing stuffed animals and blankets from a baby's bed is to prevent the baby's face from being covered, which would result in the baby re-breathing stale air. It is believed that re-breathing stale air triggers a complex series of biochemical processes in an infant that increases the risk of SIDS.

Startle reflex: See Moro reflex.

Stem cells: The bone marrow components that are responsible for producing red cells, white cells, and platelets.

Stork bites: Pinkish, irregularly shaped patches of skin that are typically found at the nape of the neck or on the face, although they can also be found on other parts of the body.

Stranger anxiety: A baby's fear of strangers.

Strawberry hemangioma: Raised reddish-blue birthmarks that occur when an area of the skin develops an abnormal blood supply.

Strep throat: A bacterial infection that is characterized by a very sore throat, a fever, and swollen glands in the neck. If a skin rash is also present, the condition is known as scarlet fever.

Stretch marks: Reddish streaks on the skin of the breasts, abdomen, legs, and buttocks that are caused by the stretching of the skin during pregnancy. Stretch marks fade over time but they don't disappear entirely.

Stridor: Noisy or laboured breathing. Stridor occurs when a baby is breathing in and may be associated with croup.

Sudden infant death syndrome (SIDS): The sudden and unexpected death of an apparently healthy infant under one year of age that remains unexplained after all known and possible causes have been ruled out through autopsy, death scene investigation, and review of the medical history.

Tetanus: A disease that can lead to muscle spasms and death.

Thrush: A breastfeeding-related yeast infection that affects both mother and baby.

Tongue-tied: A condition that occurs when the stringy, fibrous membrane that connects the lower part of the tongue to the floor of the mouth (see frenulum) may be too tight to allow the baby's tongue to extend far enough forward to take hold of the nipple during breastfeeding.

Tonic neck reflex: A newborn baby's instinctive tendency to turn his head to one side and extend the arm and leg on that same side in a classic fencing position if placed on his back. Sometimes referred to as the fencer's reflex.

Toxoplasmosis: A parasitic infection that can cause stillbirth or miscarriage in pregnant women and congenital defects in babies.

Transitional milk: The milk that your breasts produce after they are finished producing colostrum but before they are ready to produce mature milk.

Tympanic temperature: A temperature reading that is taken using a tympanic (ear) thermometer.

Umbilical cord: The cord that connects the placenta to the developing baby, removing waste products and carbon dioxide from the baby and bringing oxygenated blood and nutrients from the mother through the placenta to the baby.

Umbilical hernia: A small swelling close to the belly button that becomes more prominent when a baby is crying.

Undescended testicles: Testicles that have not yet descended from the abdomen into the scrotum by the time a baby boy is born.

Uterus: The mother's hollow muscular organ that protects and nourishes the fetus prior to birth.

Vacuum extraction: A process in which a suction cup is attached to a vacuum pump placed on a baby's head to aid in delivery.

Varicella zoster immune globulin: A type of immune globulin that is given to prevent or minimize the severity of chicken pox.

Vascular disease: Heart disease.

Ventricular septum: The dividing wall between the right and left pumping chambers of the heart.

Vernix caseosa: A greasy white substance that coats and protects the baby's skin before birth.

Whooping cough: A disease that is characterized by a severe cough that makes it difficult to breathe, eat, or drink. Whooping cough can lead to pneumonia, convulsions, brain damage, and death.

Appendix B
ONLINE RESOURCES

Here's a list of reputable websites that you can turn to for support and information during your first year of motherhood. You will find articles and additional helpful resources on the official website for this book: www.having-a-baby.com.

Note: ♣ indicates a Canadian resource

Baby Growth Charts	
♣ Dietitians of Canada: World Health Organization Growth Charts Adapted for Canada (printable)	www.dietitians.ca/Secondary-Pages/Public/Who-Growth-Charts.aspx

Breastfeeding	
Australian Breastfeeding Association: Breastfeeding Information	www.breastfeeding.asn.au/bfinfo/index.html
♣ Breastfeeding Committee for Canada	www.breastfeedingcanada.ca
Breastfeeding Pharmacology Page: Thomas W. Hale, R.Ph. Ph.D.	www.infantrisk.org/category/breastfeeding
♣ Infact Canada: Infant Feeding Action Coalition	www.infactcanada.ca
The International Code of Marketing of Breast-Milk Substitutes: Frequently Asked Questions (brochure)	http://whqlibdoc.who.int/publications/2008/9789241594295_eng.pdf
International Lactation Consultant Association	www.ilca.org
KellyMom: Breastfeeding and Parenting	www.kellymom.com
♣ La Leche League Canada	www.lllc.ca
La Leche League International	www.llli.org
Motherisk Clinic at The Hospital for Sick Children	www.motherisk.org

♣ Newman Breastfeeding Clinic and Institute	www.breastfeedinginc.ca
♣ PhD in Parenting	www.phdinparenting.com
World Health Organization: Evidence for the Ten Steps to Successful Breastfeeding (book)	www.who.int/nutrition/publications/evidence_ten_step_eng.pdf

Infant Development, Play, and Learning

The Association for the Study of Play (TASP)	www.tasplay.org
♣ Canadian Child Care Federation	www.cccf-fcsge.ca
♣ Canadian Library Association	www.cla.ca
♣ Centre of Excellence for Early Childhood Development	www.excellence-earlychildhood.ca
♣ Centre of Knowledge on Healthy Child Development	www.knowledge.offordcentre.com
♣ Child and Family Canada	www.cfc-efc.ca
♣ Child Care Advocacy Association of Canada	www.ccaac.ca
♣ Childcare Resource and Research Unit	www.childcarecanada.org
♣ Handbook of Language and Literacy Development: A Roadmap from 0 to 60 Months	www.theroadmap.ualberta.ca
♣ Nipissing District Developmental Screen	www.ndds.ca
No Time for Flash Cards	www.notimeforflashcards.com
♣ Ontario Coalition for Better Child Care	www.childcareontario.org
Zero to Three	www.zerotothree.org

Infant Health and Safety

♣ Canada Safety Council	http://canadasafetycouncil.org
♣ Canadian Red Cross	www.redcross.ca
♣ Canadian Toy Testing Council	www.toy-testing.org
♣ CanChild Centre for Childhood Disability Research	www.canchild.ca
Centers for Disease Control and Prevention: Parent Portal	www.cdc.gov/parents/
♣ Health Canada: Healthy Babies	www.hc-sc.gc.ca/hl-vs/babies-bebes/index-eng.php
♣ Infant and Toddler Safety Association	www.infantandtoddlersafety.ca
Juvenile Products Manufacturers Association	www.jpma.org

National Association for the Education of Young Children	www.naeyc.org
♣ Safe Kids Canada	www.safekidscanada.com
♣ Safe Start	www.bcchildrens.ca/KidsTeensFam/ChildSafety/SafeStart
St. John Ambulance	www.sja.ca

Postpartum Health

♣ Canadian Association of Midwives (links to all Provincial/Territorial associations)	www.canadianmidwives.org
♣ Childbirth and Postpartum Professional Association	www.cappacanada.ca
Childbirth Connection	www.childbirthconnection.org
Coalition for Improving Maternity Services	www.motherfriendly.org
Consumers Supporting Midwifery Care	www.midwiferyconsumers.org
DONA International (doulas)	www.dona.org
International Childbirth Education Association	www.icea.org
Lamaze International: Science and Sensibility	www.scienceandsensibility.org
♣ Mothers of Change	www.mothersofchange.com
National Advocates for Pregnant Women	http://advocatesforpregnantwomen.org
♣ Power to Push Campaign	www.powertopush.ca
♣ Public Health Agency of Canada: The Maternity Experiences Survey	www.phac-aspc.gc.ca/rhs-ssg/survey-eng.php
♣ Society of Obstetricians and Gynaecologists of Canada	www.sogc.org

Perinatal Mood Disorders (including Postpartum Depression and Anxiety)

♣ Here to Help	http://heretohelp.bc.ca/publications/factsheets/postpartum
MGH Women's Mental Health Center	www.womensmentalhealth.org
♣ Mood Disorders Society of Canada	www.mooddisorderscanada.ca
♣ Mother Reach: Perinatal Mood and Anxiety Disorders	www.helpformom.ca
♣ Pacific Post Partum Support Society	www.postpartum.org
Postpartum Men	www.postpartummen.com
Postpartum Progress	www.postpartumprogress.com
Postpartum Support International	www.postpartum.net

Perinatal Loss and Birth Trauma

♣ Bereaved Families of Ontario	www.bereavedfamilies.net
♣ Birth Trauma Canada	www.birthtraumacanada.org
♣ Canadian Foundation for the Study of Infant Deaths	www.sidscanada.org
♣ The Compassionate Friends of Canada	www.tcfcanada.net
♣ Glow in the Woods: For Babylost Parents	www.glowinthewoods.com
Hygeia Foundation	http://hygeiafoundation.org/resources
♣ Pregnancy and Infant Loss Network	www.pailnetwork.ca
Share Pregnancy and Infant Loss Support	www.nationalshare.org
Subsequent Pregnancy After a Loss Support	www.spals.com

Women's Health

♣ Canadian Association for the Advancement of Women and Sport: Mothers in Motion	www.caaws.ca/mothersinmotion/e/index.cfm
♣ Canadian Federation for Sexual Health	www.cfsh.ca
♣ Canadian Foundation for Women's Health	www.cfwh.org
♣ Canadian Women's Health Network	www.cwhn.ca
♣ Centres for Excellence for Women's Health	www.cewh-cesf.ca
♣ The Fat Nutritionist	www.fatnutritionist.com
♣ National Eating Disorder Information Centre	www.nedic.ca
♣ National Network on Environments and Women's Health	www.nnewh.org
♣ Serena Canada: Mastering the Menstrual Cycle	www.serena.ca
Uppity Science Chick	www.uppitysciencechick.com
♣ Women's Health Data Directory	www.womenshealthdata.ca
♣ Women's Health Matters	www.womenshealthmatters.ca
♣ YWCA Canada	www.ywcacanada.ca

Work-Life and Parental Leave

♣ Canadian Centre for Occupational Health and Safety	www.ccohs.ca
♣ Childcare Resource and Research Unit	www.childcarecanada.org
Family and Parenting Institute	www.familyandparenting.org

Parenting in the Workplace Institute	www.parentingatwork.org
❖ Service Canada: Having a Baby (guide to government services)	www.servicecanada.gc.ca/eng/lifeevents/baby.shtml
Sloan Work and Family Research Network	http://wfnetwork.bc.edu
❖ Work-Life Harmony	www.worklifeharmony.ca

Family Health and Wellness

❖ Canadian Centre on Substance Abuse	www.ccsa.ca
❖ Canadian Fitness and Lifestyle Research Institute	www.cflri.ca
❖ Canadian Mental Health Association	www.cmha.ca
❖ Dietitians of Canada	www.dietitians.ca
EWG's Skin Deep Cosmetics Database	www.ewg.org/skindeep/
❖ Health Canada: Licensed Natural Health Products Database	www.hc-sc.gc.ca/dhp-mps/prodnatur/applications/licen-prod/lnhpd-bdpsnh-eng.php
❖ Healthy Canadians	www.healthycanadians.gc.ca
HealthyChildren.org	www.healthychildren.org
National Center for Complementary and Alternative Medicine	http://nccam.nih.gov
National Institutes of Health: PubMed.gov research database search tool	www.ncbi.nlm.nih.gov/pubmed

Health Associations

❖ Aboriginal Nurses Association of Canada	www.anac.on.ca
❖ Canadian Association of Paediatric Health Centres	www.caphc.org
❖ Canadian Association of Speech-Language Pathologists and Audiologists (CASLPA)	www.caslpa.ca
❖ Canadian Dental Association	www.cda-adc.ca
❖ Canadian Dermatology Association	www.dermatology.ca
❖ Canadian Immunization Awareness Program	www.immunize.ca
❖ Canadian Institute of Child Health	www.cich.ca
❖ Canadian Medical Association	www.cma.ca
❖ Canadian Nurses Association	www.cna-nurses.ca
❖ Canadian Paediatric Society: Caring for Kids	www.caringforkids.cps.ca
❖ Canadian Pharmacists Association	www.pharmacists.ca

♣ Canadian Public Health Association	www.cpha.ca
♣ Canadian Society for Exercise Physiology	www.csep.ca
♣ College of Family Physicians of Canada	www.cfpc.ca
♣ Community Health Nurses of Canada	www.chnc.ca
♣ Health Canada	www.hc-sc.gc.ca
♣ Public Health Agency of Canada	www.phac-aspc.gc.ca

Specific Health and Medical Conditions

About Face International	www.aboutfaceinternational.org
♣ Allergy/Asthma Information Association	www.aaia.ca
♣ Asthma Society of Canada	www.asthma.ca
♣ Canadian AIDS Society	www.cdnaids.ca
♣ Canadian Cancer Society	www.cancer.ca
♣ Canadian Diabetes Association	www.diabetes.ca
♣ Canadian Association of the Deaf	www.cad.ca
♣ Canadian Directory of Genetic Support Groups	www.lhsc.on.ca/programs/medgenet/support.htm
♣ Canadian Down Syndrome Society	www.cdss.ca
♣ Canadian Hemophilia Society	www.hemophilia.ca
♣ Canadian Liver Foundation	www.liver.ca
♣ Canadian Lung Association	www.lung.ca
♣ Canadian National Institute for the Blind (CNIB)	www.cnib.ca
♣ Canadian Organization for Rare Disorders	www.cord.ca
♣ Canadian Spinal Research Organization	www.csro.com
♣ Crohn's and Colitis Foundation of Canada	www.ccfc.ca
♣ Cystic Fibrosis Canada	www.cysticfibrosis.ca
♣ Easter Seals Canada	www.easterseals.ca
♣ Epilepsy Canada	www.epilepsy.ca
♣ The Kidney Foundation of Canada	www.kidney.ca
♣ Lupus Canada	www.lupuscanada.org
♣ Multiple Sclerosis Society of Canada	www.mssociety.ca
♣ Muscular Dystrophy Canada	www.mdac.ca

APPENDIX B — ONLINE RESOURCES | 425

♦ Ontario Association of Children's Rehabilitation Services	www.oacrs.com/en/usefullinks
♦ Spina Bifida and Hydrocephalus Canada	www.sbhac.ca
♦ Thyroid Foundation of Canada	www.thyroid.ca
♦ Turner Syndrome Society of Canada	www.turnersyndrome.ca
Parenting Resources	
♦ Adoption Council of Canada	www.adoption.ca
♦ About Kids Health	www.aboutkidshealth.ca
Ask Moxie	www.askmoxie.org
♦ Best Start: My Child and I: Attachment for Life (booklet)	www.beststart.org/resources/hlthy_chld_dev/pdf/parent_attachment_eng.pdf
Brain, Child: The Magazine for Thinking Mothers	www.brainchildmag.com
Campaign for a Commercial-Free Childhood	www.commercialfreechildhood.org
♦ Canadian Association of Family Resource Programs	www.frp.ca
♦ Canadian Family	www.canadianfamily.ca
♦ The Canadian Fatherhood Involvement Initiative	www.cfii.ca
Doing Good Together: Family Volunteering and Caring Kids	http://doinggoodtogether.org
♦ FamilyDoctor.org	www.familydoctor.org
Fathering: A Journal of Theory, Research, and Practice About Men as Fathers	www.mensstudies.com
♦ Father Involvement Research Alliance	www.fira.ca
Literary Mama	http://literarymama.com
♦ Motherhood Initiative for Research and Community Involvement	www.motherhoodinitiative.org
The Mothers Movement Online	www.mothersmovement.org
Mothering	www.mothering.com
♦ Multiple Births Canada	www.multiplebirthscanada.org
Museum of Motherhood	www.mommuseum.org
Natural Child Magazine	www.naturalchildmagazine.com
New American Dream	www.newdream.org
Search Institute: Developmental Assets Lists	www.search-institute.org/developmental-assets/lists

Sustainable Mothering	www.sustainablemothering.com
♣ 24 Hour Cribside Assistance for New Dads	www.newdadmanual.ca
♣ Vanier Institute of the Family	www.vifamily.ca
Healthy Communities	
♣ Atkinson Centre for Society and Child Development	www.oise.utoronto.ca/atkinson/Main/index.html
♣ Campaign 2000: End Child and Family Poverty in Canada	www.campaign2000.ca
♣ Canadian Centre for Policy Alternatives	www.policyalternatives.ca
♣ Canadian Coalition for the Rights of Children	www.rightsofchildren.ca
♣ Canadian Council on Social Development	www.ccsd.ca
♣ Canadian Index of Wellbeing	www.ciw.ca
♣ Canadian Partnership for Children's Health & Environment	www.healthyenvironmentforkids.ca
♣ Roots of Empathy	www.rootsofempathy.org
♣ Vanier Institute of the Family	www.vifamily.ca

Index

A

abdominal muscle separation, 53
abdominal pain, 42, 264, 276, 290, 294, 297
About Face International, 424
abscess, breast, 204, 409
acetaminophen, 57, 203, 216, 263, 264, 272, 273–75, 278, 279, 281, 282, 283, 285, 291, 292, 293, 294, 296, 316
Adamec, Christine, 130
adoption, 130, 209
Adoption Council of Canada, 425
advice, coping with unwanted, 79, 80, 141–42
afterpains, 52–53, 153
Agency for Healthcare Research and Quality, 273
AIDS, 424
alcohol, 93, 104, 112, 185–86, 265, 334, 338
Allergy/Asthma Information Association, 424
amniotic fluid, 8, 11, 16, 29, 35, 164, 329, 409
anemia, 32, 33, 34, 71, 281
  during postpartum period, 58
  sickle-cell, 281
anencephaly, 329, 409, 414
Angiers, Natalie, 127
announcements, baby, 6
antibiotics, 45, 204, 206, 220, 262–63, 272, 273, 274–75, 276, 277, 278, 296, 297, 412

anus, 32, 286, 296
  imperforate, 412
Apgar, Virginia, 28
apgar test, 27, 28, 409
areola, 23, 99, 107, 153, 155, 189, 197, 198, 199, 201, 205, 409
arms, 12, 18, 20, 23, 25, 31, 99, 146, 159, 214, 215, 236, 242, 260, 278, 316, 372, 374, 376, 378, 394, 397, 413
asphyxia, perinatal, 34–35
Asthma Society of Canada, 424
axillary temperature, 259, 260, 409

B

baby blues, 11, 133
baby care, 3, 77, 93, 120, 139, 213–42
baby carriers, 67, 108, 116, 174, 310
baby food, making your own, 3, 343, 346, 347, 348–51
baby gate, 301
baby lotion, 239
baby oil, 226, 280
baby powder, 219, 221, 267
baby sling, 106, 115, 174, 237–38
baby swing, 325
baby walkers, 307
baby wipes, 215, 220
baby's room, decorating, 302–03
babyproofing, 298–303, 309, 389–90
balanoposthitis, 409
bassinets, 7–8, 301, 325

bathing, 119–20, 213, 223, 235, 237, 239, 240, 280, 304, 330
  sponge baths, 223, 235, 237, 238, 265
bathtub, baby, 46, 119, 120, 223, 237–40, 303, 352, 397
Bereaved Families of Ontario, 422
bibs, 231, 345
bilirubin, 36–38, 409, 414
Bing, Elisabeth, 142
birth, first minutes after, 28–29, 177, 222, 334, 409
birth control, 74, 75
  breastfeeding moms, 73–74
birth defects, 250
birth experiences, 88
birth registration, 38–39
birthing doula, 88, 93, 410, 415, 421
birthmarks, 12, 18, 19, 413, 417
birthweight, low, 272
biting, 135, 178–179, 318
bleeding, 8, 32–33, 44–45, 49, 62, 70, 223, 227, 288, 314–15
  vaginal, 41–42, 68
blindness, 33
body image, postpartum, 54, 70
boils, 277–78, 409
bonding, 6, 8, 10, 82, 144, 145, 321, 388
bottlefeeding, 70, 93, 103, 181, 182, 186–87, 188, 189, 192, 207, 230, 266, 342, 352, 353, 354
bottles, 305
bowel movements (see also stools; illnesses, diarrhea), 38, 43, 51, 52, 101, 107, 176, 220, 255, 286, 286, 288–89, 294, 359
breast cancer, 180
breast care, 56
breast changes, 54–57, 191, 415
breast milk, 56, 63, 64–65, 84, 104, 106, 109, 110, 137, 162, 174, 180, 181, 182, 183, 185–86, 187, 188, 189, 192, 194–95, 202, 208, 227, 228, 251, 285, 288, 289–90, 339, 342, 353, 356
  appearance, 102, 164
  colostrum, 54, 101, 151, 152, 153, 159, 161, 185, 288, 410, 417

expressing, 187, 198, 201, 207, 208, 209
foremilk, 411
hindmilk, 412
premature babies, 206–07
pumping, 106, 107, 109, 157, 164, 193, 194, 198, 207, 322, 418
supply, 63, 99–100, 101, 102, 151, 165, 166, 186, 321,
taste, 64, 169, 177–78
transitional milk, 101, 152, 417
breastfeeding,
  after adoption, 206, 209
  after breast reduction, 206, 209–10
  after breast surgery, 206, 209–10
  after Caesarean, 161
  alcohol and, 104, 185–86
  and working, 189, 191–92
  as birth control, 73–74
  benefits, 8–9, 62–63, 65, 81, 93, 98, 100, 101–04, 110, 115, 135, 145, 149–79
  biting, 178, 179
  breast abscess, 204, 409
  breast infection, 105, 106, 108, 177–78, 199, 201, 202, 203, 204, 334
  breast pad, 55, 56, 99, 105, 200, 201, 202, 204
  breast pumps, 55, 105, 107, 109, 192, 193, 194, 197, 205, 322
  breast shells, 200
  caffeine, 103, 356
  cleft lip, 109, 162, 208, 410
  cleft palate, 31, 109, 162, 208, 410
  common questions, 158–91
  congenital problems, 13, 208
  cystic fibrosis, 209
  diarrhea and, 152, 255
  domperidone, 163–64
  Down Syndrome, 208–09
  ducts, plugged, 185, 190, 202–03
  engorgement, 43, 54–55, 196, 197, 199, 334, 409
  expressing breastmilk, 54, 55, 106, 107, 193, 194, 197, 198, 201, 322, 332, 334, 398
  frequency, 161–62, 175, 203
  fussy baby, 173–74
  growth spurts, 100

INDEX | 429

herbal products, 104, 186
hormones, 73, 110, 115, 151, 166
lactation consultant, 56, 81, 105, 109, 157, 163, 177, 200, 201, 322, 412, 419
lactation device, 181, 186
lactation failure, primary, 162, 181, 415
Lactational Amenorrhoea Method, 73
latch, 9, 24, 26, 31, 56, 98, 99, 105-09, 126, 155, 156, 157, 162, 175, 177-79, 181, 186, 187, 189, 197, 199, 200, 201, 207, 208, 298, 301, 302, 304, 415
leaking, 55, 73, 191, 201-02, 334
length of feedings, 160-62, 170
let-down reflex, 153, 157, 176, 413
mastitis, 108, 190, 197, 202, 203-204, 413
maternal lifestyle, 185
maternal weight, 62-63, 64
medications, 57, 91, 104, 108, 177, 179-80, 185, 197, 199
menstruation while, 72, 210
milk supply, 63, 99, 102, 103, 106, 107, 109, 153, 158, 161, 162, 163, 164, 166, 167, 176, 178, 186, 192, 196, 200, 210, 321, 322, 402
milk-ejection reflex, 204, 413, 414
multiples, 206, 210-11
nipple confusion, 188
nipple shields, 200
nipples, cracked, 196, 199, 203
nipples, flat, 43, 107, 196, 200, 201
nipples, sore, 56, 105, 106, 107, 157, 165, 185, 189, 199, 200, 201, 204
nursing bras, 56, 67, 105
nursing strike, 106, 177, 178, 191, 203, 414
phenylketonuria, 181
placental fragments, 162
plugged ducts, 185, 190, 202-03,
positioning, 107, 162, 372
premature baby, 206-07
problems, 55-56, 100, 105, 196, 201, 286

protection against SIDS, 103, 104, 112, 185-86, 294, 324, 327
pumping, 106, 107, 109, 157, 164, 193, 194, 198, 207, 322, 418
rooting reflex, 24-25, 26, 98, 146, 158, 415
science of, 151-55
sleepy baby, 9, 38, 105, 106, 158, 165, 178, 179, 186
smoking, 104, 112, 186
special circumstances, 206-11
supplementing, 151, 154, 162, 165, 170, 181, 182, 183, 184, 186
switching sides, 160, 210
thrush, 108, 199, 204-06, 417
vaginal dryness, 49, 73
vs. bottlefeeding, 102, 103, 104, 110, 154, 180-81, 182, 184, 202, 205, 208, 220, 228, 272, 285, 288, 326, 353
weaning, 142, 149, 170, 190, 191
weight gain, 167, 169, 184, 208, 240, 321
Breastfeeding Committee for Canada, 419
burns, 46, 48, 56, 182, 220, 224, 225, 226, 284, 305, 306, 314, 316, 371
burping, 159, 174, 175, 294

C

Caesarean, 12, 14, 409, 411, 415
breastfeeding after, 161
gas pains, 61
incision, 43, 54
recovery, 42, 43, 44, 45, 50, 52, 60-62, 68, 128
Caesarean, scar, 41, 62, 71
café au lait marks, 18, 410
campylobacteriosis, 285
Canada Safety Council, 420
Canada's Food Guide to Healthy Eating, 172-73
Canadian AIDS Society, 424
Canadian Association of Family Resource Programs, 425
Canadian Association of Speech-Language Pathologists and Audiologists, 423
Canadian Association of the Deaf, 424
Canadian Cancer Society, 424

Canadian Child Care Federation, 420
Canadian Dental Association, 227, 229, 423
Canadian Dermatology Association, 225, 423
Canadian Diabetes Association, 424
Canadian Down Syndrome Society, 424
Canadian Hemophilia Society, 424
Canadian Institute of Child Health, 188, 207, 267, 423
Canadian Liver Foundation, 424
Canadian Lung Association, 424
Canadian Medical Association, 51, 423
Canadian Mental Health Association, 423
Canadion National Institute for the Blind, 424
Canadian Nurses Association, 423
Canadian Organization for Rare Disorders, 424
Canadian Paediatric Society, 2, 34, 166, 168, 182, 183, 189, 235, 245, 262–63, 270, 325, 327, 356, 390, 423
Canadian Red Cross, 314, 420
Canadian Toy Testing Council, 420
Canadian Women's Health Network, 422
cancer, 104, 179, 180, 250, 251, 424
car safety, 311–13
car seats, 60, 225, 238, 310–13, 325
car travel, 243
cardiorespiratory distress, 35
career, 139, 402, 404
caregivers (see health care practitioners)
carotenoids, 153
cavernous hemangioma, 18, 410
cellulitis, 278, 410
cerebral palsy, 37
checkup, newborn, 36
chicken pox vaccine, 250–51, 418
child care, 70, 401
    caregiver-child ratios, 401, 420
Child Care Advocacy Association, 420
Childbirth and Postpartum Professional Association, 421
Childcare Resource and Research Unit, 401, 420, 422
Children's National Medical Center, 327
chloasma (see mask of pregnancy)

choking, 113, 168, 182, 227, 233, 246, 302, 305–07, 314, 315, 316–17, 338, 342, 343, 351, 355, 412
chromosomal anomalies, 329, 410
circumcision, 21, 222–23, 410
clothes, 70, 104, 201, 202, 224, 231, 232, 233, 234, 300
clubfoot, 31, 410
colic, 67, 103, 104, 114, 115, 116, 117, 118
collarbone, broken, 31
College of Family Physicians of Canada, 221, 222, 260, 261, 272, 290, 424
Colman, Libby, 127, 142
colostrum, 54, 101, 151, 152, 153, 159, 161, 185, 288, 410, 417
congenital anomalies, 30, 128, 329
congenital pigmented nevi, 19, 410
contraceptives (see birth control)
contraceptives, oral, 75
corn syrup, 168
co-sleeping, 186, 410
coughing, 254, 268–69, 274, 278, 319, 379
cradles, 131, 210–11, 301, 325, 330, 335
crawling reflex, 26
crib sheets, 231
cribs, 298
Crohn's and Colitis Foundation of Canada, 424
crying, 1, 23, 29, 32, 45, 55, 80, 97, 114, 115, 116, 117, 118, 120, 121, 127, 129, 137, 143, 145, 146, 151, 155, 158, 160, 168, 175, 177, 199, 243, 262, 290, 294, 321, 329, 372, 373, 387, 417

D

d'Harcourt, Claire, 338
Davis, Deborah, 131, 132, 320, 324, 329, 330, 333
deafness, 37, 424
death (see infant death)
demand feeding (see feeding)
dental care, 227
dental problems, 167
Depo-Provera, 75
detergent, 221, 224, 300, 306

INDEX | 431

developmental milestones, 80, 244, 367–68, 385
  cognitive, 369–84, 385
  physical, 385
  social, 369, 426
diabetes, 424
  gestational, 13, 329, 412
diaper rash, 204, 218, 220, 221, 222, 320, 359
diapering, 213, 215, 217, 222
diapers, 106, 107, 119, 125, 126, 165, 176, 215–16, 217, 219, 221, 222, 359
  number of wet, 106, 165, 359
diastasis recti abdominis, 53, 410
dislocatable hip, 31
disorders, rare, 33, 424
dizziness, 45, 68, 258
doctor, 2, 15, 18, 19, 27, 45, 52, 68, 71, 73, 86, 89, 104, 118, 130, 140, 142, 189, 203, 205, 208, 209, 230, 237, 243, 244, 253, 258, 262, 265, 268, 269, 286, 287, 289, 290, 315, 316, 333, 339, 344, 385, 425
  newborn checkup, 28–36
  when to call, 16, 19, 44, 49, 114, 120, 131, 163–64, 174, 176, 185, 203–04, 221, 223, 224, 227, 243, 245, 249, 254, 261, 264, 266, 270–86, 287, 288, 290, 291–97, 314, 318, 319–20, 328, 331, 334, 340, 368, 369, 385, 387
doll's eye reflex, 26
domperidone, 163–64
Doron, Mia Wescher, 24
doulas,
  birthing, 88, 410
  postpartum, 93, 410, 415
Down Syndrome, 109, 162, 208, 385, 410, 424
dressing a baby, 231, 234–35
drooling, 262, 271, 319
drugs, 22, 35, 49, 185, 259, 280, 324, 334

E

ears, 11, 16, 24, 30, 60, 92, 236, 242, 252, 258, 273, 279, 284 (*see also* hearing)
Easter Seal, 424

Eberlein, Tamara, 207, 210
eclampsia, 13, 329, 411, 415
epidural, 411
Epilepsy Canada, 424
episiotomy, 43, 45, 46, 47, 49, 51, 72, 411
epispadias, 21, 411
erythromycin ointment, 33, 411
eyes, 7, 11, 15, 22, 24, 26, 30, 33, 38, 60, 105, 146, 225, 236, 249, 252, 255, 256, 260, 266, 267, 282, 290, 292, 318, 319, 369, 373, 375, 380, 393 (*see also* vision)

F

falls, 301, 303
family resource programs, 406, 425
father's experience, 10, 71, 80, 83, 128, 133, 134, 137, 139, 140, 333, 405, 411, 425
feeding, (*see also* bottlefeeding, breastfeeding)
  demand, 99–100, 153, 286
  feeding, frequency, 161, 162, 175, 203
  growth spurts, 100
  hunger signals, 146, 158, 178
  weight gain, 167, 184, 208, 353–54
feet, 12, 16, 20, 25–26, 27, 29, 30, 69, 78, 101, 159, 281, 383, 394, 410, 412
femoral pulse, 32
fencer's reflex, 26, 417
fertility, 21
fever, strips, 260
fever, treating a, 203–04, 262–65, 278, 279, 282, 283, 291, 292, 293, 294
fingernails, 20, 227, 279, 280, 282, 296
first aid, 314–19
fluoride, 230
Fontanel, Béatrice, 338
fontanelles, 14, 30, 214, 238, 255, 262, 290, 295, 411, 416
food, solid, 3, 52, 74, 166, 169, 183, 188, 189, 219, 228, 229, 266, 276, 284, 290, 337, 338, 339–45, 253, 256
food guide, 65, 171, 172
forceps, 12, 51, 411

foremilk, 411
foreskin, 21, 218, 409, 410, 414
formula, 74, 102, 103, 104, 110, 151, 154, 175, 176, 180, 181, 182, 183, 184, 186, 189, 202, 205, 208, 209, 220, 228, 231, 272, 285, 288, 289, 290, 294, 326, 353, 356
frenulum, 31, 109, 208, 411, 417
frostbite, 226
fundus, 42, 53
fussiness, 103, 250, 272, 273, 278, 320 (see also crying, colic)

G
galactosemia, 180, 181, 182
genitals, 11, 20, 22, 30, 32, 222
Gentian violet, 205
gestational age, 29, 35, 324, 338, 385, 412
grandparents, 117, 330, 332, 379
grasping reflex, 25
grief, 52, 61, 82, 131, 132, 323, 329, 330, 332, 333, 334, 335
groin, 32, 279
growth charts, 184, 419
growth spurts, 100

H
hair, 11, 14, 16, 19, 23, 59, 196, 226, 237, 238, 331, 394, 413
  loss, 59
handling a baby, 214–15
hands, 8, 12, 16, 20, 23, 27, 29, 146, 165
Harvard School of Public Health, 201
head, 10, 11, 12, 13–14, 30
head injury, 318–19
Health Canada, 2, 33, 164, 172, 172, 183, 233, 240, 264, 310, 313, 327, 338, 353, 420, 423, 424
health care practitioners, 189, 333
health, infant, 3, 42 (see also illness)
health insurance, 2, 39
hearing, 22, 34, 135, 272, 273, 329, 333, 370, 373, 375, 379
heartrate, 27, 28, 29, 36, 82, 269, 321, 409
hemangioma,
  capillary, 18, 410
  cavernous, 18, 410
  strawberry, 18, 351, 410, 417
hemorrhage, postpartum, 43, 44, 45, 50, 415
hemorrhoids, 46, 48
herbal teas, 356
hernia, umbilical, 19, 32, 417
high blood pressure, 13, 35, 412, 415
high chair, 298, 304, 306, 340, 341, 345, 352, 392, 396
high-risk pregnancy, 130
  adjustment after, 72
hindmilk, 412
HIV, 180, 249
honey, 168, 328, 356
hormonal changes, 11, 57, 71, 87, 151, 210
hospital, 6, 8, 9, 33, 35, 36, 37, 38, 39, 58, 62, 81, 84, 132, 163, 166, 193, 220, 243, 267, 270, 275, 291, 296, 301, 314, 315, 316, 319, 321, 322, 323, 330, 331, 333
Hospital for Sick Children, 185, 209, 344, 419
hospitalization, baby, 319–32
Human Resources Development Canada, 39
humidifier, 226, 267–68
hydrocephalus, 329, 412, 414, 416, 425
hypertension, 13, 35, 411, 412, 415
hypoglycemia, 29, 180, 412
hypospadis, 21, 412
hypothyroidism, 33, 412

I
Ikramuddin, Aisha, 302–03
illness,
  abdominal pain, 42, 264, 276, 290, 294, 297
  allergies, 173, 254, 267, 280, 339, 341, 354
  asthma, 262, 268, 269, 360, 409, 424
  behavioural changes, 256, 319
  bloody stools, 288
  boils, 277, 278, 409
  breathing, noisy, 267, 274
  breathing difficulties, 271, 417
  bronchiolitis, 269, 409
  bronchitis, 269, 409

INDEX | 433

campylobacteriosis, 285
caring for a sick baby, 243
cellulitis, 278, 410
chicken pox, 180, 181, 250, 278, 279, 284
chlamydia, 33
cold, common, 253, 254, 258, 270, 274, 277
conjunctivitis, 274
constipation, 51, 52, 58, 65, 285, 286, 288, 415
convulsions, 246, 250, 260, 261, 262, 283, 297, 318, 319, 411, 418
coughing, 154, 268–69, 274, 278, 319, 379
cradle cap, 14, 279, 410, 416
cramps, 255, 258, 285, 291, 292, 293, 354
croup, 254, 271, 410, 417
cystic fibrosis, 209, 424
cytomegalovirus (CMV), 34–35, 410
dehydration, 57, 181, 224, 255, 263, 264, 269, 275, 276, 282, 283, 284, 289, 290, 291, 293, 295, 415
diarrhea, 57, 152, 252, 255, 258, 262, 282, 285, 286, 289, 290, 291–95, 353, 354
difficulty swallowing, 281, 282, 412
dizziness, 45, 68, 258
drooling, 262, 271, 319
e. coli, 291
ear infections, 167, 190, 245, 249, 252, 257, 258, 267, 272–273, 276, 283, 286, 295, 360, 414
eczema, 14, 227, 280, 360, 411
encephalitis, 250, 283, 411
encephalopathy, 35
epiglottitis, 262, 411, 412
erythema infectiosum, 281, 411
escherichia coli, 291
eye infections, 11, 237
febrile convulsions, 260, 261, 283, 411
fever, 42, 45, 61, 106, 108, 203, 204, 221, 241, 243, 249, 250, 251, 252, 253, 255, 256, 257, 258, 261, 262, 263, 270, 271,

272, 273, 274–76, 279, 281, 282, 284, 285, 290, 291, 293, 295, 296, 297, 315, 334, 411, 412, 414, 415, 416, 417
fifth disease, 281, 411
flu, 252–53, 296
food poisoning, 291, 295
gas, 60, 61, 292
gastroesophageal reflux, 108, 114, 174, 178, 294, 295, 360, 411
gastrointestinal conditions, 285–86
gastrointestinal illness, 255, 285, 286, 288, 339
giardia, 291, 292, 412
gonorrhea, 33
group B streptococcus, 412
hand, foot, and mouth disease, 412
headache, 45, 242, 262, 270
heart disease, congenital, 22
heat stroke, 256
hemophilia, 424
hepatitis A, 292
herpangina, 281, 412
herpes, 35, 180, 410
impetigo, 271, 275, 282, 412
influenza, 252–53, 296
jaundice, 32, 35, 36–37, 38, 105, 159, 256, 292, 329, 414
kidney disease, 22, 276, 415
lockjaw, 297
measles, 246, 247, 248, 249, 250, 282, 283, 412, 416
meningitis, 35, 246, 249, 250, 252, 261, 261, 262, 275, 295, 296, 412, 413
milia, 17, 413
miliaria, 17, 413
mumps, 247, 248, 249, 250, 296, 413
muscle spasms, 57, 246, 297, 417
nausea, 45, 68, 252, 258, 291, 292
Norwalk virus, 292
pertussis, 246, 247, 414
pink eye, 256, 274
pinworms, 296, 360, 414
pneumonia, 246, 249, 250, 252, 255, 261, 262, 274, 275, 276, 283, 412, 414, 418
polio, 246, 247, 414

projectile vomiting, 102, 174, 294, 295, 415
pyloric stenosis, 295, 415
rashes, 38, 222, 256
respiratory syncytial virus (RSV), 275, 415
Reye's syndrome, 279
rheumatic fever, 276, 415
ringworm, 415
roseola, 283, 416
rotavirus, 247, 251, 293, 416
rubella, 35, 247, 248, 249, 250, 283, 284, 412, 416
runny nose, 60, 249, 252, 253, 254, 258, 267, 269, 270, 274
salmonella, 293
scarlet fever, 276, 284, 416, 417
seborrhoeic dermatitis, 416
sepsis, 35, 416
shigella, 293, 416
shingles, 278, 284, 416
sinusitis, 276
skin and scalp conditions, 277–78
skin blotches, 12, 251, 262
skin changes, 256, 331
skin infections, 276
sore joints, 281
sore muscles, 258
sore throat, 252, 257, 258, 270, 271, 276, 281, 412, 417
stiff neck, 262, 295, 296
strep throat, 275, 276, 284, 416, 417
stridor, 271, 417
swollen glands, 258, 276, 284, 296, 413, 417
syphilis, 34–35
tetanus, 246, 247, 297, 417
thrush, 108, 199, 204–206, 417
tonsillitis, 258, 276, 284
urinary tract infection, 50, 69, 297
vomiting, 45, 49, 102, 174, 252, 255, 256, 258, 262, 264, 274, 284, 286, 289, 291, 292, 293, 294, 295, 296, 319, 354, 415
wheezing, 249, 251, 254, 268, 269, 275, 314, 354, 415
whooping cough, 246, 277, 414, 418
yeast infections, 206, 222

immunities, 54, 251
immunization, 152, 243, 244, 245, 246, 247, 248, 249, 250, 251, 252, 253, 256, 423
incision, 43, 45, 54, 60, 61, 409, 411
incontinence, 48, 49, 50, 51, 66, 67, 68
INFACT Canada, 419
Infant and Toddler Safety Association, 298, 420
infant care (*see* baby care)
infant death, 113, 130, 168, 243, 267, 306, 310, 327, 328, 329, 417
infant massage, 118, 240–41
infertility, 130
injuries, birth-related, 30, 31
intestinal protrusions, 32
intrauterine growth restriction, 412

J
Jackson, Marni, 1, 143
joint laxity, 60, 68
joint soreness, 281

K
kangaroo care, 156, 167, 207, 321, 412
Kegels, 50, 69, 412
kidney disease, 22, 276, 415
Kidney Foundation of Canada, 424
kidneys, 32
Kitzinger, Sheila, 97

L
La Leche League, 104, 110, 162, 163, 175, 193, 200, 322, 419
lactiferous sinuses, 412
lactogen, 151
Landsberg, Michele, 149
lanugo, 11, 16, 23, 30, 30, 413
Lee, Valerie, 298
learning disabilities, 22
legs, 12, 18, 20, 31
let-down reflex, 153, 157, 413
Linden, Dana Weschler, 24
linea nigra, 54
linens, baby, 231
liver, 32, 36, 37, 170, 180, 251, 279, 288, 292, 414, 424

INDEX | 435

lochia, 42–45, 62, 413
Luke, Barbara, 210
lungs, 7, 23, 209, 250, 254, 268, 269, 287, 409, 414
Lupus Canada, 424

M
mask of pregnancy, 54
maternal health, 13
maternal instinct, 79, 97, 131, 142, 256, 389
maternity leave 333, 342, 404–405
McMaster University, 223
meconium 32, 37–38, 152, 287, 288, 413 (*see also* bowel movements, stools)
medications,
    ear drops, 266
    eye drops/ointments, 266, 274
    how to administer, 265
    oral, 265, 266, 283
    skin ointments or creams, 266
melanosis, pustular, 17, 415
menstruation, resumption of, 72
mental health, 94, 100, 151, 421, 423
miscarriage, 130, 417
mongolian spots, 18, 413
Moro reflex, 25, 387, 413, 416
motherhood, 1, 56, 66, 70, 71, 82, 84, 86, 87, 88, 89, 91, 93, 94, 95, 129, 143, 144, 154, 191, 201, 419, 425
Motherisk Clinic, 104, 180, 185, 419
moulding, 13–14, 413
mouth, 31, 228, 229, 230
mucous, 30, 176, 286, 288
Multiple Births Canada/Naissances Multiples Canada, 232, 245
Multiple Sclerosis Society of Canada, 424
multiples, 13, 22, 206, 210, 232, 323, 324
muscle tone, 23, 27, 28, 51, 73, 208, 285, 376, 395, 409
Muscular Dystrophy Association of Canada, 424

N
nasal drops, 263, 270
nasal sprays, 253, 270
nasogastric tube, 207, 413

National Advisory Committee on Immunization, 245, 251, 253
National Eating Disorder Information Centre, 422
neck, 31
    stiff, 262, 295, 296
necrotizing enterocolitis, 207, 413
neonatal death, 328–29, 413
    early, 411
    late, 413
neonatal intensive care unit (NICU), 207, 319, 320, 321, 322, 413, 414
neonatal urticaria, 413
neural-tube defects, 414
nevi, congenital pigmented, 19, 410
nevi, spider, 19, 416
newborn,
    appearance, 10–16
    appearance, premature baby, 22–23
    behaviour, 7–10
    exam, 28–36
    hearing, 34–35
    jaundice (*see* illnesses, jaundice)
    reflexes, 8, 24–26
    senses, 8
    sleep patterns, 111
    smell, 8, 30, 178, 187,
    taste, 8, 31, 177–78, 184, 189
    vision, 30
Newman, Jack, 108, 109, 420
Norwalk virus, 292
nose, 16, 17
nursing (*see* breastfeeding)
nursing pillow, 211
nursing strike, 106, 177, 178, 191, 203, 414

O
Ontario Coalition for Better Child Care, 420
oral contraceptives, 75
oral electrolyte solution, 263, 286, 289, 295
oral hygiene, 227, 228
osteoporosis, 170, 171
otitis media, 252, 272, 414
oxytocin, 8, 36–37, 45, 52, 73, 115, 137, 147, 153, 156, 161, 164, 202, 413, 414

P

play, 3, 125, 142, 146, 240, 306, 308, 352, 375, 383, 389–92, 394, 395, 397, 398, 399–400, 401, 407, 420
playpen, 307
port wine stains, 18, 414
postpartum blues, 66, 89, 94, 414
postpartum body, 6, 41, 59, 60, 71, 135
    abdominal flabbiness, 53, 54
    afterpains, 52–53, 153
    anemia, 58
    body image, 54, 70
    breast changes, 54, 191, 415
    chills, 45
    constipation, 51–52, 57–58, 65
    episiotomy, 43, 45, 46, 47, 49, 51, 72, 411
    exercise, 68–69
    faintness, 58, 68
    fitness, 70
    hair loss, 59
    hemorrhage, 43, 44, 45, 50, 329, 415
    hormonal changes, 57, 71, 87
    incontinence, 67–68
    infection, 42, 43, 45, 47
    joint laxity, 60, 68
    Kegels, 50, 69, 412
    linea nigra, 54
    lochia, 42, 43, 44, 45, 62, 413
    mask of pregnancy, 54
    menstruation, 72, 210
    perineum, 43, 46, 47, 48, 49, 50, 51, 52, 70, 72, 220, 414
    physical changes, 127–28
    sex after baby, 70–75
    stretch marks, 41, 54, 59, 62, 191, 417
    sweating, 59
    urination, 45, 49–50
    vagina, 48–49
    vaginal bleeding, 41–42
    vaginal dryness, 49, 73
    weight loss, 62–63, 64, 170
postpartum depression, 3, 65, 66, 77, 89–95, 111, 128, 133, 145, 415, 421
postpartum doula, 93, 415
pregnancy complications, 12, 19, 43, 329

pregnancy-induced hypertension, 35, 415
premature baby, 22–24
prolactin, 9, 104, 115, 135, 137, 151, 153–54, 180, 358, 415
pustular melanosis, 17, 415

R

rare disorders, 33, 424
rash creams, 220
Registered Educational Savings Plan, 39
renal disease, 13, 415
reproductive health, 44
respiratory secretions, 30
Rh-incompatibility, 414
RhoGAM, 43
Rich, Adrienne, 124
rocking chair, 302

S

Safe Kids Canada, 303, 421
Safe Start, 421
safety, 124, 167, 233, 239, 253–336, 420, 421, 422
Satter, Ellyn, 344
scrotum, 20, 21, 32, 416, 417
seborrhoeic dermatitis, 416
sedatives, 154
self-soothing behaviours, 156, 359, 363, 374, 382
separation anxiety, 359, 360, 382, 416
Serena Canada, 422
shampoo, 216, 226, 237, 238, 280, 304
shoes, 231, 233, 235
shopping for baby, 231–35
    moneysaving tips, 231–35
    secondhand, 232
Short, R.V., 153
single gene abnormality, 416
skin,
    blotches, 12, 262
    care, 167
    changes, 256, 331
    conditions, 17, 227, 279, 410
    infections, 276
    tags, 19, 416

sleep,
    deprivation, 70, 71, 83, 87, 92, 95, 97, 111, 113, 126, 133, 140, 144, 388
    habits, 244
    hygiene, 93
    patterns, 78, 387
    position, 113, 175, 325
sleeping through the night, 111, 337, 356–64, 365
sling (*see* baby carriers)
Small, Meredith, 153
smell, 8, 117, 178, 187, 195
smoking, 104, 112, 186
soap, 19, 61, 105, 119, 167, 184, 196, 199, 216, 217, 221, 226, 236, 237, 260, 280, 238, 259, 300, 316, 396
social development, 369, 426
Social Insurance Number, 39
social referencing, 382, 416
soft spot (*see* fontanelles)
solid food,
    age-appropriate foods, 337–46
    allergies and, 339, 341, 354–55
    readiness for, 337–46
    when to introduce, 337–46
soothing techniques, 97, 115, 117, 118, 139, 167, 168, 179, 192, 215, 241, 362, 363, 398
special needs, 130, 386
speech problems, 228
spinal column, 32, 416
spitting up, 81, 102, 174, 175, 256
spleen, 32
stale air, 416
Stanford University, 70
startle reflex, 25, 214–15, 387, 413, 416
stem cells, 416
stepping reflex, 25–26, 372
sterilization, 205
stillbirth, 130, 131, 409, 417
stools, (*see also* bowel movements)
    bloody, 288, 290, 291
    bottlefed baby, 165, 288
    breastfed baby, 288
    meconium, 32, 37–38, 152, 287, 288, 413
    starvation, 290

    transitional, 287, 288
stork bites, 18, 416
stranger anxiety, 380, 381, 417
strollers, 67, 86, 225, 304, 309, 325
Sudden Infant Death Syndrome (SIDS), 113, 168, 243, 267, 328, 329, 417
sun exposure, 220, 225
swollen glands, 258, 276, 283–84, 296, 413, 417

T

taste, 8, 31, 177–78, 184, 189
teeth, 31, 208, 227, 228, 229, 230, 258, 259, 284
teething, 179, 258, 358, 359, 360, 391
temperature,
    axillary, 259, 260, 409
    rectal, 259, 261
    tympanic, 29, 259, 260, 417
The Compassionate Friends of Canada, 422
thermometers, 259–60
thumbsucking, 20
thyroid, 33, 34, 412
Thyroid Foundation of Canada, 425
tongue, 25, 31, 98, 159, 168, 179, 204, 205, 208, 265, 282, 315, 317, 318, 340, 343, 377, 411
tongue-tied, 109, 177, 208, 417
tonic neck reflex, 26, 387, 417
toxins, 173, 299, 300, 306
toxoplasmosis, 35, 417
toys, 3, 246, 270, 300, 305, 306, 307, 308, 309, 373, 375, 377, 378, 381, 383, 384, 386, 389, 390, 391, 392, 394, 397, 398
    stuffed animals, 371, 391, 416
Transport Canada, 313

U

umbilical,
    cord, 19, 31, 32, 34, 223, 224, 235, 237, 329, 417
    cord blood, 32, 34
    cord care, 19, 223–24
undescended testicles, 21, 417
University of Wisconsin, 70–71
urination,
    baby, 38, 45, 290, 297

uterus, 8, 11, 13, 41, 42, 43, 44, 45, 50, 52, 53, 67, 202, 213, 409, 413, 414, 417

V
vacuum extraction, 411, 417
Vanier Institute of the Family, 404, 426
varicella zoster immune globulin, 181, 418
vascular disease, 418
ventricular septum, 418
vernix, 11, 16, 29, 418

vision, 18, 33, 45, 68, 369, 373, 377
vitamin D, 183, 216, 353
vitamin K, 32–33
vitamins, 48, 74, 171, 304

W
walker, 307
well-baby visits (*see* doctor)
working outside the home, 143
World Health Organization, 19, 22, 103, 152, 184, 338, 419, 420
worry, 3, 10, 71, 81, 85, 86, 131

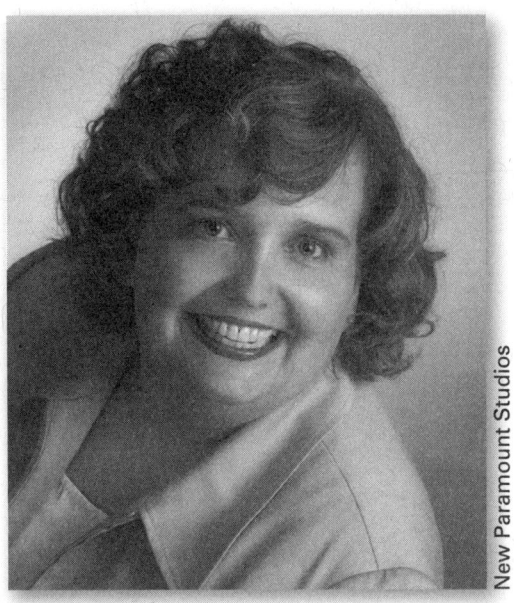

New Paramount Studios

Ann Douglas has been Canada's go-to pregnancy expert since the first edition of *The Mother of All Pregnancy Books* was published in 2000. She is the author of the other books in the bestselling The Mother of All® series: *The Mother of All Baby Books, The Mother of All Toddler Books, The Mother of All Parenting Books, and The Mother of All Pregnancy Organizers*; as well as the two titles in The Mother of All Solutions® series: *Sleep Solutions for Your Baby, Toddler, and Preschooler* and *Mealtime Solutions for Your Baby, Toddler, and Preschooler*.

Ann appears regularly in broadcast and print media. She has conducted pregnancy and parenting courses online and has led workshops for and delivered keynote addresses to groups across the country. She is a columnist for *The Toronto Star*.

Ann Douglas can be contacted via www.anndouglas.ca and www.having-a-baby.com.